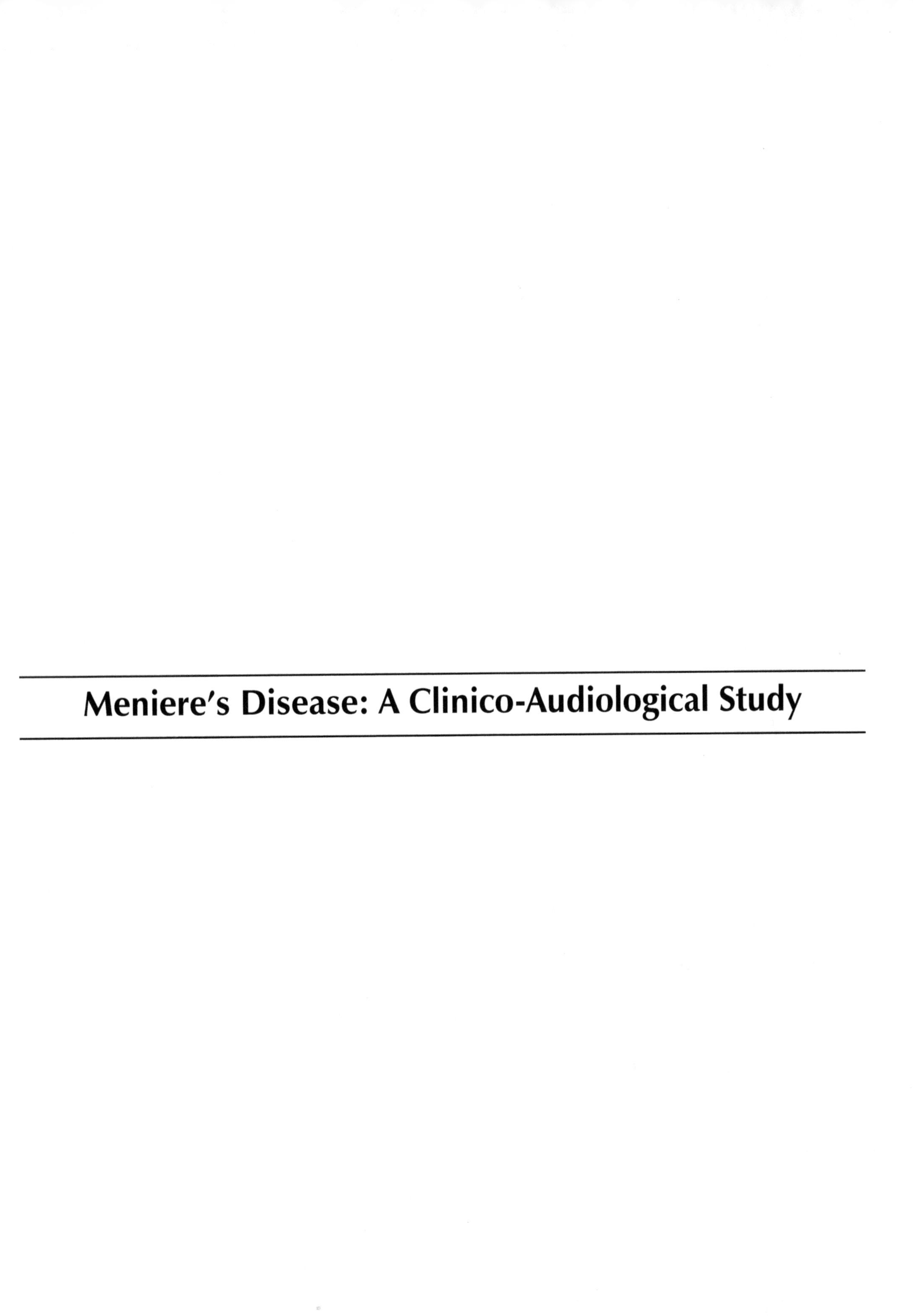

Meniere's Disease: A Clinico-Audiological Study

Meniere's Disease: A Clinico-Audiological Study

Editor: Emily Norton

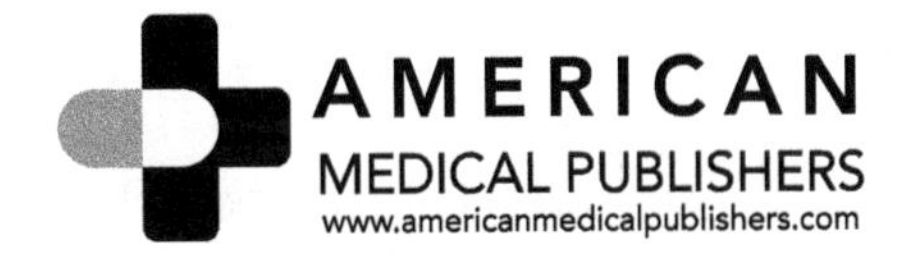

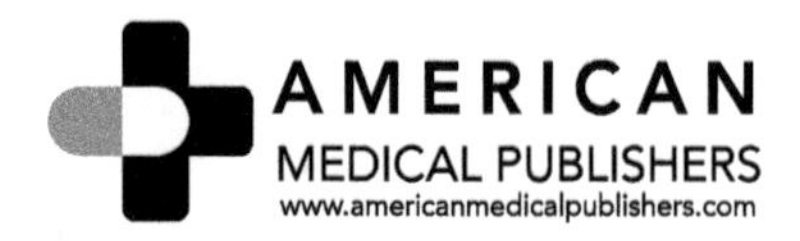

Cataloging-in-Publication Data

Meniere's disease : a clinico-audiological study / edited by Emily Norton.
p. cm.
Includes bibliographical references and index.
ISBN 978-1-63927-569-4
1. Ménière's disease. 2. Ménière's disease--Treatment. 3. Ménière's disease--Diagnosis.
4. Audiology. I. Norton, Emily.
RF275 .M46 2023
617.882--dc23

© American Medical Publishers, 2023

American Medical Publishers,
41 Flatbush Avenue,
1st Floor, New York,
NY 11217, USA

ISBN 978-1-63927-569-4 (Hardback)

This book contains information obtained from authentic and highly regarded sources. Copyright for all individual chapters remain with the respective authors as indicated. All chapters are published with permission under the Creative Commons Attribution License or equivalent. A wide variety of references are listed. Permission and sources are indicated; for detailed attributions, please refer to the permissions page and list of contributors. Reasonable efforts have been made to publish reliable data and information, but the authors, editors and publisher cannot assume any responsibility for the validity of all materials or the consequences of their use.

Trademark Notice: Registered trademark of products or corporate names are used only for explanation and identification without intent to infringe.

Contents

Preface

Every book is initially just a concept; it takes months of research and hard work to give it the final shape in which the readers receive it. In its early stages, this book also went through rigorous reviewing. The notable contributions made by experts from across the globe were first molded into patterned chapters and then arranged in a sensibly sequential manner to bring out the best results.

Meniere's disease, also called idiopathic endolymphatic hydrops, is a chronic disorder of the inner ear that affects both hearing and balance. It can occur at any age, but it usually starts between young and middle-aged adulthood, and generally affects only one ear. The exact cause of Meniere's disease is unknown but it can be caused due to genetic and environmental factors. The major symptoms of the disease are repeated events of vertigo, fluctuating hearing loss and tinnitus. Hypersensitivity to sound is an important symptom that can be diagnosed by checking the loudness discomfort levels. The symptoms of this condition are often preceded by a headache, nausea, and sweating. Treatment and management of Meniere's disease requires a combination of medications, physical therapy, counseling and surgical methods, which help in relieving the symptoms and minimizing the long-term impact on life. This book covers in detail the clinico-audiological studies on Meniere's disease. It is appropriate for students seeking detailed information on this disease as well as for medical professionals.

It has been my immense pleasure to be a part of this project and to contribute my years of learning in such a meaningful form. I would like to take this opportunity to thank all the people who have been associated with the completion of this book at any step.

Editor

1

Mental Health, Well-Being and Ménière's Disease

Jess Tyrrell[1]*, Sarah Bell[1] and Cassandra Phoenix[2]

*Address all correspondence to: j.tyrrell@exeter.ac.uk

[1]University of Exeter, Exeter, United Kingdom

[2]University of Bath, Bath, United Kingdoms

ABSTRACT

This chapter will discuss the current knowledge of the mental health and wellbeing impact of Ménière's. To date, our understanding is limited, with small sample sizes, no controls, and the inability to account for confounding factors. Our work in the UK Biobank aimed to further our understanding of the impacts of Ménière's at the population level.

Secondly we will consider the patient perspective of what it means to live with Ménière's. This is essential to develop appropriate healthcare pathways and ensure patients are able to lead fulfilling lives. There is very limited information about how the patient experiences and makes sense of the disease (or not) including its triggers and physical sensations in everyday life.

Our findings suggest that Ménière's adversely impacts on mental health, an individual's emotional state and their life satisfaction. We demonstrate the complex processes of adjustment (physical, social and emotional) following a diagnosis of Ménière's. Although a cure is not currently available, our study illustrates that much can be learnt from the adaptation strategies developed by long-term sufferers in order to help individuals with new diagnoses; an experience that is both daunting and disruptive to patients' everyday lives.

Keywords: Ménière's disease, UK Biobank, Qualitative, mental health, well-being, interdisciplinary

INTRODUCTION

Ménière's disease is a complex multifactorial disorder of the inner ear, consisting of several concurrent symptoms (e.g. aural pressure, hearing loss, tinnitus and vertigo). Patients with Ménière's range from minimally symptomatic highly functional individuals to severely affected disabled patients. Each of the main triad of Ménière's symptoms can impact on quality of life. Tinnitus may be associated with sleep disturbance, depression, irritability, reduced concentration and auditory difficulties [1]. Hearing loss can result in communication difficulties, which can cause problems in work and social life. Vertigo is known to cause anxiety and restrict physical and social activities, therefore significantly impacting on patients' health and well-being [1]. Vertigo is often considered to be the most detrimental and debilitating symptom of Ménière's [2].

Research on the mental health and well-being impact of Ménière's disease is limited. Moreover, quantitative studies in this area are negatively influenced by small sample sizes (often with fewer than 500 participants), a lack of groups to compare the mental health impacts with (i.e. no control groups), and an inability to account for confounding factors. Furthermore, our understanding of how the mental health impact of Ménière's may shift over time is partial at best.

The patient perspective of what it is like to live with this disease within the context of their day-to-day life is critically important for developing appropriate healthcare pathways and ensuring that patients are able to lead as fulfilling lives as possible [3]. While some studies have considered the adverse impact of Ménière's on quality of life, along with patients' perspectives regarding triggers and symptoms of the disease [4], there is very limited information about how patients experience and manage the disease (or not), including its triggers and symptoms in everyday life. In addition, we are currently unaware of the role that other people may play in this process [5–7] or how these issues impact on the sense of mental health and well-being amongst people with Ménière's.

This chapter will build upon existing research in this area, describing a comprehensive, multilayered two-phase analysis of the impact of Ménière's on patients' mental health and wellbeing. First, epidemiological analysis from the most powerful Ménière's resource currently available (the UK Biobank, www.biobank.ac.uk) will provide insights on the mental health and well-being impacts of Ménière's at a population level (Phase I). Secondly, qualitative research (Phase II) will provide deeper insights into patients' experiences of living with and negotiating the triggers and symptoms of Ménière's disease on a day-to-day basis, including the role of significant others in this process.

Ménière's and mental health at the population level

In Phase I, the UK Biobank dataset was utilised to understand how Ménière's influences mental health and well-being at the population level. This study contained 1376 individuals with self-reported Ménière's and included comprehensive phenotypic data (e.g. anthropometric measures, early life, lifestyle, family history, medical history, general health and well-being and diet). The aim of this population-level research was to investigate whether people with Ménière's have different mental health and subjective well-being than individuals without the condition. The impact of disease duration on mental health and level of subjective well-being was also investigated within cases.

Phase I methods

The UK Biobank, Ménière's diagnosis and mental health

The UK Biobank is a phenotypically rich study of over 500,000 individuals aged between 37 and 73 years in 2006–2010 [8]. All participants were interviewed by a nurse, who collated a list of health conditions for each participant. There were several options for ear/vestibular disorders, including tinnitus, vertigo, labyrinthitis, Ménière's disease, otosclerosis or a generic ear/vestibular disorder. The 1376 individuals who reported symptoms of Ménière's disease were selected. An investigation of prescribed medications and key symptom data (e.g. tinnitus and hearing loss) was utilised to validate the variable. For each individual reporting Ménière's, an age of diagnosis was also available and this was utilised to determine disease duration.

The UK Biobank incorporated extensive questions on mental health and subjective well-being. A subsection of questions asked participants to record the frequency of depressed mood, unenthusiasm, tiredness and tenseness within the 2 weeks prior to recruitment. Further questions focused on the number and duration of depression episodes over each participant's life. Participants rated their overall happiness and their satisfaction with health, work, friends and family and finances to provide a range of measures of subjective well-being. Participants were also asked to complete the Eysenck Personality Inventory (EPI) [9].

The participants also reported regular prescription medications, and use of the major antidepressant class—the selective serotonin reuptake inhibitors (SSRIs)—was monitored.

Statistical analysis

The mental health impact of individuals with Ménière's was compared to the whole control population of non-Ménière's sufferers. Linear regression models were utilised to investigate whether a diagnosis of Ménière's influenced the frequency of depression, tiredness, tenseness or unenthusiasm experienced in the 2 weeks prior to recruitment. Similar models were utilised to: (a) investigate how Ménière's influenced subjective well-being; (b) compare the frequency of family contact for cases and controls; and (c) examine the longest duration of depression in cases and controls.

Logistic regression models were used to investigate the odds of: (a) reporting depression; (b) reporting an episode of depression lasting over a week; and (c) utilising SSRIs in Ménière's cases compared to controls.

The role of disease duration on mental health and well-being was investigated. Individuals diagnosed for 5 or more years were compared to those diagnosed within the past 5 years.

Models were adjusted for potential confounders, including participants' age, sex, socioeconomic status, waist circumference, home location (urban versus rural as defined by the UK Biobank using the participant's postcodes and the 2001 census data) and ethnicity as covariates. Further adjustment for tinnitus severity was carried out to determine whether this symptom significantly contributed to any mental health associations. Personality is one of the biggest predictors of happiness [10] and therefore the EPI was included as a covariate in the statistical models. All analyses were conducted using STATA/SE Version 12.1 (College Station, USA). Statistical significance was denoted by $P < 0.05$ unless otherwise stated; Bonferroni correction methodology was utilised where appropriate.

Phase I results

The demographics of the 1376 Ménière's cases and controls are summarised in **Table 1**. As noted in previous studies, there was a preponderance of females (62% versus 54%). The data suggested that individuals with Ménière's had higher proportions of disability benefit than controls (5.3% versus 2.2%, $P < 0.001$) and were more likely to hold disabled badges than controls (8.7% versus 3.6%, $P < 0.001$). Ménière's cases were more likely to be unable to work because of illness (7.4% versus 3.8%, $\chi 2$ $P < 0.001$), although it should be noted that the large majority of individuals did work.

Demographics	**All MD sufferers**	**All controls**
N	1376	501,306
Sex		
Male (%)	517 (37.6)	228,677 (45.6)
Female (%)	859 (62.4)	272,629 (54.4)
Mean age at recruitment in years (95% CI)	63.4 (63.0–63.8)	60.4 (60.4–60.5)
Ethnicity (%)		
White	1333 (96.9)	471,525 (94.1)
Mixed	7 (0.5)	2951 (0.6)
Asian	14 (1.0)	9869 (2.0)
Black	2 (0.1)	8065 (1.6)
Chinese	2 (0.1)	1572 (0.3)
Other	7 (0.5)	4554 (0.9)

Missing/unknown	11 (0.8)	2770 (0.5)
Household income		
Less than £18,000	351 (25.5)	96,874 (19.3)
£18,000–£30,999	319 (23.2)	107,891 (21.5)
£31,000–£51,999	250 (18.2)	110,546 (22.0)
£52,000–£100,000	171 (12.4)	86,124 (17.2)
More than £100,000	34 (2.5)	22,900 (4.6)
Missing/unknown	251 (18.2)	76,971 (15.4)
Home location		
Urban	1154 (83.9)	427,775 (85.3)
Rural	222 (16.1)	73,513 (14.7)
Disability benefit		
None	1155 (85.5)	465,963 (94.0)
Attendance	6 (0.5)	1150 (0.2)
Disability benefit	72 (5.3)	10,810 (2.2)
Blue badge holder	118 (8.7)	17,871 (3.6)
Employment		
None	8 (0.6)	2795 (0.6)
Employed or self-employed	534 (39.0)	265,185 (53.2)
Retired	588 (43.0)	160,550 (32.2)
Look after home	50 (3.7)	20,032 (4.0)
Don't work because of illness	101 (7.4)	18,940 (3.8)
Unemployed	16 (1.2)	8817 (1.8)
Voluntary	62 (4.5)	17,481 (3.5)
Student	9 (0.7)	4553 (0.9)

Table 1. Demographics of the 1376 Ménière's sufferers and the 501,306 controls in the UK Biobank.

Depression

Participants with Ménière's were at higher odds of reporting:

Doctor diagnosed depression odds ratio (OR): 1.53 (95% confidence intervals (CI) 1.32, 1.70, $P < 0.001$, **Figure 1**).

A week long period of depression (OR: 1.33; 95% CI: 1.07, 1.65; $P = 0.011$).

The use of SSRIs (OR: 1.32; 95% CI: 1.01, 1.71; $P = 0.041$).

Ménière's was associated with longer durations of depression—on average this was 10 weeks longer than controls (95% CI: 5.2, 15.2, $P < 0.001$, **Figure 1**).

Mental health impact

Ménière's was associated with increased frequency of depression, tiredness, tenseness and unenthusiasm in the 2 weeks prior to recruitment, although adjustment for the participant's neuroticism subscale of the EPI attenuated the regression coefficients with only tiredness remaining significant (**Figure 2**).

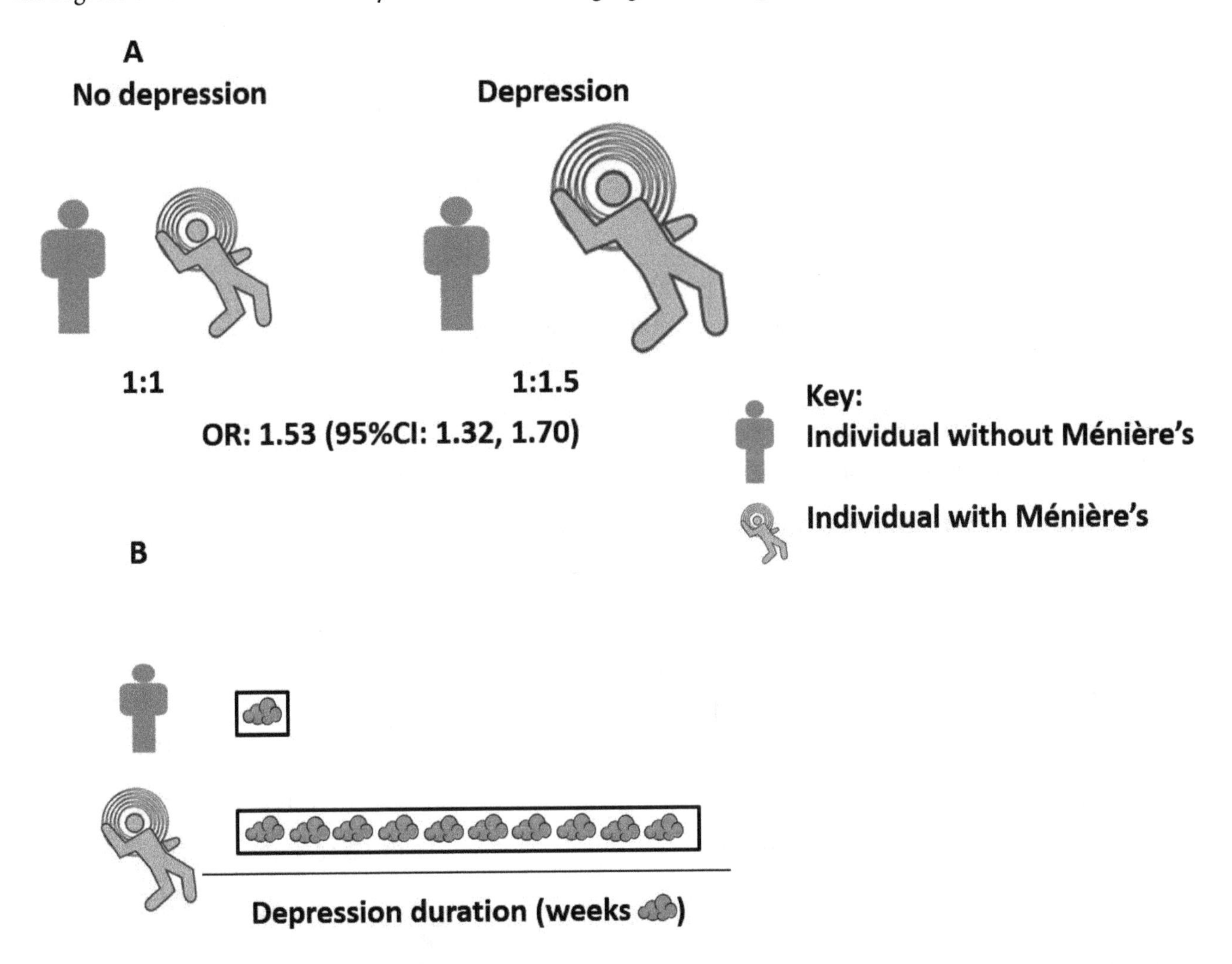

Figure 1. Graphic demonstrating the association between Ménière's and (A) depression and (B) the duration of depression.

Tinnitus, a major symptom of Meniere's, is linked to mental health. Adjustment for tinnitus severity in a subset of the population (n = 168,341), with a similar prevalence of Ménière's (0.25% versus 0.27%), attenuated all the mental health associations.

Subjective well-being

Individuals with Ménière's had lower health satisfaction scores than controls and were on average less happy overall. However, there was no difference between cases and controls in terms of satisfaction with their family relationships, friendships and financial situation (**Figure 3**). Higher odds of having social interaction with family and friends on a daily basis (odds ratio 1.5; 95% CI: 1.3, 1.8, $P < 0.001$) or 2–4 times per week (1.2; 1.0, 1.4, $P < 0.01$) was noted for Ménière's cases when compared to controls. The frequency of social interaction predicted individual satisfaction with friends and family.

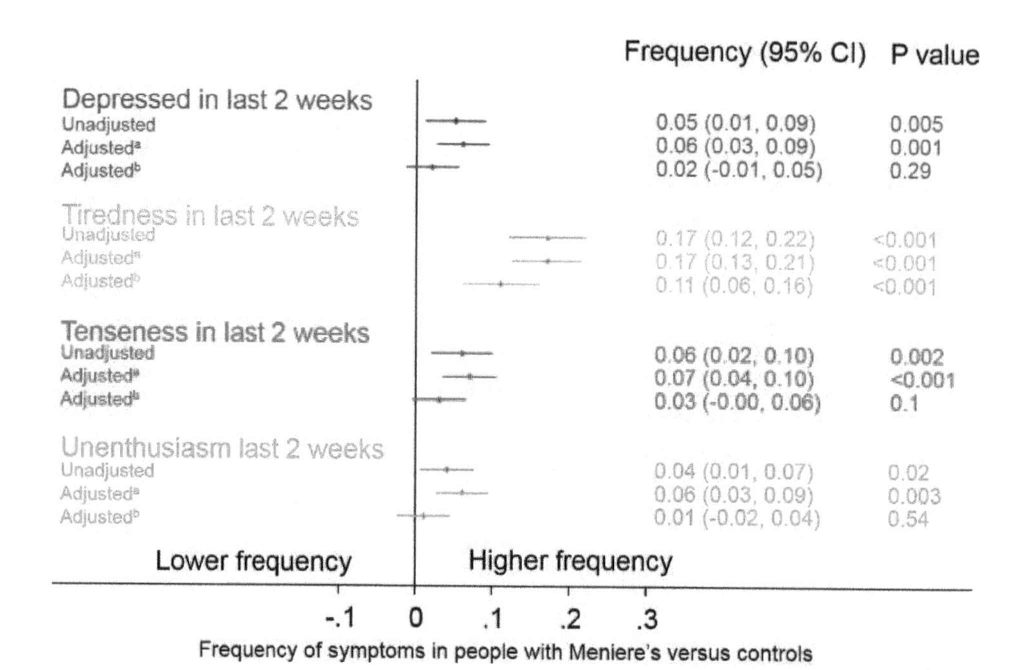

Figure 2. Change in frequency of depression, tiredness, tenseness and unenthusiasm in cases compared to controls.

Adjusteda accounts for common covariates and Adjustedb includes the EPI.

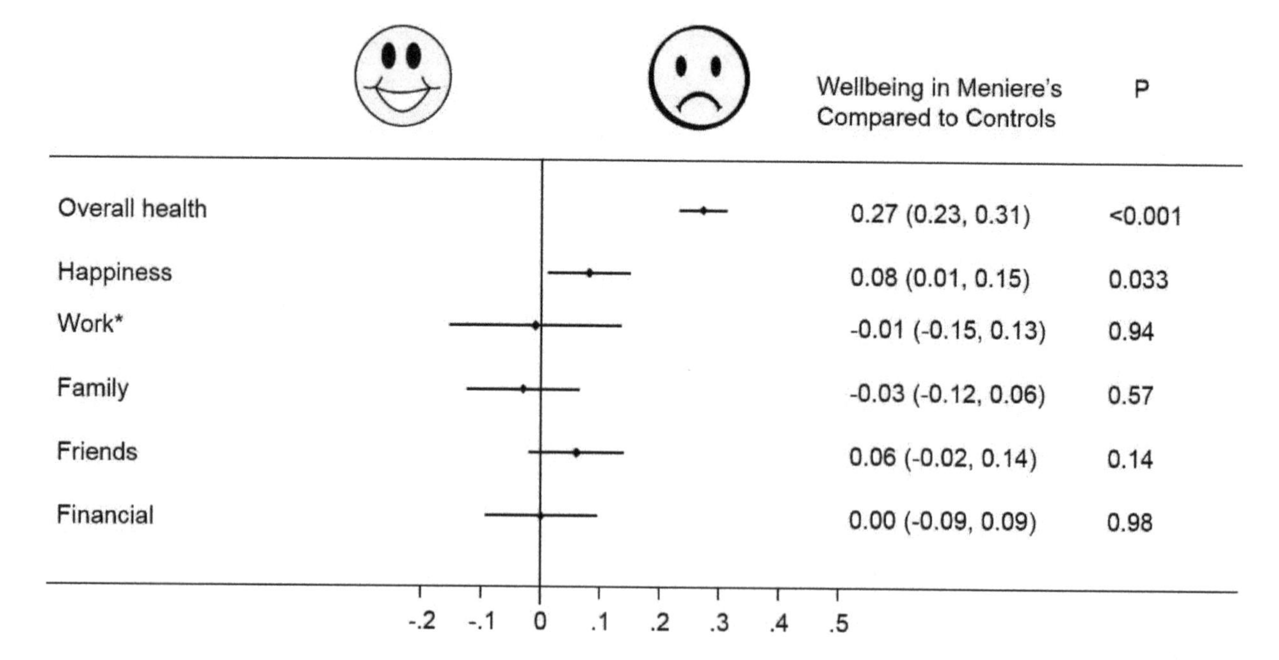

Figure 3. Differences in well-being in cases and controls. *Work satisfaction only asked in individuals with a job.

Disease duration

Within the Ménière's cohort, disease duration was associated with lower levels of depression in the 2 weeks prior to recruitment ($P < 0.05$). Furthermore, individuals diagnosed for more than 5 years were at lower odds of visiting a doctor about depression 0.60 (0.41, 0.90) than recently diagnosed individuals. Longer disease duration was also associated with improved health satisfaction ($P < 0.01$, **Figure 4**).

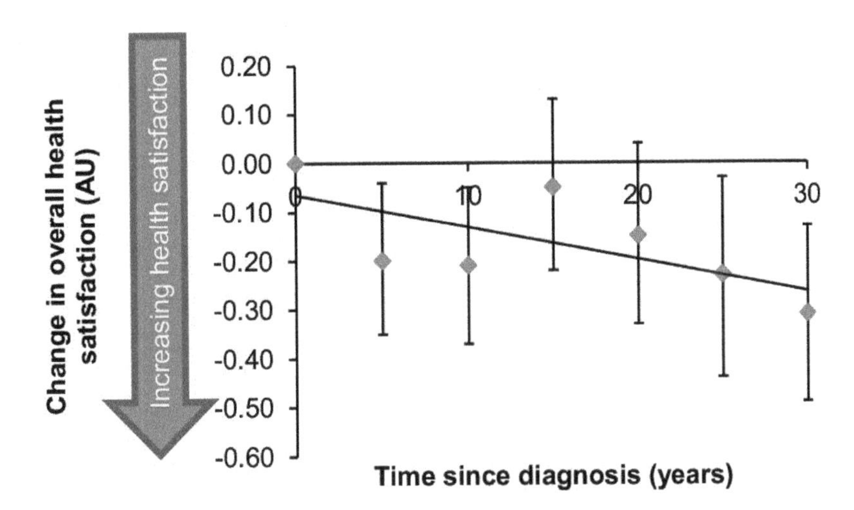

Figure 4. Scatter plot representing how health satisfaction within the Ménière's sufferers changes with time since diagnosis. Regression analysis indicated a significant relationship between overall health satisfaction and disease duration ($P<0.01$).

Ménière's and mental health at the individual level

Complementing the population-level analyses, Phase II adopted an in-depth qualitative approach to understand and contextualise people's experiences of Ménière's in their everyday lives. Ethical approval for this phase of the study was secured from the University of Exeter Medical School Research Ethics Committee (Approval Reference 13/09/029).

Phase II method

With the assistance of the Ménière's Society UK, a purposive sample of 20 Ménière's patients was recruited from across south west England, focusing on individuals diagnosed by an Ear Nose and Throat consultant, reporting symptoms within the previous 12 months (see **Table 2** for sample composition). Purposive sampling allowed information-rich views to be shared by individuals at different stages of the condition, offering insights into the variability of the condition rather than focusing only on the 'typical' or average case [11]. Four participants requested that their partners be present during their interviews, offering emotional support and also providing valuable perspectives on the shared effort of managing and adapting to the onset and progression of Ménière's [12]. A further eight semi-structured interviews were undertaken with partners of other participants to examine these shared and relational impacts in more detail.

Data collection commenced in June 2015, with interviews lasting between 1 and 3.5 hours, all conducted at a time and place of participants' choosing. A flexible interview guide was developed to inform the interview process, using open questions and active listening techniques to facilitate participant-led, open-ended responses. All of the interviews began by giving participants an opportunity to reflect (in their own words) on what was happening in their lives when they first started experiencing symptoms and how things had progressed from there. Follow-up questions focused on: participant interpretations, perceptions of their everyday experiences of the condition; the perceived impacts of the condition on their mental health, social roles and identities, friendships and relationships; interactions with the medical profession; the mechanisms by which they tried to self-manage and adapt to the condition over time; and the role of social support in this process.

Pseudonym	Age bracket (yrs)	Ménière's duration	Unilateral/bilateral symptoms?	Employment status	Presence of others during interview?
Participants with Ménière's					
Maggie	51–60	<5 yrs	Unilateral	Full time	–
Nicola	31–40	<5 yrs	Unilateral	Full time	–
Jane	61–70	<5 yrs	Unilateral	Retired	–
Louisa	51–60	<5 yrs	Unilateral	Full time	–
Susan	61–70	<5 yrs	Unilateral	Retired	–
Melissa	31–40	<5 yrs	Unilateral	Full time	–
Tom	41–50	<5 yrs	Unilateral	Full time	–
Debbie	61–70	>5 yrs	Unilateral	Non-working	Husband (Mick)
Becky	31–40	>5 yrs	Bilateral	Non-working	Daughter (toddler)
Dawn	51–60	>5 yrs	Unilateral	Early retirement	–
Angus	61–70	>5 yrs	Bilateral	Early retirement	–
Chloe	51–60	>5 yrs	Unilateral	Part time	–
Yvonne	61–70	>5 yrs	Unilateral	Early retirement	–
Caroline	51–60	>5 yrs	Shifting to bilateral	Nonworking	Husband for last half hour
Jennie	41–50	>5 yrs	Bilateral	Part time	Teenage daughter for last half hour
Emily	51–60	>5 yrs	Unilateral	Nonworking	Husband, teenage daughter
Richard	61–70	>5 yrs	Unilateral	Retired	–
Elaine	71–80	>5 yrs	Unilateral	Retired	Husband
John	71–80	>5 yrs	Unilateral	Early retirement	Grandson (periodically through interview)
Emma	51–60	>5 yrs	Unilateral	Self-employed	–
Participants supporting someone with Ménière's					
Karen	62–70	N/A	N/A	Full time	–
David	61–70	N/A	N/A	Self-employed	–
Magda	61–70	N/A	N/A	Part time	–
Matt	61–70	N/A	N/A	Self-employed	-
Sandy	61–70	N/A	N/A	Retired	Wife (Dawn) for last half hour
Mick	71–80	N/A	N/A	Retired	Wife (Debbie)
Toby	51–60	N/A	N/A	Full time	–
Tessa	41–50	N/A	N/A	Part time	Daughter (toddler)

Table 2. Sample composition for the qualitative study.

Interview transcripts were anonymised, checked against the original interview recordings and copies sent back to participants for member-checking purposes [13]. After a period of data immersion, listening back to recordings and annotating transcripts with initial codes and themes, a copy of each transcript and an initial thematic coding framework were uploaded to NVivo 10 (qualitative data management software). Each transcript was then subject to further thematic narrative analysis [14], with the aim of situating emerging themes within each participant's life story, and identifying more subtle, intersecting themes within the data [15]. In order to ensure the analysis and interpretations resonated with individuals living with Ménière's, the early findings were shared and discussed with members of a Ménière's support group in August 2015.

3.2. Phase II results

A key aim of Phase II was to understand more about the adverse mental health impacts observed with the onset and progression of Ménière's, and how participants experienced and negotiated these impacts during their everyday lives. We explore this further in what follows, focusing particularly on the strategies used to adapt to a life of uncertainty in the face of Ménière's, and the roles of supportive partners, family and friends in this process.

Recurring throughout participants' narratives were anxieties linked to the sudden onset of symptoms (vertigo in particular), their varying severity and the unpredictable progression of the condition [16–18]. The accumulation of these anxieties over time resulted in a significant loss of confidence, independence and a deep sense of frustration amongst participants, who likened it to 'driving a car with a dodgy break' and serving a 'prison sentence' with no clear release date. Given the limited efficacy of medication or surgery in treating the condition, participants (and their families) felt powerless in many respects, with even long-term sufferers describing it as 'an alien being' sitting in the body. Throughout participants' interviews, it was apparent that the process of adjusting to life with Ménière's was experienced as a steep and emotionally challenging learning curve, often requiring significant compromises to everyday practices and pleasures.

Participants described lifestyle shifts made in an effort to regain some semblance of control over Ménière's, be they diet-related, or focused more on physical activity, rest and relaxation. Some of these were in response to recommendations from their Ear Nose and Throat consultants (e.g. reducing salt, caffeine and alcohol), whereas others were strategies they had identified through trial and error in the process of learning to 'read' their body as the condition progressed. These included, for example, the use of specific vitamin supplements, postural adjustments, finding activities that would build their core strength without aggravating symptoms (e.g. modified versions of yoga, pilates, tai chi) and maximising sleep and rest where possible. However, participants warned against being overly simplistic in drawing links between stress, relaxation and vertigo severity. Many identified occasions when they had been under significant stress and not had a vertigo attack, or at their most relaxed and still had an attack. As such, although participants engaged in efforts to minimise stress and maximise opportunities for rest and relaxation, they indicated these stress pathways to be complex, inconsistent and intertwined with other factors going on in their lives at the time.

Managing anxiety was highlighted as particularly challenging, even amongst those who had lived with the condition for over 10 years, with many describing a 'shrinking world', loss of spontaneity and sense of isolation. While participants perceived varied potential in counselling, cognitive behavioural therapy and mindfulness interventions, many called for improved access to tailored psychological support from therapists able to appreciate and work with the tangible physical underpinnings of their anxieties. Some conveyed a 'ride the storm' mentality, combining determination with careful contingency strategies in order to cope with the unpredictability of the condition. These participants often described strategies used to distract themselves during less acute, but nonetheless destabilising, stages of an att be it watching the clouds through the bedroom window, listening to the radio or taking comfort from the companionship of a quiet cat or dog (reflecting wider literature on the value of companion animals in coping with long-term chronic illness [19, 20]).

Debbie: *'I find having a dog helps, especially this one… I find that touching her does make me feel better… it makes me feel like life's worth living really… She lays still – if she was jumping about I wouldn't be able to stand it, but she seems to sense when I'm not very well and she stays so close to me and still that it does make a difference'.*

Contingency strategies ranged from keeping anti-sickness medication in every pocket/bag, carrying sick bags, tissues, a torch (in winter with shorter hours of daylight), using ear defenders (in noisy settings), wearing sunglasses (to avoid bright light triggers, particularly those living with Ménière's and migraine) and wearing a medical bracelet to convey their emergency contact details if out alone. Perhaps the most important contingency strategy discussed by participants was the role of a reliable support network, be it partners, family or friends, as illustrated in the extract from Dawn's interview below.

Dawn: *'You don't ever feel like "Oh I'm better now, I'll move on." Not completely. There's a little, small percentage of you that's thinking, "Am I going to be okay doing this?"… I have to have a back-up plan. Like, my back-up plan now is that I've trained my husband to actually have his mobile phone with him all the time, which is a massive breakthrough, trust me!'*

Once 'rescued' and brought back to the familiarity of home (described by one participant as their 'cave'), participants explained that they preferred to be left alone to ride out the attack, knowing that someone would be there if needed. In part, this links to feelings of social embarrassment about one's physical state during an attack, but also to the sense that others cannot do much to help at that stage anyway. The increased reliance on partners, family and friends to fulfil this support role was upsetting for some participants, particularly when they felt their condition was compromising the independence of others as well as their own. As one partner commented (the husband of a participant with long-term Ménière's), 'it's not a disease one person gets – if it's a couple, it's a disease that two people get'. Participants, including those with Ménière's and the partners interviewed, explained the need to find a balance between being stoic whilst also recognising limitations. This is illustrated in the extract from Toby's interview below (husband of a participant trying to adapt to bilateral Ménière's).

Toby: *'I mean she probably thinks it's bothered me more than it actually has. The bit that bothers me is to see her suffering. I don't care that I can't go to a pub or cinema… I really don't care about that. She's very stoic, I say this to people – she wouldn't have any gas and air when she had the children. She's a right little tough nut… I mean she won't let it beat her. She'll just, you know, she'll do different-, we'll just do different things'.*

In this extract, Toby draws on an earlier biographical experience (childbirth) to emphasise and show respect for his wife's strength and determination, noting the shared process of finding alternative activities to do together that better accommodate the needs of the condition. Although this was recognised as difficult in particularly active phases of vertigo, several participants described positive examples, including going on outdoor walks, finding quiet pubs/ restaurants for lunch or dinner (sitting outside weather-permitting or eating early indoors to avoid crowds and noise), people watching by the coast and visiting nature-based/heritage attractions at quiet times of the day/year. Although this process of finding compensations— be it alone or with a partner, family or friends—often took time, it was deemed particularly important amongst longer-term sufferers:

Emma: *'With the gap that's created by perhaps not being able to do what you would normally do, try and fill it with something else that brings you happiness and pleasure… I've done loads of sewing… and I make these little bags – this is my therapy – I like to have something to show for my day… I've chosen fabrics which are nice and tactile, and in fact I've got a delivery coming today of really amazing bright coloured velvets with velvet silk!'*

Finding these personal 'havens' [21] sometimes required significant (and ongoing) shifts in aspirations and outlook over time, with participants coming to value pleasures and activities they had previously taken for granted. This is indicated in the interview extract below from a participant who had lived with severe symptoms for over 12 years:

> ***Emily:*** *'I was sort of going along, going along, going along, going along, and then somewhere along this path, I thought "Hang on, we don't do anything. I haven't got a life". I, I, I existed, but I hadn't got a life... But now we have found little places where we can go, so we have got a bit of a life now'.*

The importance of 'counting blessings' came through as particularly important in the interviews of longer-term sufferers. Participants talked about trying to focus on the 'good' things in their lives, making the most of remission phases and cherishing the support networks they have in place to co-navigate the condition. This is conveyed in the extract from Becky's interview below; Becky had lived with Ménière's since she was 17 years old. In her early thirties at the time of the interview, and having recently become a parent, she described the changes in her att to the condition since starting to experience bilateral symptoms of tinnitus and imbalance:

> ***Becky:*** *'I've changed so much in how I've dealt with it. Because before I would have been like, "Oh just get on with it!" to other Ménière's people, you know, "I did". But now I completely understand how devastating an illness it can be... So I just, I'm grateful for each day of normality... I still appreciate living in the now, and living when like my balance is good, and my hearing is good, and the tinnitus isn't so bad... just very much, counting my blessings... focusing on what's good rather than what might happen'.*

Several participants used hope to maintain a sense of morale during the most challenging phases of the condition, particularly with regards to the potential for future medical and technological advances (e.g. stem cells, refi hearing aid and directional microphone technology, etc.) to bring greater understanding of, and predictability to, their condition. Indeed, two participants expressed a reluctance to undergo any of the (albeit limited) surgical procedures currently available for fear of compromising their eligibility for any bett more appealing options emerging further down the line. This touches on the recognition in the wider long-term illness literature that 'absolute faith in medicine may be problematic, prohibit change and be constraining to live by' [22]. As such, it seems important for participants to fi a balance between taking comfort from those hopes while also allowing themselves to use all the resources available in the present to fully accept and adapt to their current situation.

Discussion

Our research demonstrates that the unpredictable and disabling symptoms of Ménière's result in sufferers experiencing prolonged periods of depression. In addition, it provides insight into how this is experienced in the context of everyday life. We strengthen and extend the evidence from a number of studies suggesting the adverse mental health impact of Ménière's [1, 2, 23], while also supporting previous evidence regarding the impact of Ménière's on fatigue, tenseness and unenthusiasm [23]. The importance of tinnitus severity and mental health outcomes was also highlighted.

Ménière's was strongly associated with lower health status satisfaction. This was unsurprising given the unpredictable nature of the condition and the known association with depression. Indeed, many of our participants lived with an ongoing sense of anxiety as symptoms caused their body to 'dys-appear', or emerge problematically into direct consciousness [24]. Moreover, this occurred in ways that were not only unpredictable but also uncontrollable. Losing control over a body that, prior to the onset of symptoms (severe or otherwise), had become disciplined and predictable through acts of routinised self-regimentation (working, exercising, eating, socialising and so forth—without the need for careful and strategic planning) further contributed to mental distress [25].

The similarity in other life domains between people with Ménière's and controls, including satisfaction with family, friends and financial status, is particularly noteworthy. It might be anticipated that because of their condition people with Ménière's would be less satisfied with all aspects of their life. However, previous work on other chronic health conditions has suggested that people do not always rate their quality of life as badly as healthy people might anticipate [26]. Further some studies have demonstrated small differences in reported life satisfaction or happiness between people with serious physical disabilities and 'normal' control subjects [27]. One explanation for this might be found in our participants' accounts of learning to find joy and happiness in activities that formed the fabric of their daily life, but had previously been taken for granted. Included here was the realisation of unwavering support and in some instances, new found closeness with the people around them. Indeed, the data suggested that individuals with Ménière's had more contact and satisfactory relationships with family and friends.

In day-to-day life, people with Ménière's can feel isolated, afraid, dependent and on some occasions embarrassed. Yet, reflecting previous literature on chronic illness [21], our research highlights the value of support networks and suggests they may enable people with Ménière's to live satisfying lives. We would, therefore, emphasise the importance of not just informing friends and family about the condition, but educating them on how they might best assist during its various manifestations. This might range from being mindful of inclusive forms of communication for those with impaired hearing, to supporting from afar during an attack. Aasbo et al.'s [28] concept of 'biographical we' is useful here in helping to understand the great effort partners of chronically ill put in to re-establish normality and continuity in everyday life; effort, that as our research signalled, can come at a cost of their own needs being overlooked. 'Ménière's is a disease that two people get' and this aspect warrants greater consideration as part of the broader patient treatment pathway.

Improvements in the frequency of depression episodes and health satisfaction were noted as disease duration increased. This may refl the disease progression pathway, which usually involves a reduction in the number of vertigo att experienced by individuals as the disease progresses [29]. Our participants' improved ability to read their bodies and recognise signs of an impending attack suggests the development of *Ménière's literacy*. Borrowing from the concept of *interactive health literacy*, whereby individuals develop an improved capacity to act independently on knowledge with motivation and confidence in an empowered way [30], *Ménière's literacy supports* adaptation by individuals to their condition and/or medical interventions and lifestyle changes reducing the frequency of vertigo attacks. Given that vertigo is considered to be the most detrimental symptom in Ménière's [2], reductions in vertigo severity should, therefore, improve mental health and well-being. All of this is not to suggest that adaptation diminishes the ongoing sensory, emotional and social challenges that people with Ménière's face in their everyday life [16]. Indeed, our research showed that at a population level, disease duration did not alter the frequency of tiredness, tenseness or a lack of enthusiasm experienced by Ménière's sufferers. While some aspects of Ménière's may improve over time and an individual may adapt to some extent, overall it continues to impact negatively on everyday life.

Conclusions

Our research findings emerged from cross-sectional data. It cannot and does not seek to determine the causal pathway of Ménière's disease. Our interpretations of the qualitative data are shaped as much by the absence of certain voices as they are by the presence of others. To that end, it is noteworthy that our sample for Phase II consisted primarily of women (16 female patients, 3 female supportive partners), with just four participants experiencing bilateral symptoms of tinnitus, imbalance and hearing loss (i.e. symptoms in both ears).

Those limitations noted, the research provides the most comprehensive study of the mental health and well-being impacts of Ménière's to date and highlights the adverse mental health effects of Ménière's. By utilising the UK Biobank, the inclusion of key confounders and sufficient numbers to investigate the role of disease duration in Phase

I has enabled us to offer a unique contribution to the field. Likewise, a combined focus on the individual everyday realities of living with Ménière's disease provides original insight into how it intersects with mental health and well-being in a number of different ways and across a variety of contexts. While offering a holistic and detailed analysis of this subject, the research also provides a working example of interdisciplinary, integrated research and the value it can bring to our attempts to understand complex health conditions like Ménière's disease in a way that respects the importance of the big picture, without ignoring the individual 'expert' voices of patient experience.

Acknowledgements

The research presented in this book chapter was funded by the UK Ménière's Society. The Phase I research was conducted using the UK Biobank resource. We would like to thank participants from the UK Biobank and those that took part in the Phase II research.

References

[1] Yardley L, Dibb B, Osborne G. Factors associated with quality of life in Meniere's disease. Clinical Otolaryngology and Allied Sciences. 2003;28(5):436-41.

[2] Arroll M, Dancey CP, Attree EA, Smith S, James T. People with symptoms of Meniere's disease: the relationship between illness intrusiveness, illness uncertainty, dizziness handicap, and depression. Otology and Neurotology. 2012;33(5):816-23.

[3] Paterson C, Britten N. Organising primary health care for people with asthma: the patient's perspective. The British Journal of General Practice : the Journal of the Royal College of General Practitioners. 2000;50(453):299-303.

[4] Kirby SE, Yardley L. Physical and psychological triggers for attacks in Meniere's disease: the patient perspective. Psychotherapy and Psychosomatics. 2012;81(6):396-8.

[5] Manchaiah VK, Pyykko I, Kentala E, Levo H, Stephens D. Positive impact of Meniere's disorder on significant others as well as on patients: our experience from eighty-eight respondents. Clinical Otolaryngology. 2013;38(6):550-4.

[6] Pyykko I, Nakashima T, Yoshida T, Zou J, Naganawa S. Meniere's disease: a reappraisal supported by a variable latency of symptoms and the MRI visualisation of endolymphatic hydrops. BMJ Open. 2013;3(2). Pii: e001555.

[7] Stephens D, Pyykko I, Kentala E, Levo H, Rasku J. The effects of Meniere's disorder on the patient's significant others. International Journal of Audiology. 2012;51(12):858-63.

[8] Collins R. What makes UK Biobank special? Lancet. 2012;379(9822):1173-4.

[9] Eysenck HJ, Eysenck SBG. Manual of Eysenck Personality Inventory. London: University of London Press; 1964.

[10] DeNeve KM, Cooper H. The happy personality: a meta-analysis of 137 personality traits and subjective well-being. Psychological Bulletin. 1998;124(2):197-229.

[11] Flyvbjerg B. Five misunderstandings about case study research. Qualitative Inquiry. 2006;12:219-45.

[12] Polak L, Green J. Using joint interviews to add analytic value. Qualitative Health Research. 2015;26(12):1638-48.

[13] Sparkes AC, Smith B. Qualitative Research Methods in Sport, Exercise and Health: From Process to Product. Abingdon: Routledge; 2014.

[14] Riessman CK. Narrative Methods for the Human Sciences. London: SAGE Publications Ltd.; 2008.

[15] Phoenix C, Smith B, Sparkes AC. Narrative analysis in aging studies: a typology for consideration. Journal of Aging Studies. 2010;24(1):1-11.

[16] Bell SL. The role of fluctuating soundscapes in shaping the emotional geographies of individuals living with Meniere's Disease. Social & Cultural Geography. 2016: 1-20.

[17] Bell SL, Tyrrell J, Phoenix C. A day in the life of Meniere's disease. Sociology of Health and Illness. 2016 In Press.

[18] Bell SL, Tyrrell J, Phoenix C. Ménière's disease and biographical disruption: Where family transitions collide. Social Science & Medicine. 2016 (166):177-85

[19] Brooks HL, Rogers A, Kapadia D, Pilgrim J, Reeves D, Vassilev I. Creature comforts: personal communities, pets and the work of managing a long-term condition. Chronic Illness. 2013;9(2):87-102.

[20] Ryan S, Ziebland S. On interviewing people with pets: reflections from qualitative research on people with long-term conditions. Sociology of Health and Illness. 2015;37(1):67-80.

[21] Lundman B, Jansson L. The meaning of living with a long-term disease. To revalue and be revalued. Journal of Clinical Nursing. 2007;16(7B):109-15.

[22] Smith B, Sparkes AC. Men, sport, spinal cord injury, and narratives of hope. Social Science & Medicine. 2005;61(5):1095-105.

[23] Levo H, Stephens D, Poe D, Kentala E, Pyykko I. Use of ICF in assessing the effects of Meniere's disorder on life. Annals of Otology, Rhinology and Laryngology. 2010;119(9):583-9.

[24] Leder D. The Absent Body. Chicago: University of Chicago Press; 1990.

[25] Frank AW. The Wounded Storyteller. Body, Illness and Ethics. Chicago: University of Chicago Press; 1995.

[26] Buick DL, Petrie KJ. "I Know Just How You Feel": The validity of healthy women's perceptions of breast-cancer patients receiving treatment. Journal of Applied Social Psychology. 2002;32(1):110-23.

[27] Riis J, Loewenstein G, Baron J, Jepson C, Fagerlin A, Ubel PA. Ignorance of hedonic adaptation to hemodialysis: a study using ecological momentary assessment. Journal of Experimental Psychology General. 2005;134(1):3-9.

[28] Aasbo G, Solbraekke KN, Kristvik E, Werner A. Between disruption and continuity: challenges in maintaining the 'biographical we' when caring for a partner with a severe, chronic illness. Sociology of Health and Illness. 2016;38(5):782-96.

[29] Huppert D, Strupp M, Brandt T. Long-term course of Meniere's disease revisited. Acta Otolaryngology. 2010;130(6):644-51.

[30] Nutbeam D. Health literacy as a public health goal: a challenge for contemporary health education and communication strategies into the 21st century. Health Promotion International. 2000;15(3):259-67.

2

Intelligent Segmentation Algorithm for Diagnosis of Meniere's Disease in the Inner Auditory Canal using MRI Images with Three Dimensional Level Set

Ting Liu,[1] Ying Xu,[1] Yujuan An,[2] and Hongzhou Ge[1]

[1]Department of Otolaryngology, Qingdao Hospital of Traditional Chinese Medicine (Qingdao Hiser Hospital), Qingdao 266034, Shandong, China

[2]Department of Intravenous Infusion Center, Qingdao Hospital of Traditional Chinese Medicine (Qingdao Hiser Hospital), Qingdao 266034, Shandong, China

Correspondence should be addressed to Hongzhou Ge; hedan2012@cau.edu.cn

Academic Editor: Yuvaraja Teekaraman

ABSTRACT

Th paper aimed to explore segmentation effects of the magnetic resonance imaging (MRI) images of the inner auditory canal of patients with Meniere's disease under the intelligent segmentation method of the inner ear based on threedimensional (3D) level set (IS3DLS). Th statistical shape model and the level set segmentation algorithm were combined to propose the IS3DLS. First, the shape training samples of the inner ear model were determined, and the results were manually segmented to further obtain region of interest (ROI) of the inner ear. Th IS3DLS was employed to accurately segment MRI images of the inner auditory canal of patients with Meniere's disease. Th segmentation performance of IS3DLS was compared with the expert manual segmentation method and the region growth level set-based segmentation algorithm. Results showed that Matthews correlation coefficient (MCC), Dice similarity coefficient (DSC), false positive rate (FPR), and false negative rate (FNR) of this algorithm were 0.9599, 0.9594, 0.0325, and 0.03655, respectively. Therefore, the IS3DLS could achieve good segmentation effect in MRI images of the inner auditory canal of patients with Meniere's disease, which was helpful for diagnosis and subsequent treatment of Meniere's disease.

INTRODUCTION

Meniere's disease is an idiopathic inner ear disease, and the inner ear mainly includes bony and membranous labyrinths, which locates between the thigh chamber and the bottom of the inner ear canal. The main pathological change of this disease is membrane labyrinth hydrops, which is clinically manifested as recurrent rotating vertigo, fluctuating hearing loss, tinnitus, and ear fullness. It mostly occurs in young and middle-aged people aged 30–50 years, and the incidence is about 0.2–0.5% [1]. Meniere's disease is mostly caused by various infections, injuries, otosclerosis, tumors, leukemia, autoimmune diseases, and genetic factors. Clinical examination often applies the imaging detection, and MRI of the inner ear membrane labyrinth under special contrast can show the narrowing of the endolymphatic vessels in some patients [2]. MRI is a type of tomography that adopts the magnetic resonance phenomena to obtain electromagnetic signals from the human body, so as to reconstruct the information of human body. It can display the distribution of a certain physical quantity in panic and weight loss and can obtain tomographic images and three-dimensional images in any direction. Besides, it is featured with the absence of ionizing radiation, clear soft tissue structure, and multisequence imaging. The shortcoming is that the spatial resolution is not high [3].

The regional growth level set segmentation algorithm is to initially determine the inner ear contour through the traditional regional growth cutting, to remove the inner ear boundary noise, and to repair the inner ear boundary by the adaptive curvature threshold method. Finally, the distance regularized level set evolution (DRLSE) model in the level set method is applied to accurately segment the inner ear region [4]. This method can effectively prevent missed detection of image edges and can process images of various types of lesions. However, the accuracy and operability of this method need to be improved [5]. Statistical shape models are the models that employ the high-resolution images as training samples and are compared with the images to be tested, so as to obtain accurate solutions through appropriate registration methods [6]. The level set segmentation algo-rithm adopts the evolution of a 3D surface to represent the evolution of a 2D curve. It means that the continuous evolution of the curve motion is applied to find the boundary of the image until the target contour is found, and then, the curve stops moving. The curve moves along each section of the image, slices are taken from different sections, and then, a closed curve is obtained. As time goes by, the level set is changed and the vision domain is calculated. The level set method can have a good image segmentation effect in order to obtain a corresponding shape for the contour extraction [7, 8].

To sum up, the statistical shape model was compared with the level set segmentation algorithm in order to improve the efficiency of doctors' diagnosis of inner auditory canal MRI images of Meniere's disease patients, so IS3DLS was put forward in this study. There was a comparison on segmentation results of different segmentation algorithms (this algorithm, the region growth level set segmentation algorithm, and the expert manual segmentation method). Therefore, the optimal segmentation method was selected and evaluated through the above.

Experimental Methods

Establishment of Research Data. 68 patients with Meniere's disease were selected as the research objects of this study, who were diagnosed and treated at hospital from October 2017 to April 2020 with symptoms of tinnitus. Th were 18–62 years old, including 38 males and 30 females. Th criteria for inclusion were defined to include patients who were in line with the diagnosis basis and efficacy evaluation of Meniere's disease of the Otolaryngology Branch of the Chinese Medical Association. (1) Th were 2 or more episodes of vertigo, each lasting from 20 minutes to 12 hours. (2) At least one hearing test confirmed low-medium and low-frequency hearing loss and fluctuating hearing loss. Th criteria for exclusion were defined to include patients who suffered from Meniere's disease and who had received endolymphatic sac surgery, cochlear implant surgery, and femoral gentamicin injection. Vertigo caused by other diseases, such as benign paroxysmal positional vertigo, labyrinthitis, and vestibular neuritis, was excluded. Th experiment had been authorized by the Ethics Committee of hospital, and all the research objects and their family members had signed the consent forms.

Establishment of the Statistical Shape Model of the Inner Ear. First, all training samples were placed in the same coordinate space. Platts analysis was used for alignment of the corresponding training sample sets with the same number of feature points. Under a 2D sample space, the sum of squared errors between each shape sample S_i and the average shape S was expressed as $D : D \ |(S_i - S)^2|$. The initial average shape was a sample image randomly specified from the training sample set. D expressed the Platts distance, which was denoted by P_d. Thus, the Platts distance between any two shapes S_i and S_j could be calculated as follows:

$$P_d = \sum_{m=1}^{n} \left|(s_i - s_j)^2\right| = \sum_{m=1}^{n} \left|(x_{im} - x_{jm})^2 + (y_{im} - y_{jm})^2\right|. \qquad (1)$$

In (1), n stood for the number of feature points contained in each shape.

Under the expansion condition of high-dimensional space, it was necessary to align any two shape samples. First, the center of each shape should be calculated, and all shapes should be unified in size and expressed by the Euclidean distance equation, as shown in

$$E(S) = \sqrt{\sum_{m=1}^{n} \left[(x_m - \overline{x})^2 + (y_m - \overline{y})^2 \right]}. \qquad (2)$$

The centers of the two shapes should be aligned, and the singular value decomposition method was applied to align the rotation direction. Then, the final aligned sample was obtained by minimizing the Platts distance.

Measurement of the Image by Three-Dimensional Registration Technology. According to the image registration process in Figure 1, the reference and floating images were first input, and the reference image was transformed into geometric coordinates according to the given initial transformation parameters. Then, the floating image was calculated through interpolation to obtain the value of the new coordinate area. The similarity of reference image and the floating images after the difference should also be calculated. If the similarity met the preset registration requirements, the change parameters were output to obtain the interpolated image of the best floating image. However, the optimization would be continued if the registration requirements were not met. The transformation parameters were changed until the final parameters that met the requirements were obtained.

Acquisition of the Region of Interest in the Inner Ear. In this study, registration technology was employed to automatically locate and acquire the ROI of the inner ear. The 3D rigid body transformation was selected as the transformation model. Furthermore, the rigid body transformation included translation and rotation.

$$(X_m, Y_m, Z_m) = A(X_f, Y_f, Z_f) + b = \mathrm{AF} + b. \qquad (3)$$

In (3), (X_m, Y_m, Z_m) represented the spatial position coordinates of the registered image and (X_f, Y_f, Z_f) stood for the spatial position coordinates of the target image to be transformed. A and b expressed the rotation matrix and the translation vector in turn, and the constraints of the matrix

were A^T = I and det$A$ 1. Besides, AT was the transpose of A, and I meant the identity matrix. Th mutual information was chosen in this study as the similarity metric. For a given image X and Y, their mutual information was expressed as follows:

$$\mathrm{MI}(X, Y)\ H(X) + H(Y) - H(X, Y). \qquad (4)$$

In (4), $H(X)$, $H(Y)$, and $H(X, Y)$ were the entropy X, entropy Y, and their joint entropy, respectively.

$$H(X, Y) \leq H(X) + H(Y). \qquad (5)$$

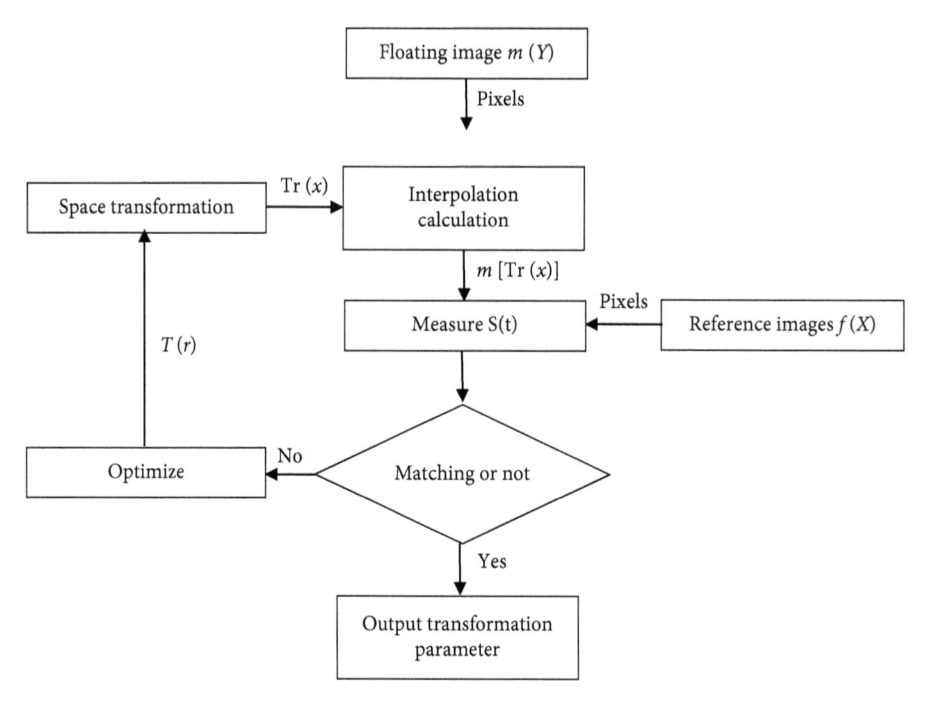

Figure 1: Flow chart of image registration.

When X and Y were independent of each other, the joint entropy was equal to the sum of their respective entropy. When X and Y were not independent of each other, the joint entropy was less than the sum of their respective entropy. The above was expressed in (5).

The gradient descent method was selected as the optimization algorithm of the registration process, and the objective function was optimized by an iterative method to achieve the best conditions. Then, the cubic polynomial interpolation method was adopted to make the nonlinear difference of the voxel points, so that the final registered image could be obtained. Thus, the ROI of inner ear could be automatically located and identified. The algorithm of the difference result could be calculated as

$$v(x, y) = \sum_{i=0}^{3} \sum_{j=0}^{3} a_{ij} x^i y^i. \qquad (6)$$

Segmentation of the Three-Dimensional Level Set Algorithm. The MRI image of the inner ear of patient with Meniere's disease was segmented through the method proposed in this study. Figure 2 indicates the segmentation process of IS3DLS. The main steps were as follows. First, the training set samples were collected to create the inner ear statistical shape model, and then, the average shape model was calculated. Second, the inner ear MRI image was for weighting and the ROI of inner ear was extracted. Third, the inner ear ROI and the average shape model were registered to obtain the initial contour. Fourth, the level set was applied to segment the initial contour and the characteristic image to get the result after the segmentation.

Evaluation Indicators of Inner Ear Segmentation Accuracy. Taking the expert manual segmentation as the standard, the true position (TP) and the false position (FP) were employed to measure the error between the regions obtained by the two segmentation algorithms. Moreover, the average minimum Euclidean distance (AMED) and Hausdorff distance (HD) were adopted to determine the difference between the algorithm segmentation contour and the manual segmentation contour.

The four indicators (MCC, DSC, FPR, and FNR) were adopted in this study to evaluate the accuracy of the segmentation results. The manual segmentation result has been forwarded as a standard. The IS3DLS, regional level set segmentation, and expert manual segmentation were compared, and the comparison results were calculated. In addition, DSC and MCC verified the similarity between the results of different algorithm segmentation and expert manual segmentation by calculating the overlap ratio of pixels. The calculation result was near 1, which meant that the calculation result of IS3DLS was closer to the result of expert manual segmentation algorithm, and the accuracy was higher. FPR and FNR represented the oversegmentation and undersegmentation in sequence. The closer the value was to 0, the lower the degree of error in segmentation was and the better the accuracy was.

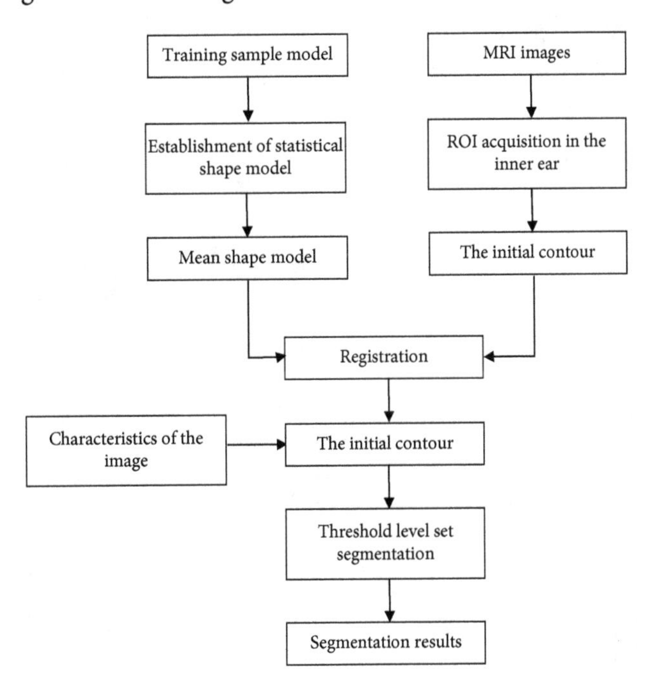

Figure 2: Flow chart of inner ear level set segmentation based on the statistical shape model.

Statistical Analysis. All measurement data were expressed as mean ± standard deviation (SD), and SPSS 21.0 software package was used for statistical processing of data. Analysis of variance (ANOVA), *t*-test, and chi-square test were used for intragroup comparison, intergroup comparison, and the count data comparison, respectively. In addition, $P < 0.05$ indicated the difference was statistically substantial.

Experimental Results

MRI Images of the Inner Auditory Canal of Patients with Meniere's Disease. Figure 3 shows the MRI and computed tomography (CT) images of the inner ear of one patient. This patient was diagnosed with enlarged vestibular aqueducts; the area indicated by the arrow presented the abnormal enlargement of endolymphatic vessels and sac, thus confirming that the patient suffered from Meniere's disease.

Experimental Results of Level Set Segmentationofthe Inner Ear Based on the Statistical Shape Model. As shown in Figure 4, the inner ear shape samples were used for statistical analysis, so that the inner ear shape model was established. Then, the average shape of the inner ear was obtained through the statistical model.

Based on the inner ear average shape model as the initial contour, the level set segmentation algorithm was used for segmentation. One of the images was arbitrarily selected as a reference, the other images were extracted through registration technology to take the inner ear ROI out, and the inner ear ROI was segmented through level set evolution to obtain the image (Figure 5). The inner ear was drawn through the segmentation algorithm proposed in this study to obtain Figure 6. Through comparison, it was found that the algorithm proposed in this study showed clear display of the vestibule, cochlea, and semicircular canal, and the segmentation was accurate. Thus, the results were basically consistent with the actual structure of the inner ear.

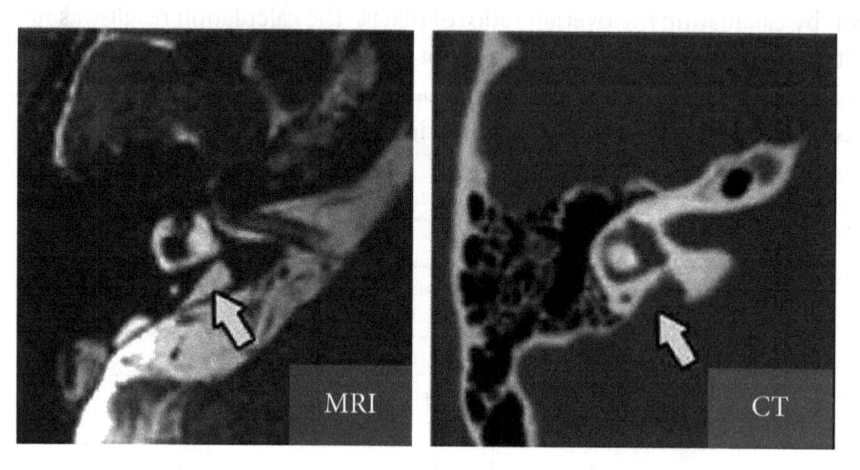

Figure 3: The images of the inner ear of one child patient with Meniere's disease.

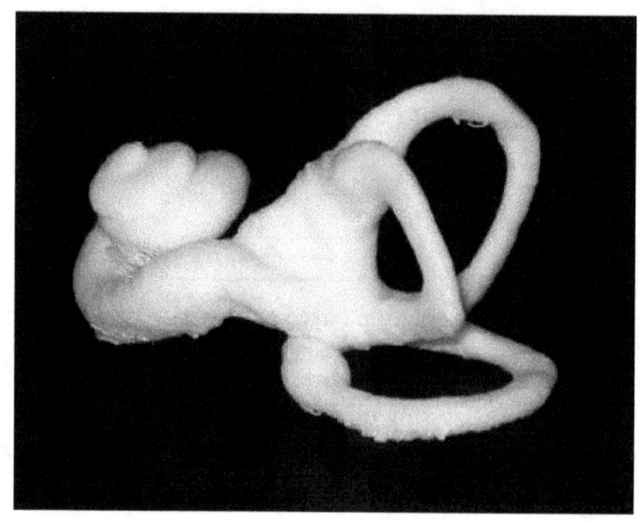

Figure 4: Modeling results of the statistical shape model of the inner ear.

The comparison results of the three segmentation methods are shown in Table 1. Th measurement indicators in Table 1 were evaluated from the accuracy and error of the segmentation results. Th results revealed that the segmentation algorithm in this study had a good segmentation effect, and the accuracy and error rates were close to 1 and 0 in turn. It indicated that the results of segmentation algorithm proposed in this study were similar to the manual result of experts.

Comparison on the Results of Different Segmentation Algorithms. Table 2 discloses that the other two segmentation algorithms had a high TP value (>90%) compared with expert manual segmentation, and the IS3DLS was higher than the region growth set segmentation. The FP value of IS3DLS was obviously smaller than that of the region growth set segmentation ($P < 0.05$). The AMED and HD values of IS3DLS decreased sharply in contrast to the region growth set segmentation. The difference in HD values *pf* patients from the two groups was statistically marked ($P < 0.05$).

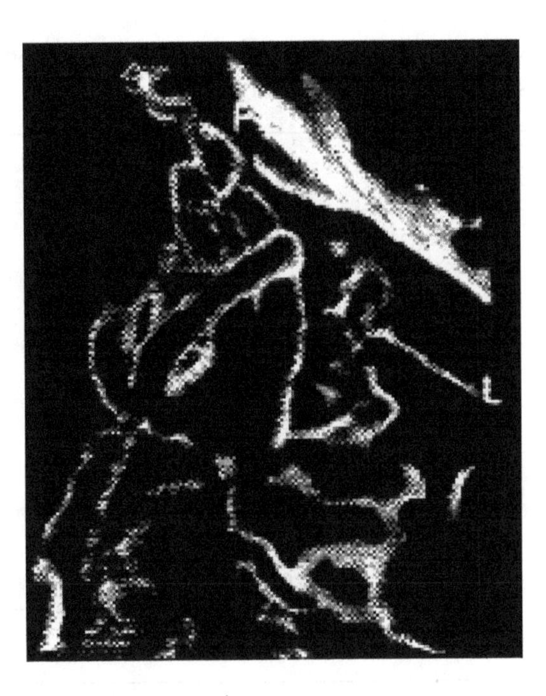

Figure 5: Drawing result of the inner ear ROI.

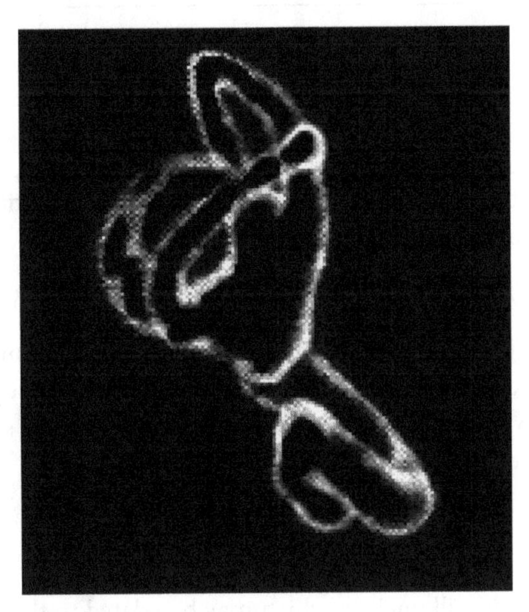

Figure 6: Result of the segmentation algorithm in this study.

Table 3 indicates the comparison results of the 3D surface gray matter of the three segmentation algorithms. By comparing with expert manual segmentation, the accuracy indicators of IS3DLS and the segmentation under the region growth level set were compared, and the results are shown in Table 3. MCC stood for the similarity of the two data. From the table, IS3DLS had a higher overlap rate and closer results with expert manual segmentation in contrast to the region growth set segmentation. DSC represented the segmentation effect. When the DSC value was greater than 0.8, the algorithm segmentation effect is considered good. From the table below, the segmentation effect of the two segmentation algorithms was good, but the segmentation effect of IS3DLS was better. PPR meant the false positive rate, which was employed to indicate undersegmentation, FNR expressed the false negative rate, which indicated oversegmentation, and FPR and FNR both showed the error of the segmentation effect. The FPR and

FNR values of IS3DLS were lower steeply than the values of region growth set segmentation ($P < 0.05$). It further demonstrated the accuracy of the segmentation method in this study.

Group	MCC	DSC	FPR	FNR	D_{mean} (mm)	D_{max} (mm)
A	0.9532	0.9483	0.0353	0.0778	0.1573	1.1144
B	0.9758	0.9629	0.0517	0.0821	0.1424	0.9151
C	0.9442	0.9535	0.0125	0.0567	0.1842	0.7846
D	0.9431	0.9723	0.0215	0.0551	0.1165	0.8782
E	0.977	0.9682	0.0419	0.0614	0.1792	1.1286
F	0.9661	0.9512	0.0321	0.0977	0.1426	1.2379
Average	0.9599	0.9594	0.0325	0.0718	0.1537	1.0098

Table 1: Performance test results of IS3DLS.

Algorithm	TP	FP	AMED	HD
IS3DLS	97.81	1.52*	0.78	2.15*
Region growth set segmentation	96.36	2.78	0.83	2.98
P	>0.05	<0.05	>0.05	<0.05

Note: the symbol * means that the difference was statistically substantial in contrast to the region growth set segmentation algorithm ($P < 0.05$).

Table 2: Comparison of results of segmentation algorithms influenced by MRI.

Analysis on Complexity of Different Segmentation Algorithms. Table 4 shows the running time of the region growth set segmentation and the segmentation algorithm proposed in this study. The running time of the region growing set segmentation was 37.15 s, and the running time of IS3DLS was 23.53 s. Thus, the running time of IS3DLS was markedly less than that of the region growth set segmentation ($P < 0.05$).

Discussion

The cause of Meniere's disease is still unclear, which may be related to the balance of endolymph production and absorption. The structure of the inner ear has complex changes [9], and 3D-weighted water imaging sequences are often used for multiplanar reconstruction. The above is adopted for MRI examinations of inner ear diseases, thin-slice scanning of auditory nerves, and water imaging of inner ear labyrinth [10]. The advantage of MRI is that it does not produce bony false shadows and is suitable for diseases of various systems throughout the body. However, the imaging time of MRI is long and the spatial resolution is low, which is only 2 mm according to statistics [11]. Medical image segmentation plays a vital role in digital medical research and the formulation and implementation of treatment plans. Noise and contrast have critical effects on image segmentation. Traditional segmentation algorithms are difficult to obtain satisfactory results and run for a long time. Although the expert manual segmentation method has a relatively high accuracy rate, it is time-consuming and challenging, and it is difficult for inexperienced doctors to accurately judge [12, 13].

Algorithm	MCC	DSC	FPR	FNR
IS3DLS	0.9599^{*}	0.9594^{*}	0.0325^{*}	0.0365^{*}
Region growth set segmentation	0.8693	0.8721	0.1402	0.0718
P	<0.05	<0.05	<0.05	<0.05

Note: the symbol * shows there was a statistically obvious difference in contrast to the region growing set segmentation algorithm ($P < 0.05$).

Table 3: Quantitative analysis results of evaluation indicators in different algorithms.

Algorithm	Running time (s)
IS3DLS	23.53^{*}
Region growth set segmentation	37.15
P	<0.05

Note: the symbol * reveals that the difference was statistically marked in contrast to the region growth set segmentation algorithm ($P < 0.05$).

Table 4: Comparison on running time of different algorithms.

There are more and more applications based on the level set method in image segmentation, which can incorporate images of different shapes into the energy function, so as to finally obtain the shape of the contour represented by the zero level function set. A level set segmentation algorithm is proposed based on differential geometry. When segmenting the images of ultrasound, CT, and MRI, this method can effectively segment the blurred area or partially missing lesions of the image boundary. The level set method has high segmentation accuracy [14, 15]. Statistical shape model is a powerful visualization and quantification tool that can connect geometric pattern with functional pattern. By testing the statistical shape model, the features of the patient image are obtained [16].

At present, the idea that the histopathologic change of Meniere's disease is endolymphatic hydrops is clinically recognized, but the cause of the hydrops is not fully understood pathologically in Meniere. Fiorino et al. [17] believed that endolymphatic hydrops was related to disease grade and VEMP, and the more severe the endolymphatic hydrops was, the worse the hearing was. However, the correlation between endolymphatic hydrops presented by MRI in Meniere's disease and other examination indicators was not confirmed yet. Th experimental results of this study showed that MRI could detect abnormal enlargement of endolymphatic vessels and sacs, thereby diagnosing patient as Meniere's disease. Through statistical analysis of all training samples, a statistical shape model of the inner ear could be obtained. Th inner ear ROI obtained by 3D registration technology was similar to the drawing results of the inner ear ROI. Compared with expert manual segmentation, the MCC and DSC values of IS3DLS were 0.9599 and 0.9594 in turn, and the values of the region growth set segmentation were 0.8693 and 0.8721, respectively. Although both segmentation methods had good segmentation results, the method proposed in this study was closer to 1, and its FPR and FNR were 0.0325 and 0.0365, respectively. Compared with the FPR and FNR of the region growth set segmentation (0.1402 and 0.0718), those of the method proposed in this study were lower, indicating that the IS3DLS was better. Moreover, the running time of IS3DLS was 23.53 s, which was extremely lower than the time of the regional growth set segmentation (37.15 s) ($P < 0.05$).

Conclusion

It was found that MRI images of the inner auditory canal could diagnose patient as Meniere's disease. The inner ear ROI obtained by the 3D registration technology was similar to the drawn inner ear ROI. The IS3DLS and the region growth set segmentation had good segmentation results. Compared with the region growth set segmentation, the segmentation effect of IS3DLS was closer to expert manual segmentation, and the error was smaller. The IS3DLS had faster speed and saved time, and its performance was related to the size of the training sample. When the training sample size is small, there is a certain error. However, it is difficult to obtain a large number of training samples in real experiments, so the error of the test is even greater when the shape of the image to be tested differs greatly from the selected training sample. It is hoped that more advanced segmentation algorithms will be introduced in the future to further improve the segmentation effect of MRI images and increase the application value of computer-assisted therapy in clinical medicine. The results of this study can provide an experimental basis for the investigation of the segmentation algorithm of MRI images of the inner auditory canal of Meniere's disease patients, thereby promoting the resolution of MRI images.

Authors' Contributions

Ting Liu and Ying Xu contributed equally to this work.

References

[1] R. Gu¨rkov, I. Pyyko¨, J. Zou et al., "What is Menie`re's disease? a contemporary re-evaluation of endolymphatic hydrops," *Journal of Neurology*, vol. 263, no. 1, pp. S71–S81, 2016.

[2] R. Quatre, A. Attye´, A. Karkas, A. Job, G. Dumas, and S. Schmerber, "Relationship between audio-vestibular functional tests and inner ear MRI in meniere's disease," *Ear and Hearing*, vol. 40, no. 1, pp. 168–176, 2019.

[3] T. Yousaf, G. Dervenoulas, and M. Politis, "Advances in MRI methodology," *International Review of Neurobiology*, vol. 141, pp. 31–76, 2018.

[4] Y. Liu, G. Captur, J. C. Moon et al., "Distance regularized two level sets for segmentation of left and right ventricles from cine-MRI," *Magnetic Resonance Imaging*, vol. 34, no. 5, pp. 699–706, 2016.

[5] S. Merino-Caviedes, M. T. Pe´rez, and M. Mart´ın-Ferna´ndez, "Multiphase level set algorithm for coupled segmentation of multiple regions. Application to MRI segmentation," *IEEE*, in *Proceedings of the 2010 Annual International Conference of the IEEE Engineering in Medicine and Biology*, pp. 5042–5045, Buenos Aires, Argentina, August 2010.

[6] C. Van Dijck, R. Wirix-Speetjens, I. Jonkers, and J. Vander Sloten, "Statistical shape model-based prediction of tibiofemoral cartilage," *Computer Methods in Biomechanics and Biomedical Engineering*, vol. 21, no. 9, pp. 568–578, 2018.

[7] X. Li, C. Li, H. Liu, and X. Yang, "A modified level set algorithm based on point distance shape constraint for lesion and organ segmentation," *Physica Medica*, vol. 57, pp. 123–136, 2019.

[8] Y. Zhao, S. Guo, M. Luo et al., "A level set method for multiple sclerosis lesion segmentation," *Magnetic Resonance Imaging*, vol. 49, pp. 94–100, 2018.

[9] E. G. Ekdale, "Form and function of the mammalian inner ear," *Journal of Anatomy*, vol. 228, no. 2, pp. 324–337, 2016. [10] F. Baselice, G. Ferraioli, and V. Pascazio, "A 3D MRI denoising algorithm based on Bayesian theory," *BioMedical Engineering OnLine*, vol. 16, no. 1, p. 25, 2017.

[11] T. Higaki, Y. Nakamura, F. Tatsugami, T. Nakaura, and K. Awai, "Improvement of image quality at CTand MRI using deep learning," *Japanese Journal of Radiology*, vol. 37, no. 1, pp. 73–80, 2019.

[12] B. Khorram and M. Yazdi, "A new optimized thresholding method using ant colony algorithm for MR brain image segmentation," *Journal of Digital Imaging*, vol. 32, no. 1, pp. 162–174, 2019.

[13] S. Zheng, B. Fang, L. Li, M. Gao, and Y. Wang, "A variational approach to liver segmentation using statistics from multiple sources," *Physics in Medicine and Biology*, vol. 63, no. 2, Article ID 025024, 2018.

[14] I. Y. Maolood, Y. E. A. Al-Salhi, and S. Lu, "Thresholding for medical image segmentation for cancer using fuzzy entropy with level set algorithm," *Open Medicine*, vol. 13, no. 1, pp. 374–383, 2018.

[15] L. Gui, C. Li, and X. Yang, "Medical image segmentation based on level set and isoperimetric constraint," *Physica Medica*, vol. 42, pp. 162–173, 2017.

[16] A. Suinesiaputra, J. Dhooge, N. Duchateau et al., "Statistical shape modeling of the left ventricle: myocardial infarct classification challenge," *IEEE Journal of Biomedical and Health Informatics*, vol. 22, no. 2, pp. 503–515, 2018.

[17] F. Fiorino, F. B. Pizzini, A. Beltramello, and F. Barbieri, "MRI performed after intratympanic gadolinium administration in patients with Me´ni`ere's disease: correlation with symptoms and signs," *European Archives of Oto-Rhino-Laryngology*, vol. 268, no. 2, pp. 181–187, 2011, Epub 2010 Aug 10. PMID:20697903.

3

Meniere’s Disease: Surgical Treatment

Yetkin Zeki Yilmaz[1]*, Begum Bahar Yilmaz[1] and Mehmet Yilmaz[2]

[1] ENT, Cerrahpasa Medical Faculty, Istanbul University, Istanbul, Turkey

[2] Yunus Emre Clinic, Turkey

*Address all correspondence to: dr_yzy@hotmail.com

Academic Editor: Yuvaraja Teekaraman

ABSTRACT

When Meniere's disease's vertigo attacks are too frequent and medical treatment options fail, surgical treatment options should be considered. Meniere's disease is progressive, and there is not a known cure, and all treatment options are symptomatic. Also the possibility of bilateral involvement is another well-known characteristic of this condition as well as its effect on hearing. Some of the patients have progressive hearing loss with vertigo attacks. In order to decide a surgical procedure for these patients, clinicians must be aware of the natural course of Meniere's disease. In order to their effects on vestibular system, there are two types of surgical procedures. Nondestructive surgeries aim to alter the course of disease, and destructive surgeries aim to control symptoms while eliminating all vestibular functions of the effected ear.

Keywords: Meniere's disease, labyrinthectomy, vestibular neurectomy, endolymphatic sac surgery, neuro-otology

INTRODUCTION

When Meniere’s disease’s vertigo attacks are too frequent and medical treatment options fail, surgical treatment options should be considered. Meniere’s disease is progressive; there is not a known cure and all treatment options are symptomatic. Also the possibility of bilateral involvement is another well-known characteristic of this condition as well as its effect on hearing. Some of the patients have progressive hearing loss with vertigo attacks. In order to decide a surgical procedure for these patients, clinicians must be aware of the natural course of Meniere’s disease.

Some authors recommend to wait 6–12 months in order to recommend surgery for intractable Meniere’s disease. However, there are different definitions of “intractability.” When medical treatment fails and patient keep experiencing severe and frequent vertigo attacks, surgery option could be evaluated. If the symptoms are resistant to medical and psychological therapy for at least 3–6 months, hearing loss and vertigo attacks are frequent, and the condition could be accepted as intractable [1]. Ten to twenty percent of Meniere’s disease patients are considered to have an intractable disease [2].

There are destructive and nondestructive surgical options; in decision process, patients’ general health condition, age, and hearing levels should be considered. Progressive and bilateral nature of the disease always should be considered.

The ideal surgery must restore remaining functions while relieving patients' severe symptoms. International Consensus (ICON) on treatment of Meniere's disease recently proposed a treatment algorithm. When conservatory treatment options were insufficient to control patient's symptoms, it is recommended to evaluate patient's remaining hearing. If the effected ear has efficient hearing, conservative surgical treatment options are recommended, but if remained hearing is not efficient, destructive surgical or medical treatment options are recommended. Conservative surgery is the third step of the treatment, while destructive surgery is the fifth and last option (**Figure 1**) [3].

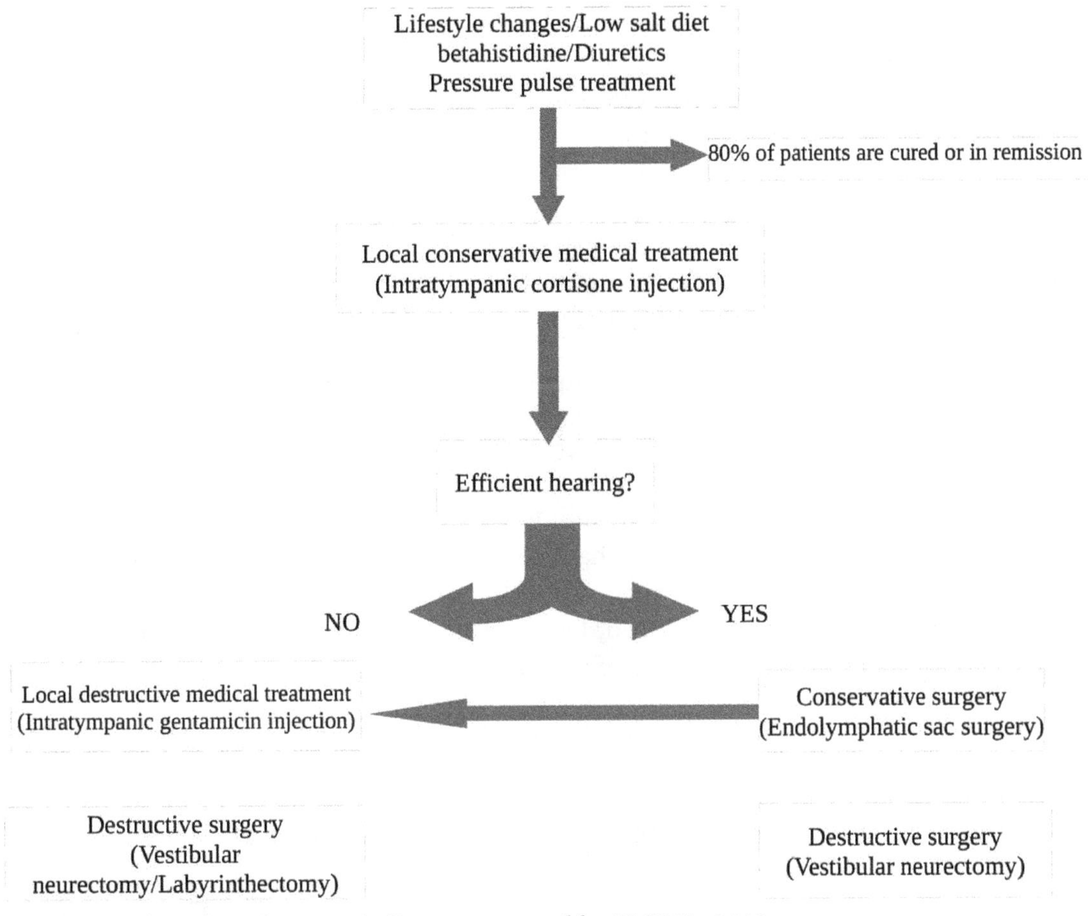

Figure 1. *Treatment algorithm of Meniere's disease, proposed by ICON in 2018.*

French Otorhinolaryngology Head and Neck Surgery Society (SFORL)'s guideline of Meniere's disease recommends surgical options after noninvasive treatment options were tried [4]. European position statement on diagnosis and treatment of Meniere's disease has similar opinions about surgery with ICON and SFORL guidelines [5].

Since local destructive medical treatment (intratympanic gentamicin) is another subject of another chapter of this book, the main focus of this chapter will be surgical procedures.

Patient selection

A successful treatment requires precise diagnosis. Typical Meniere's disease causes fluctuating hearing loss and episodic vertigo that could last minutes to hours with tinnitus and ear fullness. For every patient who describes one or more of these symptoms, clinician should consider Meniere's disease in differential diagnosis. Even nowadays, diagnosis of Meniere's disease is clinical. Detailed history and complete physical examination should be taken. After routine exam, there are some diagnostic tests that should be ordered like complete audiometric assessment, vestibular test battery, and imaging studies. Differential diagnosis of unilateral vestibular disorders is summarized in **Table 1**.

MR imaging studies should be ordered in all unilateral cases of Meniere's disease. It is helpful to exclude retrocochlear pathologies, endolymphatic sac tumors, vestibular schwannomas, or any other conditions that could mimic the symptoms of Meniere's disease. Also Nakashima et al. managed to visualize endolymphatic hydrops in Meniere's disease after administrating the contrast substance gadolinium intratympanically [6]. Miyagawa et al. visualized the endolymphatic hydrops with intravenous administered gadolinium MRI [7]. Naganawa and Nakashima evaluated the imaging for Meniere's disease and its correlation with vestibular tests of Meniere's disease patients. They reported that endolymphatic hydrops could be observed with MRI, and also all patients with Meniere's disease had endolymphatic hydrops in imaging studies, but not all patients who had endolymphatic hydrops were diagnosed with Meniere's disease [8]. If patient is unable to go under MRI, auditory brainstem response audiometry could be helpful to evaluate retrocochlear pathologies [9]. Nevertheless imaging studies are important part of differential diagnosis; also if surgery is going to be performed, computed tomography should be ordered for surgery plan.

Serial audiograms are helpful to document fluctuating hearing loss. Most specific pattern is sensorineural hearing loss of low frequency and its reversibility. Most authors reported sensorineural hearing loss at low frequencies with better hearing at 2000 Hz, called peak pattern [10, 11].

Unilateral vestibular hypofunction is most common finding of unilateral Meniere's disease, although it is reported that half of the Meniere's disease patients have completely normal responses in bithermal caloric tests [12]. Video head impulse test (VHIT) is a significant parameter to evaluate peripheral vestibular system since it evaluates semicircular canals individually. In order to evaluate utricule and saccule functions, vestibular evoked myogenic potentials (VEMPs) are very useful [13].

Electrocochleography is considered to be the most valuable test to diagnose Meniere's disease. Summation and action potentials that arise from cochlea are:

Autosomal dominant sensorineural hearing loss type 9 (DFNA9) caused by COCH gene
Autosomal dominant sensorineural hearing loss type 6/14 (DFNA6/14) caused by WSF1 gene
Autoimmune inner ear disease
Cerebrovascular disease (stroke or transient ischemic attack in the vertebrobasilar system, bleeding)
Cogan's syndrome
Endolymphatic sac tumor
Cerebellopontine tumors (such as meningioma) Neuroborreliosis
Otosyphilis
Susac syndrome
Third window syndromes (perilymph fistula, canal dehiscence, enlarged vestibular aqueduct)
Vestibular migraine
Vestibular schwannoma
Vogt-Koyanagi-Harada syndrome

Table 1. *Differential diagnosis of unilateral vestibular disorders.*

Peripheral labyrinth dysfunction	• Unilateral caloric weakness • Spontaneous or positional nystagmus (although oculomotor findings are normal) • Nystagmus could be provoked with specific maneuvers (DixHallpike, Roll, etc.) • Asymmetric or abnormal rotational chair phase • Reduced gain on rotational chair phase (bilateral weakness)
Central nervous system pathology	• Vertical or perverted nystagmus • Abnormal oculomotor test results • Nystagmus would not be suppressed with visual fixation
Uncompensation	• Persistent nystagmus (positional or spontaneous) • Post head-shaking nystagmus • Asymmetric rotational chair phase • Abnormal dynamic posturography
Compensation	• Resolution of nystagmus • Resolution of asymmetric rotational chair phase • Improvement of performance on dynamic posturography

Table 2. *Clinical interpretations of vestibular tests.*

evaluated. Summation potential/action potential ratio increases in order of endolymphatic hydrops [14]. It is not diagnostic for Meniere's disease; the ratio is found to be elevated at 62% of Meniere's disease patients as well as 21% of control subjects [15].

Sixty to eighty-seven percent of patients with Meniere's disease reported to be able to continue their normal life style with medical treatment [16, 17]. If medical treatment tried for 3–6 months and attacks of patient was not able to be controlled with medical treatment, surgical options must be considered [18, 19]. Character of the surgery is decided upon patient's remaining hearing. If hearing levels are 50 dB or higher or speech discrimination scores are 80% or higher, conservative surgeries should be offered, but if hearing is not functional, destructive options must be considered [20].

The interpretation of vestibular test results was summarized in **Table 2**.

Surgical procedures

In order to their effects on vestibular system, there are two types of surgical procedures. Nondestructive surgeries aim to alter the course of disease, and destructive surgeries aim to control symptoms while eliminating all vestibular functions of the effected ear.

Nondestructive procedures are endolymphatic sac decompression or shunt in order to increase endolymph drainage, ventilation tube insertion in order to equalize increased pressure of inner and middle ear, and lateral semicircular canal plugging to block the movement of endolymph into the effected canal [21].

Destructive procedures aim to abolish the end vestibular organs. Most of these procedures have high risk to harm the cochlea. Selective vestibular neurectomy aims to cut all the inputs coming from vestibular organs, cochleovestibular nerve section aims to stop all vestibular and audiologic input from the effected ear, labyrinthectomy aims to destruct the labyrinth which also leads to total hearing loss of the operated side, and chemical ablation aims to abolish vestibular inputs, which also has a risk to cause hearing loss and will be evaluated in another chapter [22].

Nondestructive procedures

Cochleosacculotomy

Cochleosacculotomy is also called "cochlear endolymphatic shunt procedure." This procedure's aim is to equalize the pressure between the perilymph and endolymph by creating a permanent shunt [23].

Definition of the procedure

Tympanomeatal flap is elevated and a round window niche is visualized. Angled pick is inserted through the round window membrane and directed to the oval window, and then osseous spiral lamina of cochlea is fractured.

Indications and complications

This procedure is rather easy when compared to other surgeries. It does not have risk of cerebrospinal fluid leakage. However, sensorineural hearing loss is expected to be 25% on high-frequency sensorineural hearing loss and 10% of profound hearing loss are reported [24]. Success rates are up to 70% with long-term vertigo relief [25]. It should be considered as an alternative of labyrinthectomy in elder patient who already had severe hearing loss [26].

Endolymphatic sac surgery

The exact pathophysiology of Meniere's disease is still unclear, but one of the most accepted theories is endolymphatic hydrops. Temporal bone studies of Meniere's disease patients reported endolymphatic hydrops [27, 28]. The AAO-HNS guideline of Meniere's disease defines "certain" Meniere's disease when endolymphatic hydrops are demonstrated histopathologically in the postmortem temporal bone specimen of the patient [29].

Endolymph is produced in stria vascularis and dark vestibular cells. It flows through the duct to the sac, and with active transport mechanisms, it is absorbed [30]. Animal study designed by Kimura et al. achieved to cause cochlear hydrops by ductus reuniens obliteration [31].

Paparella suggested that inadequate absorption of endolymph leads to endolymphatic hydrops. He described his theory with "lake-river-pond" comparison while endolymphatic sac is the pond, vestibular aqueduct is the river, and endolymphatic space is the lake. Any obstruction or overproduction leads to hydrops [32].

Perisaccular fibrosis, endolymphatic sac atrophy, loss of epithelial integrity of endolymphatic sac, vestibular aqueduct hypoplasia, and narrowing of endolymphatic duct lumen were observed in the pathological findings in temporal bone studies [30, 33–35].

Also some anatomic abnormalities were observed during endolymphatic sac procedures and proposed as a cause of hydrops. Some of the patient's lateral semicircular canal are located anteriorly and observed in many of the patients. It was suggested to cause vascular compression of endolymphatic sac that leads to hydrops [36, 37].

The findings of revision endolymphatic sac surgeries are another source that used to gather information about the pathophysiology of the disease. Hypoplastic mastoid air cell system with perisaccular fibrosis, discoloration of silastic tube that is inserted at primer surgery, incomplete decompression of sigmoid sinus and mastoid cavity, granulation formation in mastoid cavity, and perisaccular space were the reported findings [36–38].

Portmann was the first surgeon who suggested endolymphatic sac surgery for Meniere's disease nearly 90 years ago and reported improvement of hearing and vestibular functions of patients [39]. In the 1960s, House suggested endolymphatic subarachnoid shunt procedure [40]. Endolymphatic sac enhancement to mastoid cavity was proposed by Paparella et al. in 1980 [41].

Definition of the procedure

First cortical mastoidectomy is performed and carried on until the mastoid antrum is visualized. Then the bony labyrinth should be identified. Horizontal and superior semicircular canals are important landmarks of this procedure. Imaginary line that parallel to the horizontal semicircular canal toward to the dome of the superior semicircular canal is called "Donaldson line" is drawn. Endolymphatic sac is always located inferior of this line.

Boundaries of the endolymphatic sac are Donaldson line in superior, sigmoid sinus in posterior, jugular bulb in anteroinferior, and mastoid segment of facial nerve in lateral. These structures are in danger during this procedure. Sigmoid sinus should be skeletonized widely and facial nerve should be followed toward the digastric ridge and stylomastoid foramen in order to avoid to harm these structures. Posterior fossa dura behind the sigmoid sinus as well as the sigmoid sinus is decompressed with a large diamond drill.

Sigmoid sinus is retracted and bony dural plate and presigmoid posterior fossa dura is dissected. The sigmoid sinus and dura are retracted, and the bony dural plate that is located inferior of the Donaldson line is removed to the jugular bulb. In order to see the endolymphatic duct's entry in to bone medial to posterior semicircular canal, dissection should be carried anteromedially into retrofacial air cells. When the endolymphatic sac is identified, it is up to the surgeon to terminate the procedure or open the lumen and place a shunt. Shunt could be placed into mastoid cavity of subarachnoid space.

This procedure has many variations, sac decompression with or without decompression of posterior fossa dura or sigmoid sinus and sac drainage or shunt placement to sac [42, 43].

The role of endolymphatic sac in development of Meniere's disease is still unknown. Inadequate absorption of endolymph by the endolymphatic sac hypothetically causes hydrops which leads to Meniere's disease. The aim of decompression of the sac is to relieve the pressure that inhibits the absorptive capacity of the sac. However, when the temporal bones of patients who underwent endolymphatic sac decompression surgery were studied histopathologically by Chung et al., they observed a diffuse hydrops of the cochlea, saccule, utricule, and ampulla and reported that the decompression is the opposite of the aim of the surgery, not efficient to relieve the hydrops [44]. Linthicum and Santos reported that complete endolymphatic sac removal does not lead to hydrops in the endolymphatic duct or cochlea [45]. According to these findings, Saliba et al. recently described a novel method, endolymphatic sac blockage. They described their procedure in their recently published paper in 2015. Procedure is similar with endolymphatic sac decompression surgery;

after the endolymphatic sac identification, they block the endolymphatic duct with two titanium clips. The results were found significantly better than the endolymphatic sac decompression [46].

Indications and complications

If medical treatment options failed and hearing function of the patient is sufficient and patient is relatively young, endolymphatic sac surgery should be recommended [3]. Its effect on hearing is minimal and recommended especially in bilateral Meniere's disease [4]. Possible complications are facial paralysis, CSF leak, and hearing loss. Also in order to reach to the endolymphatic sac, the drilling is close to the posterior semicircular canal, so surgery could stimulate the otolith displacement that leads to benign paroxysmal vertigo.

Results

The results of this procedure are mostly from retrospective or observational studies. It is usually reported as an efficient and relatively safe procedure. However most of the studies lack randomization or placebo control.

The rate of complete control of vertigo after endolymphatic sac surgery is reported to be 30–72% in literature [47–52].

Thomsen, Bretlau et al. designed a randomized controlled trial to observe the efficacy of endolymphatic sac surgery. They performed endolymphatic sac surgery and cortical mastoidectomy as placebo procedure on intractable Meniere's disease patients. The results were like a milestone in otology society. Endolymphatic sac surgery results were the same with placebo surgery [2]. This paper decreased the popularity of the procedure. Twenty years later, Welling and Nagaraja re-examined their results. They found that patients who underwent placebo procedure had a complete cortical mastoidectomy when the Trautmann triangle was decompressed. Thomsen and colleagues had completed the most important step of successful decompression surgery, a complete mastoidectomy, in placebo group. After these findings, data was re-analyzed, and it was reported that endolymphatic sac surgery results on vertigo control and hearing preservation in short term were significantly better than the placebo procedure [53].

Ostrowski et al. reported that 72% of their patients were significantly improved in long term [43]. Very large group of patients, 3000, had over 90% complete or substantial control of vertigo after 3 years of endolymphatic sac decompression [54].

Kitahara et al. reported that vertigo attacks of patients who received endolymphatic sac surgery, with intraendolymphatic sac steroid injection, had significantly declined, compared to the patients who refused surgery, after 12 years of observation [55].

Cochrane review on surgery for Meniere's disease in 2013 analyzed the literature. Only two studies were suitable for inclusion. Neither of these studies' results were significantly effective on Meniere's disease symptom control, and they reported that the recent data was insufficient in order to demonstrate the benefits of endolymphatic sac surgery [56].

Sood et al. published a meta-analysis on endolymphatic sac surgery procedures. They compared the results of decompression, mastoid shunt with silastic tube and without silastic tube, in shortand long term. Decompression or shunt procedures were found to have similar vertigo control rates in short term, and the same results were observed in long term. Also no significant difference was reported between shunting procedures with or without silastic tube usage. Rates of vertigo control or hearing preservation were found similar between these procedures in short and long term. However hearing preservation results were significantly better in shunting without silastic in shortand long term.

Shunting and decompression have similar effects, but the usage of silastic tube for shunting procedure is not advised [57].

Silverstein compared the results of 83 patients who received endolymphatic sac surgery, vestibular neurectomy, and labyrinthectomy to 50 patients who were surgical candidates but refused the intervention. About 70% of patients who refused the surgery found to be freed of their vertigo attacks in 8.3 years [48].

Saliba et al. described a new approach by blocking the endolymphatic duct. They randomly distributed patients in to two groups, and endolymphatic sac decompression and endolymphatic blockage were performed. They compared the results of endolymphatic sac decompression and endolymphatic duct blockage. After 24 months of follow-up endolymphatic duct blockage group's vertigo spells were significantly improved. Also tinnitus and aural fullness were improved significantly [46].

The results of these procedures may vary between authors, but due to its relatively conservative nature and low complication rates, endolymphatic sac procedures were advised as first line of surgical treatment of intractable Meniere's disease.

Destructive surgical procedures

When the medical or nondestructive surgical procedures are not able to control the vertigo or after these interventions vertigo is recurrent destruction of the effected side must be considered. Destruction of the labyrinth is the gold standard procedure in order to relieve the patient whose vertigo is caused by an inner ear problem. Remaining hearing is lost completely after labyrinthectomy. If hearing must be preserved, selective vestibular neurectomy should be considered. Both of these procedures' aim is to block any input that come from the defective side.

While blocking the input from the periphery, it is important to prepare the central for better compensation. Before offering any surgical intervention to the vestibular system, adequate vestibular rehabilitation should be tried. After labyrinthectomy or neurectomy, complete unilateral vestibular loss is created. It has been reported that early vestibular rehabilitation after vestibular neurectomy for acoustic neuroma showed improved results to adapt [58–60]. The pathology is different with Meniere's disease, but the result of the ablative procedures is similar. It is an accepted practice to improve the daily functions of the patients. The program should be customized for each patient. Somatosensory sensation is found to be adapted earlier, and within 3 weeks, the sensation of disequilibrium resolves, but gaining of postural stability may take months [61].

Patients' mental state is another important factor that affects the success of the treatment. Patients who had no mental stress found to have better results, compared to stressed ones. Also surgical interventions are found to have better results that nonsurgical treatment in psychologically affected group. The patients' state of mind is an important factor to be considered, and psychological support should be advised to all Meniere's disease effected patients [62]. Patients who have psychological stress like depression, vestibular rehabilitation might be helpful in diagnostic process. This program could help compensation of the remaining vestibular disorder as well as coping with its effects on their psychology. If rehabilitation fails after 4–6 weeks of trial, an unstable vestibular lesion should be added in the differential diagnosis list [63].

Ablative procedures are irreversible, and surgeon must carefully evaluate the patient. Documentation of the symptoms is important to guide the patient to the most appropriate treatment option. Further vestibular investigation should be performed with every patient. These tests provide very useful information on the location of the pathology, labyrinth dysfunction, and compensation statuses.

The observation of spontaneous, positional nystagmus with electronystagmography or videonystagmography means failure of central compensation. In case of an uncompensated peripheral vestibular lesion, vestibuloocular reflex results are persistently asymmetric after several tests. Resolation of this asymmetry is a clue of compensation. Dynamic posturography could provide additional information about all systems that contribute to balance, like vision and somatosensory sense. When the test results are indicating a peripheral vestibular pathology, the offended side must be identified.

Unilateral caloric weakness, under normal oculomotor condition if spontaneous or positional nystagmus is observed, positional nystagmus that provoked with DixHallpike maneuver, asymmetric findings on vestibular tests are indicate to a peripheral labyrinth dysfunction. If nystagmus is persistent, asymmetric results are present rotational chair test or dynamic posturography results indicate an abnormal sensory organization, patient is in an uncompensated status, however if nystagmus, asymmetrics results resolve or posturography performance is improving, compensation status of the patient is improving with the advised treatment method.

Asymmetric sensorineural hearing loss is the best indicator to identify the affected side [64]. The other helpful but less reliable findings are tinnitus, aural fullness, the side that trigger the nystagmus, or asymmetric results from vestibular test batteries. Sometimes patients could describe tinnitus and aural fullness at the unsuspected ear, and this may be a clue of a beginning of a bilateral involvement. In this case if surgery is considered to be offered, the procedures that preserve the hearing should be advised [26].

If vertical or perverted nystagmus is present, oculomotor test results are abnormal, or in order to suppress the nystagmus visual fixation fails, it indicates the central nervous system involvement. Intracranial lesion of posterior fossa lesions could mimic the symptoms of peripheral pathologies; in order to eliminate these conditions, gadolinium-enhanced MRI studies must be performed [65]. If the patients are at high risk of general anesthesia or surgery due to their general health problem, nonsurgical destructive treatment options should be considered.

If surgery is the decided treatment method, the next step is to decide on the procedure. The most important factor in decision process is hearing function of the patients and his perception of their hearing. If patient has a residual hearing and he/ she finds it useful, then vestibular neurectomy, which is aimed to preserve hearing, should be advised. If no evidence of remaining hearing or patient cannot acknowledge the hearing on the affected side, labyrinthectomy, which destructs the remaining hearing function completely, should be advised.

French Otorhinolaryngology Head and Neck Surgery Society guideline of Meniere's disease management advises to start with less invasive and destructive procedures, such as ventilation tube placement and endolymphatic sac surgery. Especially in bilateral cases, clinician is advised to avoid from any destructive procedures. If these approaches are insufficient, destructive procedures should be considered according to the hearing function of the patient [4]. European position statement on Meniere's disease management advise the destructive procedures as the fifth and last line of treatment [5]. International Consensus (ICON) on treatment of Meniere's disease also keeps the destructive surgical options as the last resort [3].

Meniere's disease's progressive nature, the risk of bilateral involvement in any time of the life and possibility of spontaneous relief of vertigo in years always have to be kept in mind. Paparella recommended that treatment should be started with less invasive and destructive options; if the current treatment method seemed to fail, more invasive and destructive procedures should be considered [1].

Destructive procedures

Labyrinthectomy

If the affected side's hearing is not functional and the labyrinthine symptoms are recurrent, labyrinthectomy could be performed for any vestibular dysfunction. If patients have profound hearing loss and have intractable vertigo or Tumarkin crisis and disease is unilateral, then labyrinthectomy should be considered [4]. It could be performed in a transcanal or transmastoid approach.

Transcanal labyrinthectomy

Tympanomeatal flap is elevated transcanally and middle ear is visualized. Stapes is removed from the oval window in order to access to the bony part of labyrinth. If visualization of the vestibule is needed, the bone from the promontory that lies below the oval window to round window could be removed. Saccule and utricule are identified and then removed. Access to the ampullae of the horizontal and superior semicircular canals is performed with a right angled instrument that is placed medial to the facial nerve and conducted with blind dissection. The bony part of the vestibule could be drilled to the round window to improve visualization and identification of the nerve that innervates the posterior semicircular canal, located to the posterior ampullae. Posterior semicircular canal nerve should be identified, and in order to not leave any residual PSCC function must be sectioned.

Some authors choose to pack the cavity with soluble packing materials that soaked with aminoglycoside, to prevent from its ototoxic effects and improve the surgery success.

Transmastoid labyrinthectomy

Transmastoid labyrinthectomy is a gold standard procedure of the vestibular function destruction. Mastoid cortex is presented in retroauricular approach. Cortical mastoidectomy is performed, and sinodural angle and middle fossa dura should be carefully dissected to have adequate visualization to facial nerve and access to the vestibule and posterior canal ampullae. The antrum is identified and the dome of horizontal semicircular canal is visualized at the depth. The largest bur that fits between middle fossa dura and horizontal semicircular canal should be chosen. The drilling must be deepened with solid angle between the three bony semicircular canals before any canal lumen is opened. Lumens of bony canals are opened from the internal surface of each canal toward the center of a deeper bony cup until the labyrinthine bone is removed completely.

Horizontal semicircular canal is an important landmark to identify the tympanic segment of the facial nerve so it usually opened first. The drill should never rise to a level that is lateral to the inferior lip of the bony cup to prevent facial nerve injury. After horizontal canal is opened, dissection is continued toward its nonampullated end until the superior canal is identified and opened. The posterior canal is followed to its ampulla end. At this site, bleeding from subarcuate artery is expected and should be controlled. Following the posterior canal, ampulla is opened which is adjacent to the horizontal canal ampulla.

Dissection stays inside the cup, and inner surface of the posterior canal must be followed to prevent the injury of the second genu of the facial nerve. By skeletonize the facial canal and removal of and bony structure to limit the visualization should be removed to protect the facial nerve. Drilling should be carried on to the parallel of the facial nerve canal. After the posterior canal ampulla is opened, the bone that connects the three ampullae is removed. All membranous labyrinth is carefully removed, and the thin bone at the lateral end of the internal acoustic canal should be preserved.

Complications

It is not a complication but an expected result, but the remaining hearing of the ipsilateral ear is lost with vestibular function. Nystagmus could persist for days, and most of the patients are able to move without any assistance in 2–3 days, but the complete vestibular compensation takes months. Disequilibrium could persist in some patients.

Possible complications are facial nerve injury, CSF leak, and chronic disequilibrium. The dura of the posterior cranial fossa or IAC must be preserved to prevent CSF leak or meningitis.

Results

Labyrinthectomy is the oldest procedure to treat Meniere's disease and gold standard. Wareing and O'Connor demonstrated that vertigo control rates of labyrinthectomy are 93–100%; however in longer follow-up 76% of the patients reported to have residual symptoms. Possible incomplete removal of the vestibular tissue might be the reason of recurrence in long term [66]. It is also reported that some patients have hard time of compensation, first 1 or 2 weeks of disequilibrium is expected but it could take months for fully compensation also inadequate removal of the vestibular tissue could cause these residual sysmptoms [67]. Vertigo control rates are superior compared to vestibular neurectomy or endolymphatic sac surgery [68].

Vestibular neurectomy

The aim of this procedure is to inhibit the inputs from peripheral vestibular system and prevent the cochlear nerve to protect remaining hearing. It has high vertigo control rates which vary from 80 to 95% but still not better than labyrinthectomy [26].

Translabyrinthine approach and transcochlear approach

For these approaches, common labyrinthectomy is performed. Then the dissection is carried on with intradural dissection of the vestibular nerve within IAC. The vestibular nerve is dissected to the medial of Scarpa's ganglion. After labyrinthectomy is performed in transmastoid approach, IAC dura is identified and opened. The division of vestibular nerve to superior and inferior is identified and sectioned.

Transcochlear approach begins with transcanal labyrinthectomy. Then the cochlea is opened and cochlear nerve is followed in IAC with vestibular nerve. This approach aims to decrease tinnitus. However these approaches contain high risk of CSF leak and meningitis, and desired results could be achieved with adequate transmastoid labyrinthectomy [69].

Middle fossa approach

House was the first surgeon to introduce middle fossa approach for vestibular neurectomy in 1961 [70]. Later it was improved by Fisch and Glasscock et al. in the 1970s [71–73].

It is a very refined surgical procedure, and vestibular nerve fibers are identified in the lateral part of IAC where the vestibular nerve separates from the cochlear nerve.

Temporal craniotomy that is centered to external auditory canal is performed. Dura is elevated from the temporal bone and the temporal lobe is retracted. Dura of IAC is skeletonized; in order to prevent further injury to the cochlea, superior semicircular canal, and facial nerve, dissection should be carried around IAC widely. First superior then inferior vestibular nerve are identified and sectioned. While sectioning of inferior vestibular nerve, labyrinthine artery must be preserved. This artery is located close to the inferior vestibular nerve at the distal part of IAC.

Retrolabyrinthine approach

Retrolabyrinthine approach for vestibular neurectomy was first described by Silverstein and Norrell [74, 75]. Retrolabyrinthine approach was developed in the 1980s, and it was reported to have lower facial nerve injury and hearing loss [75– 77]. This procedure is also simpler than middle fossa approach. The eighth cranial nerve is only exposed between the brainstem and IAC; therefore it may be harder to identify auditory nerve than vestibular nerve specifically.

Dandy reported eighth cranial nerve section for vertigo treatment with suboccipital craniotomy in the 1930s, and long-term follow-up results were reported at 90% rate of complete vertigo control [78, 79]. This approach is named "retrosigmoid approach" nowadays.

The middle and posterior dura should be decompressed widely to get an ideal exposure, and retrosigmoid dura should be uncovered at least 1.5 cm posterior to the sigmoid sinus. This should allow enough extradural retraction. The bone that covers sigmoid sinus anteriorly is removed to the bony labyrinth's outline. Jugular bulb is the inferior limit of the dissection. Appropriate precautions should be taken to prevent the bone dust to enter the middle ear space.

The presigmoid dura and endolymphatic sac are incised parallel to sigmoid sinus to expose the posterior fossa dura. The cerebellum is retracted to visualize the cerebellopontine angle. Tentorium cerebelli and trigeminal nerve are identified superiorly, and the eighth cranial nerve is located inferiorly. This angle allows to visualize the posterior side of the petrous bone, so the internal acoustic canal is not visible. With minor retraction of the eighth cranial nerve, facial nerve could be visualized and advised to be controlled with electrostimulation. Vestibular fibers of the eighth nerve are located caudally (superiorly); this portion should be divided from the inferior portion of the nerve and separated with sharp dissection.

Musculus temporalis fascia is advised to be used for dural closure in order to prevent cerebrospinal fluid leak. The aditus ad antrum is blocked with fascia, and mastoidectomy defect is filled with harvested abdominal fat graft.

Retrosigmoid approach has some disadvantages such as the restricted recognition of vestibular and cochlear nerve, incomplete section of vestibular nerve, and possible damage to the cochlear nerve. However the hearing results of this approach were reported the same with other approaches. Postoperative headache is another significant trouble due to the intradural retraction of the cerebellum. Fukuhara et al. suggested the use of lumbar drainage for decompression of posterior fossa before the operation and reported that their operation time shortened, no CSF leakage occurred, and postoperative headache incidence is lowered [80].

Retrolabyrinthine-retrosigmoid combined approach was modified by Silverstein and his team in 1985. This modification allows effective access to cerebellopontine angle, and distinction of vestibular and cochlear nerve is clearer. Later they reported 85% of the patients had complete vertigo control, and the hearing preservation results were called "excellent." Only 20% of the patients had minor change at hearing, and only 4% of them experienced serious sensorineural hearing loss [81].

In order to identify cochlear and vestibular nerve clearer, some surgeons combine retrolabyrinthine approach with retrosigmoid approach. This procedure allows to remove the bone behind internal acoustic canal for better distinction of the nerve bundles [81, 82]. Retrolabyrinthine-retrosigmoid combined approach is still a gold standard in vestibular neurectomy procedure [83].

Infralabyrinthine approach

This technique is rarely used for vestibular neurectomy. The posterior semicircular canal is outlined, and the retrofacial air cells are tracted inferiorly. Internal acoustic canal is located inferiorly to the bony labyrinth.

Intradural dissection is limited to the internal acoustic canal's distal part, and vestibular nerve could be clearly identified while preserving the facial nerve. However poorly pneumatized temporal bones are hard to be dissected with this technique [84].

Intradural approaches for vestibular neurectomy could have serious complications such as stroke, subdural hematoma, and meningitis. Another life-changing complication is facial nerve paralysis, but rarely reported. Sensorineural hearing loss is another complication, reported in less than 10% of the cases [85].

Results

Most of the patients return to their daily lifestyle 2–4 months after the surgery. Vertigo control rates of vestibular neurectomy is slightly worse than labyrinthectomy, reported 80–95% [86].

Comparison of surgical interventions

Surgery is the last resort for Meniere's disease. Most of the patients' symptoms could be taken under control with less invasive methods. If surgery is on the table, it is decided upon the patients hearing and general health performance. The ideal result of the surgery must control the vestibular symptoms completely while, if present, hearing should be preserved.

Endolymphatic sac decompression is frequently performed procedure if patient has remaining hearing function. Recent Cochrane review investigated the results of endolymphatic sac decompression with other procedures. Two randomized controlled studies were included. Bretlau et al. compared endolymphatic sac shunt to placebo procedure. Placebo procedure was simple mastoidectomy. The second study was by Thomsen et al.; they compared endolymphatic sac shunt to ventilation tube insertion. Vertigo control and hearing preservation were found the same at both studies. Bretlau reported the tinnitus was improved in both groups; however, Thomsen did not find any difference between the two groups. Both of the studies used different procedures as placebo and reported that 70% of their patients had been relieved of their symptoms regardless the procedure. However it is emphasized that the blinding of the studies were poor and methodic quality is low [22].

Moffat [87], Huang and Lin [88], Gibson [89], and Gianoli et al. [90] reported their 2-year results after endolymphatic sac surgery and reported that their vertigo control rates were 43.0, 84.4, 56.8, and 60.0%, while their hearing preservation with less than 10 dB loss or improvement 10 dB or more were reported 74.0, 83.4, 44.2, and 82.0%. However these studies were lack of comparison groups.

Kitahara et al. suggested that high dose of steroid administration during endolymphatic sac drainage to improve the effectiveness of the procedure. While the endolymphatic sac was opened in to mastoidectomy cavity, steroid was applied around the sac. All of their patients had intractable disease and are grouped blindly into two groups, while the group 1 was administered steroids during surgery and group 2 did not. Patients who had intractable disease but refused surgical intervention were used as control group, Group 3. Surgery group was reported to have better vertigo control rates than nonsurgery group after 7-year follow-up, while there was no significant difference between group 1 and group 2. Steroid-administered group 1's hearing function results were significantly better than group 2. Later they reported their findings in 2013 while including group 1 and nonsurgical group 3. Group 1 reported to have significantly better hearing and vertigo control rates [91].

Paparella and Fina investigated over 2000 patients who went through endolymphatic sac enhancement surgery. Seventy-five percent of the patients had complete relief from vertigo, and over 90% of them reported that their vertigo was improved. Only 5% of the patients had revision usually 3–4 years after the first procedure. They reported that hearing preservation was achieved over 98% of the patients, and 40% of the patients hearing were improved. Serious sensorineural hearing loss after endolymphatic sac procedure was reported only to be 2% [92].

Endolymphatic sac shunt and endolymphatic sac decompression are similar operations, and both of them have similar results like more than 70% of vertigo control [93]. Further investigations of shunt procedures according to their choice on silastic placement and direct shunting to mastoidectomy cavity. Patients' hearing functions were reported better when silastic tube had not been placed, but vertigo control rates were found similar (75.0–76.9%) [55, 91].

Endolymphatic sac surgery's safety in elder population is also investigated and established as safe. Sajjadi et al. presented their results in elder Meniere's disease patients aged 65 years and older. Seventy-seven percent of their patients reported to have complete relieve of vertigo in 2-year follow-up, and no significant complications, sequels, or deaths were reported. The most major complication that reported was cardiac arrhythmia which was recorded on 1.6% of the patients [94].

Vestibular neurectomy is another option while residual hearing presents. Vestibular neurectomy with middle cranial fossa approach had 90% or above at vertigo control while hearing preservation rates are reported to be 76–92% in 2-year followup. However the long-term results showed that vestibular neurectomy did not prevent the hearing loss progression, and 5–10 years after the procedure, nearly 50% of the patients had hearing loss [95, 96].

Quaranta et al. reported their findings on hearing preservation of patients who had vestibular neurectomy, another group who had endolymphatic sac surgery, and the group who refused to had any surgical interventions. Hearing preservation rates were 58.6% in vestibular neurectomy group, 58.8% in endolymphatic sac surgery group, and 50.0% of nonsurgical group in long-term follow-up, and no significant difference was found [97].

Recent review of Kitahara et al. reviewed the results of different surgical intervention results for intractable Meniere's disease in 5–10 years. They also included nonsurgical destructive treatment and intratympanic gentamicin administration's results. Over 90% of vestibular neurectomy cases, complete vertigo control achieved while intratympanic gentamicin control rates were over 80%, endolymphatic sac surgery control rates were 70–80% and nonsurgical group vertigo control rates were 25–70%. They also evaluated the hearing function preservation (10 dB or higher) [93]. Their results were summarized in **Table 3**.

While vestibular neurectomy is superior to control vertigo attacks, endolymphatic sac surgery has better hearing preservation rates.

Labyrinthectomy is still the gold standard to control peripheral vertigo. However it is a highly destructive procedure. It destroys peripheral vestibular organ as well as the remaining hearing function. It is advised for patients who had total hearing loss at the affected ear. Selective vestibular neurectomy has advantages on this subject. Vestibular neurectomy interrupts the vestibular input while preserving the hearing functions. Both of these procedures have very successful vertigo control rates (98.8% for labyrinthectomy and 97.8% for vestibular neurectomy) [98–101].

	Complete vertigo control (%)	Hearing preservation >10 dB (%)
Vestibular neurectomy	>90	50–60
Intratympanicgentamicin	>80	50–60
Endolymphatic sac surgery	70–80	60–80
Nonsurgical	25–70	25–50

Table 3. *Results of interventions to intractable Meniere's disease in 5–10 years.*

De la Cruz et al. conducted a study to investigate the efficacy of surgical treatment modalities. They evaluated 3637 procedures that were performed on 30-year period, such as endolymphatic sac shunt, vestibular nerve section (translabyrinthine, retrolabyrinthine, retrosigmoid, and middle fossa approaches), and labyrinthectomy. They assessed the outcomes of these procedures with a questionnaire. Vertigo characteristics were reported to be improved at each group; endolymphatic sac shunt and vestibular neurectomy groups also had stated that their balance was improved. Some of the patients who had labyrinthectomy reported that their imbalance worsened after surgery. All groups reported that they still have some balance problems, while endolymphatic sac shunt group had less problems, and labyrinthectomy group's balance problems were worse than the other groups [102]. Glasscock et al. [103], Schuknecht [104], and Kemink et al. [105] also reported similar results.

It is reported that some patients' vertigo attacks were recurred after vestibular neurectomy. Incomplete nerve section, neuroma formation, inadequate compensation, vestibular disorder at the contralateral side, and unwanted nerve regeneration were suggested as an explanation for these cases [106].

Vestibular neurectomy with translabyrinthine approach and labyrinthectomy results is expected to be similar. De la Cruz et al. also compared these sub-groups with each other and found that over 80% of each group had complete control of vertigo; however labyrinthectomy groups stated that their current imbalance is more severe than the translabyrinthine vestibular neurectomy group [102]; similar results were reported by different authors [103–105].

Surgical outcomes are also related with preoperative factors. Teufert et al. designed a study to assess the prognostic factors that could affect surgical outcomes. They assessed patients with the AAO-HNS vertigo score and class, number of vertigo attacks per month, current and change in AAO-HNS disability rating, and vertigo and imbalance severity ratings and imbalance frequency. AAO-HNS disability rating, imbalance frequency and duration of symptoms were found related to outcome. Higher disability ratings and more frequent imbalance are related with poorer outcomes. Longer the symptoms had been presented, related with better outcome. The characteristic of the vertigo was not associated with outcome. Also patients who had contralateral tinnitus had worse outcome. If the first symptom was vertigo, tinnitus was present at contralateral side, and poor visual function is also found to be related with poor outcome [107].

In conclusion, there are many surgical procedures present nowadays, and each one of them has advantages as well as disadvantages. Some of the results were predictable, like hearing loss after labyrinthectomy. However surgeon must assess the patient thoroughly and choose the most appropriate procedure for him/her. The outcome has a very close relationship with patients' psychological state. Patients who did not have any psychological problems were reported to have better outcomes from treatment (surgical or nonsurgical). Surgical procedures found to be more effective than nonsurgical treatment at the patients with psychological problems [62].

Vestibular compensation after the surgery

It could take months to compensate the loss of unilateral vestibular input. Thirty percent of the patients were reported to have disequilibrium after the vestibular surgery. Pereira and Kerr demonstrated that most patients after labyrinthectomy reported that their vertigo had been relieved completely, but only 50% of them were able to return to their routine lifestyles [108]. Vertigo control is the first goal of the surgery, but compensation after surgery should not be underestimated.

The recovery after vestibular neurectomy is reported longer than labyrinthectomy and usually more incomplete; it is reported that postoperative ataxia incidence of vestibular neurectomy is 11%, but labyrinthectomy rates are reported 2% [109].

Vestibular rehabilitation is mandatory for all patients before and after the surgery. The rehabilitation program should be customized for each patient. Patients who had additional sensory deficit, visual problems, or neurologic conditions are candidates for delayed recovery. Psychological factors also play an important role in recovery phase.

Labyrinthectomy failures could occur if the diagnosis had been wrong or the neuroepithelium removal had been performed incompletely. Vestibular compensation of these patients was inadequate. Late failures of this procedure could be a result of central decompensation, but it responds to vestibular rehabilitation [110].

Vestibular neurectomy failures are usually associated with incomplete section of the vestibular nerve fibers. If the condition worsens, revision surgery should be considered.

Vestibular rehabilitation has a very important role after vestibular neurectomy and labyrinthectomy. Both procedures cause a complete loss of unilateral vestibular function. Vestibular rehabilitation is accepted as the best way to improve imbalance problems and regenerate patients' daily functions. The rehabilitation program must be customized. The somatosensory system is the first one to adapt, disequilibrium reduces within 3 weeks, and postural stability prevails months after [111].

References

[1] Sajjadi H, Paparella MM. Meniere's disease. Lancet. 2008. DOI: 10.1016/ S0140-6736(08)61161-7

[2] Arenberg I. Proposition for endolymphatic sac and duct surgery. In: Arenberg I, Graham MD, editors. Treatment Options for Meniere's Disease. Singular Publishing; 1998. pp. 19-23

[3] Nevoux J, Barbara M, Dornhoffer J, Gibson W, Kitahara T, Darrouzet V. International consensus (ICON) on treatment of Ménière's disease. European Annals of Otorhinolaryngology, Head and Neck Diseases. 2018. DOI: 10.1016/j. anorl.2017.12.006

[4] Nevoux J, Franco-Vidal V, Bouccara D, et al. Diagnostic and therapeutic strategy in Menière's disease. Guidelines of the French Otorhinolaryngology-Head and Neck Surgery Society (SFORL). European Annals of Otorhinolaryngology, Head and Neck Diseases. 2017. DOI: 10.1016/j. anorl.2016.12.003

[5] Magnan J, Ozgirgin ON, Trabalzini F, et al. European position statement on diagnosis, and treatment of Meniere's disease. The Journal of International Advanced Otology. 2018;**14**(2):317-321. DOI: 10.5152/iao.2018.140818

[6] Nakashima T, Naganawa S, Sugiura M, et al. Visualization of endolymphatic hydrops in patients with Meniere's disease. The Laryngoscope. 2007;**117**(3):415-420. DOI: 10.1097/ MLG.0b013e31802c300c

[7] Naganawa S, Yamazaki M, Kawai H, Bokura K, Sone M, Nakashima T. Visualization of endolymphatic hydrops in Ménière's disease with single-dose intravenous gadolinium-based contrast media using heavily T2-weighted 3DFLAIR. Magnetic Resonance in Medical Sciences. 2010. DOI: 10.2463/ mrms.9.237

[8] Naganawa S, Nakashima T. Visualization of endolymphatic hydrops with MR imaging in patients with Ménière's disease and related pathologies: Current status of its methods and clinical significance. Japanese Journal of Radiology. 2014. DOI: 10.1007/ s11604-014-0290-4

[9] De Sousa LCA, De Toledo Piza MR, Da Costa SS. Diagnosis of Meniere's disease: Routine and extended tests. Otolaryngologic Clinics of North America. 2002. DOI: 10.1016/ S0030-6665(02)00029-4

[10] Paparella MM. Methods of diagnosis and treatment of Meniere's disease. Acta Oto-Laryngologica. 1991. DOI: 10.3109/ 00016489109128050

[11] Paparella MM, Mcdermott JC, Sousa LCA. Meniere's disease and the peak audiogram. Archives of Otolaryngology. 1982. DOI: 10.1001/ archotol.1982.00790570021005

[12] Dobie RA, Snyder JM, Donaldson JA. Electronystagmographic and audiologic findings in patients with Meniere's disease. Acta OtoLaryngologica. 1982. DOI: 10.3109/ 00016488209128885

[13] Young Y-H, Huang T-W, Cheng P-W. Vestibular evoked myogenic potentials in delayed endolymphatic hydrops. The Laryngoscope. 2002; **112**(9):1623-1626. DOI: 10.1097/ 00005537-200209000-00018

[14] Nedzelski JM, Schessel DA, Bryce GE, Pfleiderer AG. Chemical labyrinthectomy: Local application of gentamicin for the treatment of unilateral Menière's disease. The American Journal of Otology. 1992

[15] Doyle KJ, Bauch C, Battista R, et al. Intratympanic steroid treatment: A review. Otology & Neurotology. 2004. DOI: 10.1097/00129492-200411000000031

[16] Claes J, Van De Heyning PH. A review of medical treatment for Ménière's disease. Acta OtoLaryngologica. 2000. DOI: 10.1080/ 000164800750044461

[17] Santos PM, Hall RA, Snyder JM, Hughes LF, Dobie RA. Diuretic and diet effect on Meniere's disease evaluated by the 1985 committee on hearing and equilibrium guidelines. Otolaryngology Head and Neck Surgery. 1993. DOI: 10.1177/ 019459989310900408

[18] Konrad HR. Intractable vertigo— When not to operate. Otolaryngology Head and Neck Surgery. 1986. DOI: 10.1177/019459988609500411

[19] Monsell EM, Brackmann DE, Linthicum FH. Why do vestibular destructive procedures sometimes fail? Otolaryngology Head and Neck Surgery. 1988. DOI: 10.1177/ 019459988809900505

[20] Wiet RJ, Kazan R, Shambaugh GEJ. An holistic approach to Meniere's disease. Medical and surgical management. The Laryngoscope. 1981

[21] Charpiot A, Rohmer D, Gentine A. Lateral semicircular canal plugging in severe Ménière's disease: A clinical prospective study about 28 patients. Otology & Neurotology. 2010. DOI: 10.1097/MAO. 0b013e3181ca85a2

[22] Pullens B, Hp V, Pp VB. Surgery for Ménière's disease (review). 2013;(2)

[23] Schuknecht HF, Bartley M. Cochlear endolymphatic shunt for Meniere's disease. The American Journal of Otology. 1985

[24] Schuknecht HF. Cochleosacculotomy for Meniere's disease: Internal endolymphatic shunt. Operative Techniques in Otolaryngology-Head and Neck Surgery. 1991. DOI: 10.1016/ S1043-1810(10)80227-1

[25] Kinney WC, Nalepa N, Hughes GB, Kinney SE. Cochleosacculotomy for the treatment of Meniere's disease in the elderly patient. The Laryngoscope. 1995. DOI: 10.1288/00005537-199509000000012

[26] Telian SA, Basura GJ. Surgery for vestibular disorders. In: Flint PW, Haughey BH, Lund VJ, et al., editors. Cummings Otolaryngology: Head and Neck Surgery. 6th ed. Saunders: Canada; 2015. pp. 2581-2593

[27] Yamakawa K. Über die pathologische Veränderung bei einem Meniere-Kranken. Journal of Otolaryngology. 1938;**44**:2310-2312

[28] Hallpike CS, Cairns H. Observations on the pathology of Ménière's syndrome. Proceedings of the Royal Society of Medicine. 1938. DOI: 10.1017/ S0022215100003947

[29] Committee on Hearing and Equilibrium guidelines for the diagnosis and evaluation of therapy in Meniere's disease. Otolaryngology Head and Neck Surgery. 1995. DOI: 10.1016/ S0194-5998(95)70102-8

[30] Kaufman AI. Viral theory for Meniere's disease and endolymphatic hydrops: Overview and new therapeutic options for viral labyrinthitis. Annals of the New York Academy of Sciences. 1997. DOI: 10.1111/j.1749-6632.1997.tb51901.x

[31] Kimura RS, Schuknecht HF, Ota CY, Jones DD. Obliteration of the ductus reuniens. Acta Oto-Laryngologica. 1980. DOI: 10.3109/00016488009127141

[32] Paparella MM. Pathogenesis and pathophysiology of Meniere's disease. Acta Oto-Laryngologica. 1991. DOI: 10.3109/00016489109128041

[33] Zechner G, Altmann F. Histological studies on the human endolymphatic duct and sac. Practica oto-Rhino-Laryngologica. 1969;**31**:65-83

[34] Sando I, Ikeda M. The vestibular aqueduct in patients with Meniere's disease: A temporal bone histopathological investigation. Acta Oto-Laryngologica. 1984. DOI: 10.3109/ 00016488409132934

[35] Ikeda M, Sando I. Endolymphatic duct and sac in patients with Meniere's disease: A temporal bone histopathological study. The Annals of Otology, Rhinology, and Laryngology. 1984. DOI: 10.1177/000348948409300603

[36] Paparella MM, Sajjadi H. Endolymphatic sac revision for recurrent Meniere's disease. The American Journal of Otology. 1988

[37] Paparella M, Sajjadi H. Endolymphatic sac procedures. In: Brackmann DE, Shelton C, Arriaga M, editors. Otologic Surgery. Philadelphia:WB Saunders; 2001. pp. 371-384

[38] Arts HA, Kileny PR, Telian SA. Diagnostic testing for endolymphatic hydrops. Otolaryngologic Clinics of North America. 1997

[39] Portmann G. Surgical treatment of vertigo by opening of the saccus endolymphaticus. Archives of Otolaryngology. 1969. DOI: 10.1001/ archotol.1969.00770020811005

[40] House W. Subarachnoid shunt for drainage of endolymphatic hydrops. The Laryngoscope. 1962;**72**:713-729

[41] Paparella MM, And CSK, Shea DA. Sac decompression for refractory luetic vertigo. Acta Oto-Laryngologica. 1980. DOI: 10.3109/00016488009127172

[42] Graham MD, Kemink JL. Surgical management of Meniere's disease with endolymphatic sac decompression by wide bony decompression of the posterior fossa dura: Technique and results. The Laryngoscope. 1984

[43] Ostrowski VB, Kartush JM. Endolymphatic sac-vein decompression for intractable Meniere's disease: Long term treatment results. Otolaryngology Head and Neck Surgery. 2003. DOI: 10.1016/ S0194-5998(03)00084-6

[44] Chung JW, Fayad J, Linthicum F, Ishiyama A, Merchant SN. Histopathology after endolymphatic sac surgery for Ménière's syndrome. Otology & Neurotology. 2011. DOI: 10.1097/MAO.0b013e31821553ce

[45] Linthicum FH, Santos F. Endolymphatic sac amputation without hydrops. Otology & Neurotology. 2011. DOI: 10.1097/MAO.0b013e3181db733e

[46] Saliba I, Gabra N, Alzahrani M, Berbiche D. Endolymphatic duct blockage: A randomized controlled trial of a novel surgical technique for Ménière's disease treatment. Otolaryngology Head and Neck Surgery. 2015. DOI: 10.1177/ 0194599814555840

[47] Sennaroglu L, Sennaroglu G, Gursel B, Dini FM. Intratympanic dexamethasone, intratympanic gentamicia and endolymphatic sac surgery for intractable vertigo in Meniere's disease. Otolaryngology Head and Neck Surgery. 2001. DOI: 10.1067/mhn.2001.119485

[48] Silverstein H, Smouha E, Jones R. Natural history vs. surgery for Meniere's disease. Otolaryngology Head and Neck Surgery. 1989. DOI: 10.1177/ 019459988910000102

[49] Jackson CG, Dickins JR, McMenomey SO, et al. Endolymphatic system shunting: A long-term profile of the Denver inner ear shunt. The American Journal of Otology. 1996

[50] Smith DR, Pyle GM. Outcomebased assessment of endolymphatic sac surgery for Meniere's disease. The Laryngoscope. 1997. DOI: 10.1097/ 00005537-199709000-00010

[51] Pensak ML, Friedman RA. The role of endolymphatic mastoid shunt surgery in the managed care era. The American Journal of Otology. 1998

[52] Huang TS, Lin CC, Chang YL. Endolymphatic sac surgery for Meniere's disease: A cumulative study of twelve years' experience. Acta OtoLaryngologica. 1991. DOI: 10.3109/ 00016489109128054

[53] Welling DB, Nagaraja HN. Endolymphatic mastoid shunt: A reevaluation of efficacy. Otolaryngology Head and Neck Surgery. 2000. DOI: 10.1067/mhn.2000.101575

[54] Huang TS. Endolymphatic sac surgery for Meniere's disease: Experience with over 3000 cases. Otolaryngologic Clinics of North America. 2002. DOI: 10.1016/ S0030-6665(02)00027-0

[55] Kitahara T, Fukushima M, Uno A, et al. Long-term results of endolymphatic sac drainage with local steroids for intractable Meniere's disease. Auris, Nasus, Larynx. 2013. DOI: 10.1016/j.anl.2012.11.008

[56] Pullens B, Verschuur HP, Van Benthem PP. Surgery for Ménière's disease. Cochrane Database of Systematic Reviews 2013. doi:10.1002/ 14651858.CD005395.pub3

[57] Sood AJ, Lambert PR, Nguyen SA, Meyer TA. Endolymphatic sac surgery for ménière's disease: A systematic review and meta-analysis. Otology & Neurotology. 2014;**35**(6):1033-1045. DOI: 10.1097/MAO.000000000 0000324

[58] Vereeck L, Wuyts FL, Truijen S, De Valck C, Van de Heyning PH. The effect of early customized vestibular rehabilitation on balance after acoustic neuroma resection. Clinical Rehabilitation. 2008. DOI: 10.1177/ 0269215508089066

[59] Enticott JC, O'Leary SJ, Briggs RJS. Effects of vestibulo-ocular reflex exercises on vestibular compensation after vestibular schwannoma surgery. Otology & Neurotology. 2005. DOI: 10.1097/00129492-200503000000024

[60] Tjernström F, Fransson PA, Kahlon B, et al. Vestibular PREHAB and gentamicin before schwannoma surgery may improve long-term postural function. Journal of Neurology, Neurosurgery, and Psychiatry. 2009. DOI: 10.1136/jnnp.2008.170878

[61] Gottshall KR, Topp SG, Hoffer ME. Early vestibular physical therapy rehabilitation for Meniere's disease. Otolaryngologic Clinics of North America. 2010;**43**(5):1113-1119. DOI: 10.1016/j.otc.2010.05.006

[62] Yokota Y, Kitahara T, Sakagami M, et al. Surgical results and psychological status in patients with intractable Ménière's disease. Auris, Nasus, Larynx. 2016;**43**(3):287-291. DOI: 10.1016/j. anl.2015.10.007

[63] Telian SASNT. Update on vestibular rehabilitation therapy. Otolaryngologic Clinics of North America. 1996

[64] Shone G, Kemink JL, Telian SA, Shone GR. Prognostic significance of hearing loss as a lateralizing indicator in the surgical treatment of vertigo. The Journal of Laryngology and Otology. 1991. DOI: 10.1017/S0022215100116834

[65] Disher M, Telian S, Kemink JL. Evaluation of acute vertigo: Unusual lesions imitating vestibular neuritis. The American Journal of Otology. 1991; **12**(3):227-231

[66] Wareing MJ, O'Connor AF. The role of labyrinthectomy and cochlear implantation in Meniere's disease. Ear, Nose, & Throat Journal. 1997

[67] Alarcón AV, Hidalgo LOV, Arévalo RJ, Diaz MP. Labyrinthectomy and vestibular neurectomy for intractable vertiginous symptoms. International Archives of Otorhinolaryngology. 2017. DOI: 10.1055/s-0037-1599242

[68] Kartush J. Endolymphatic sac surgery. In: Arriaga M, editor. Essentials of Neurotology. London: Thieme; 2002

[69] Langman AW, Lindeman RC. Surgery for vertigo in the nonserviceable hearing ear: Transmastoid labyrinthectomy or translabyrinthine vestibular nerve section. The Laryngoscope. 1993. DOI: 10.1288/00005537-199312000000001

[70] House W. Surgical exposure of the internal auditory canal and its contents through the middle cranial fossa. The Laryngoscope. 1961;**71**:1363

[71] Fisch U. Vestibular and cochlear neurectomy. Transactions of the American Academy of Ophthalmology and Otolaryngology. 1974;**78**(4):252-255

[72] Glasscock M 3rd. Vestibular nerve section. Middle fossa and translabyrinthine. Archives of Otolaryngology. 1973;**97**(2):112-114

[73] Glasscock ME, Kveton JF, Christiansen SG. Middle fossa vestibular neurectomy: An update. Otolaryngology Head and Neck Surgery. 1984. DOI: 10.1177/019459988409200215

[74] Silverstein H, Norrell H. Retrolabyrinthine surgery: A direct approach to the cerebellopontine angle. In: Silverstein H, Norrell H, editors. Neurological Surgery of the Ear. Birmingham, AL: Aesculapius; 1979. pp. 318-322

[75] Silverstein H, Norrell H. Retrolabyrinthine surgery: A direct approach to the cerebellopontine angle. Otolaryngology Head and Neck Surgery. 1980. DOI: 10.1177/ 019459988008800425

[76] House JW, Hitselberger WE, Mcelveen J, Brackmann DE. Retrolabyrinthine section of the vestibular nerve. Otolaryngology Head and Neck Surgery. 1984. DOI: 10.1177/ 019459988409200214

[77] Kemink JL, Hoff JT. Retrolabyrinthine vestibular nerve section: Analysis of results. The Laryngoscope. 1986

[78] Dandy WE. Benign, encapsulated tumors in the lateral ventricles of the brain. The Journal of Nervous and Mental Disease. 2006. DOI: 10.1097/ 00005053-193510000-00042

[79] Green R. Surgical treatment of vertigo with follow up on Walter Dandy's cases. In: Proceedings of the Congress of Neurological Surgeons. Baltimore: Williams and Williams; 1958. p. 141

[80] Fukuhara T, Silverman DA, Hughes GB, et al. Vestibular nerve sectioning for intractable vertigo: Efficacy of simplified retrosigmoid approach. Otology & Neurotology. 2002. DOI: 10.1097/00129492-200201000-00016

[81] Silverstein H, Norrell H, Smouha EE. Retrosigmoid-internal auditory canal approach vs. retrolabyrinthine approach for vestibular neurectomy. Otolaryngology Head and Neck Surgery. 1987. DOI: 10.1177/ 019459988709700309

[82] McKenna MJ, Nadol JB Jr, Ojemann RG, Halpin C. Vestibular neurectomy: Retrosigmoid-intracanalicular versus retrolabyrinthine approach. The American Journal of Otology. 1996

[83] Silverstein H, Norrell H, Smouha E, Jones R. Combined retrolabretrosigmoid vestibular neurectomy. An evolution in approach. The American Journal of Otology. 1989

[84] Vernick DM. Infralabyrinthine approach to the internal auditory canal. Otolaryngology Head and Neck Surgery. 1990. DOI: 10.1177/ 019459989010200401

[85] Moody-Antonio S, House JW. Hearing outcome after concurrent endolymphatic shunt and vestibular nerve section. Otology & Neurotology. 2003. DOI: 10.1097/00129492-200305000-00016

[86] Green JD, Shelton C, Brackmann DE. Middle fossa vestibular neurectomy in retrolabyrinthine neurectomy failures. Archives of Otolaryngology Head and Neck Surgery. 1992. DOI: 10.1001/ archotol.1992.01880100048012

[87] Moffat DA. Endolymphatic sac surgery: Analysis of 100 operations. Clinical Otolaryngology and Allied Sciences. 1994. DOI: 10.1111/j.1365-2273.1994.tb01228.x

[88] Huang TS, Lin CC. Endolymphatic sac ballooning surgery for Meniere's disease. The Annals of Otology, Rhinology, and Laryngology. 1994. DOI: 10.1177/000348949410300509

[89] Gibson WPR. The effect of surgical removal of the extraosseous portion of the endolymphatic sac in patients suffering from Meniere's disease. The Journal of Laryngology and Otology. 1996. DOI: 10.1017/ S0022215100135637

[90] Gianou GJ, Larouere MJ, Kartush JM, Wayman J. Sac-vein decompression for intractable Meniere's disease: Two-year treatment results. Otolaryngology Head and Neck Surgery. 1998. DOI: 10.1016/S0194-5998 (98)70370-5

[91] Kitahara T, Kubo T, Okumura SI, Kitahara M. Effects of endolymphatic sac drainage with steroids for intractable Ménière's disease: A long-term followup and randomized controlled study. The Laryngoscope. 2008. DOI: 10.1097/ MLG.0b013e3181651c4a

[92] Paparella M. Revision of endolymphatic sac surgery for recurrent Meniere's disease. Otolaryngologic Clinics of North America. 2002;**35**(3): 607-619. DOI: 10.1016/S0030-6665(02)00032-4

[93] Kitahara T. Evidence of surgical treatments for intractable Meniere's disease. Auris, Nasus, Larynx. 2018; **45**(3):393-398. DOI: 10.1016/j. anl.2017.07.016

[94] Sajjadi H, Paparella MM, Williams T. Endolymphatic sac enhancement surgery in elderly patients with Meniere's disease. Ear, Nose, & Throat Journal. 1998

[95] Silverstein H, Rosenberg S, Arruda J, Isaacson JE. Surgical ablation of the vestibular system in the treatment of Meniere's disease. Otolaryngologic Clinics of North America. 1997

[96] Tewary AK, Riley N, Kerr AG. Long-term results of vestibular nerve section. The Journal of Laryngology and Otology. 1998. DOI: 10.1017/ S0022215100142719

[97] Quaranta A, Onofri M, Sallustio V, Iurato S. Comparison of long-term hearing results after vestibular neurectomy, endolymphatic mastoid shunt, and medical therapy. The American Journal of Otology. 1997

[98] Fisch U. Middle fossa vestibular neurectomy. In: Silverstein H, Norrell H, editors. Neurological Surgery of the Ear. Aesculapius; 1977

[99] Hammerschlag PE, Schuknecht HF. Transcanal labyrinthectomy for intractable vertigo. Archives of Otolaryngology. 1981. DOI: 10.1001/ archotol.1981.00790390018006

[100] Levine SC, Glasscock M, McKennan KX. Long-term results of labyrinthectomy. The Laryngoscope. 2006. DOI: 10.1288/00005537-199002000-00003

[101] Iurato S, Onofri M. A five to thirteen year follow-up of thirty-one consecutive cases of vestibular neurectomy for Meniere's disease. In: Nadol JBJ, editor. Second International Symposium on Meniere's Disease. Cambridge; 1988. pp. 563-566

[102] De la Cruz A, Teufert KB, Berliner KI. Surgical treatment for vertigo: Patient survey of vertigo, imbalance, and time course for recovery. Otolaryngology Head and Neck Surgery. 2006. DOI: 10.1016/j. otohns.2006.05.011

[103] Glasscock ME, Davis WE, Hughes GB, Jackson CG. Labyrinthectomy versus middle fossa vestibular nerve section in Menière's disease; a critical evaluation of relief of vertigo. The Annals of Otology, Rhinology, and Laryngology. 1980. DOI: 10.1177/000348948008900405

[104] Schuknecht HF. Behavior of the vestibular nerve following labyrinthectomy. The Annals of Otology, Rhinology, and Laryngology. 1982

[105] Kemink JL, Telian SA, Graham MD, Joynt L. Transmastoid labyrinthectomy: Reliable surgical management of vertigo. Otolaryngology Head and Neck Surgery. 1989. DOI: 10.1177/019459988910100102

[106] Thedinger BS, Thedinger BA. Analysis of patients with persistent dizziness after vestibular nerve section. Ear, Nose, & Throat Journal. 1998

[107] Teufert KB, Berliner KI, De La Cruz A. Persistent dizziness after surgical treatment of vertigo: An exploratory study of prognostic factors. Otology & Neurotology. 2007. DOI: 10.1097/MAO.0b013e318157fdd0

[108] Pereira KD, Kerr AG. Disabililty after labyrinthectomy. The Journal of Laryngology and Otology. 2007. DOI: 10.1017/s0022215100133237

[109] Gacek RR, Gacek MR. Comparison of labyrinthectomy and vestibular neurectomy in the control of vertigo. The Laryngoscope. 1996;**106**(2): 225-230. DOI: 10.1097/00005537-199602000-00023

[110] Katsarkas A, Segal BN. Unilateral loss of peripheral vestibular function in patients: Degree of compensation and factors causing decompensation. Otolaryngology Head and Neck Surgery. 1988. DOI: 10.1177/019459988809800108

[111] Magnusson M, Kahlon B, Karlberg M, Lindberg S, Siesjö P, Tjernström F. Vestibular "pREHAB.". Annals of the New York Academy of Sciences. 2009. DOI: 10.1111/j.1749-6632.2009.03778.x

4

Relative Efficiency of Cochlear Hydrops Analysis Masking Procedure and Cervical Vestibular Evoked Myogenic Potential in Identification of Meniere's Disease

Niraj Kumar Singh, Rahul Krishnamurthy, and Priya Karimuddanahally Premkumar

All India Institute of Speech and Hearing, Mysore 570006, India

Correspondence should be addressed to Niraj Kumar Singh; niraj6@gmail.com

Academic Editor: Neil Bhattacharyya

ABSTRACT

Cervical vestibular evoked myogenic potential (cVEMP) and cochlear hydrops analysis masking procedure (CHAMP) have both shown sensitivity in identifying Meniere's disease. However none of the previous reports have compared the two tests for their relative efficacy in identifying Meniere's disease. Hence the present study aimed to compare the efficiency of cVEMP and CHAMP in evaluating Meniere's disease. The study included 58 individuals with unilateral definite Meniere's disease and an equal number of age and gender matched healthy individuals. cVEMP corresponding to 500 Hz tone burst was recorded from ipsilateral sternocleidomastoid muscle and CHAMP was acquired from the conventional electrode sites for single channel auditory brainstem response recording using a default protocol of the Biologic Navigator Pro evoked potential system. Both cVEMP and CHAMP showed statistically significant differences between the groups ($p < 0.05$). The receiver operating curves revealed 100% sensitivity and specificity for CHAMP as against 70.7% sensitivity and 100% specificity for cVEMP in identifying Meniere's disease. Therefore, CHAMP appears to be the test of choice provided the degree of hearing loss does not exceed a moderate degree. cVEMP could be used for all degrees of hearing losses, but with slight constraint on the sensitivity.

INTRODUCTION

Meniere's disease is a progressive idiopathic disorder of the inner ear, which may result in degeneration of cochlear and vestibular hair cells. It was first described by Prosper Meniere in 1861 and since then it has been noted as one of the most common disorders of the vestibular system [1]. It is characterized by the symptom triad of fluctuating sensorineural hearing loss, tinnitus, and vertigo [2]. The other symptoms include aural fullness, nausea, and vomiting [3].

The cause of Meniere's disease is a source of curiosity and still remains controversial. Trauma [4], viral vestibular ganglionitis [5], and genetic predisposition [6] are among the most popular theories explaining the cause of Meniere's disease. Other researchers suspect pathologies of the stria vascularis to be responsible for the symptom complex in Meniere's disease [7]. Still others believe it to be a possible autoimmune disorder [8]. Irrespective of the beliefs regarding the causative factors, the etiology of Meniere's symptoms has been shown to be an abnormal increase in endolymph volumes in the inner ear [9–12].

The disagreement among the scholars regarding a definitive causative factor for Meniere's disease adds up to the complex nature of the disease and increases the challenges posed upon clinicians towards its accurate identification. This, in addition to the high prevalence, has probably led to the trial of several tests for identifying Meniere's disease ever since its identification. These include pure-tone audiometry, immittance, posturography, glycerol test, and electrocochleography (ECochG). The sensitivity of these tests ranges from 37% to 61%, whereas the specificity ranges from 51% to 89%, with most falling below 65%, except posturography at 89% [13, 14]. Lower sensitivity and specificity than desired make the above mentioned tests erratic for diagnosis, thus making the administration of appropriate diagnostic tools a challenging task. This has resulted in continued exploration of new tests for diagnosing Meniere's disease. More recently, cervical vestibular evoked myogenic potentials [15, 16] and cochlear hydrops analysis masking procedure [17] have been reported as promising tests for the identification of Meniere's disease induced changes in the audiovestibular periphery.

Cervical vestibular evoked myogenic potential (cVEMP) is a test for evaluating the functional integrity of the saccule [18]. This sound-induced potential is produced along the sacculocolic reflex pathway [18–20]. The sound-induced electrical impulses, which predominantly originate in the saccule with some contributions from utricle and the semicircular canal, move along the vestibular apparatus through the inferior vestibular nerve and reach the sternocleidomastoid (SCM) muscle via the vestibulospinal tract [18–20]. The recorded response from the sternocleidomastoid muscle is a biphasic potential consisting of both positive and negative waves, where the positive wave is termed as P13 or P1 and the negative one as N23 or N1 [18]. cVEMP has been found to be useful in the identification of several vestibular pathologies including Meniere's disease. Findings such as reduced amplitude [21–27] and increased asymmetry ratio [25, 28] of cVEMP have been reported in individuals with Meniere's disease.

The endolymphatic hydrops, the most widely accepted etiologic factor behind Meniere's disease, has been reported to alter the stiffness properties of the basilar membrane and increased fluid column height which is believed to cause increased propagation speed of the travelling wave within the cochlea [29, 30]. Based on these unique changes in the inner ear dynamics, a noninvasive procedure known as cochlear hydrops analysis masking procedure (CHAMP) was introduced as a clinical tool to differentiate Meniere's disease from other vestibular pathologies [17]. CHAMP assesses the cochlear properties, especially of the basilar membrane, by using the principle of latency changes in ABR to click stimuli caused by the presence of progressively reduced cutoff frequency of high-pass masking noise. The undermasking caused by presence of Meniere's disease results in a much lesser difference in wave V latency of ABR between unmasked (response to click alone) and masked (response to clicks in the presence of high-pass masking with cut-off at 500 Hz) conditions of responses [17].

CHAMP and cVEMP have both been extensively explored and largely reported to be useful in identifying Meniere's disease. The sensitivity of cVEMP in identifying Meniere's disease has been reported to range from 53% to 94% [24, 31]. In terms of CHAMP, Don et al. reported 100% sensitivity and specificity in identifying Meniere's disease [17]. However, some of the other studies have questioned these findings by reporting significantly lower sensitivity and specificity values [32, 33]. While de Valck et al. reported 31% sensitivity and 28% specificity, Kingma and Wit showed 32% sensitivity using the standard criteria of <0.3 ms latency difference between click alone and click + 500 Hz high-pass masking noise [31, 32]. Thus there appears to bea wide range of sensitivity and specificity values for both the potentials. This indicates a need for continued exploration of these tests in order to establish the usefulness or lack of it in the diagnosis of Meniere's disease using these tests. Further, these studies have been conducted at different places using variable protocols and subjects. Therefore the sensitivity and specificity values for the two potentials cannot be compared directly. There is also a dearth of studies comparing these procedures on the same set of individuals for examining their relative efficacy in identifying Meniere's disease. Therefore, the present study is aimed at comparing cVEMP and CHAMP for evaluating their efficiency in identifying Meniere's disease on the same group of individuals.

Method

Participants. The present study was conducted in accordance with the declaration of Helsinki [34]. The study used 58 participants (30 males and 28 females) in the age range of 20 to 50 years (mean age = 35.2 years, standard deviation = 4.6) diagnosed with unilateral definite Meniere's disease as participants of the clinical group. Diagnosis of definite Meniere's disease was based on the criteria laid out by the Committee on Hearing and Equilibrium of the American Academy of Otolaryngology-Head and Neck Surgery [35]. As per these criteria, the diagnosis of definite Meniere's disease requires an individual to experience two or more definitive spontaneous episodes of vertigo lasting over 20 minutes, documented hearing loss using audiometric procedures on at least one occasion, tinnitus, or aural fullness in the affected ear with other causes of such precipitations ruled out. The control group consisted of 58 healthy individuals (30 males and 28 females) in the age range of 20 to 50 years (mean age = 35.2 years, standard deviation = 4.6) with normal audiovestibular system which was ascertained by normal results on pure-tone audiometry (hearing thresholds within 15 dB HL for both airand bone-conduction modes), type "A" tympanogram with acoustic reflex threshold within 100 dB HL at octave frequencies from 500 to 2000 Hz, presence of otoacoustic emissions, and indication of no retrocochlear pathology on auditory brainstem responses.

Procedure. Biologic Navigator Pro (version 7.0.0) evoked potential system (Illinois, USA) was used for recording CHAMP and cVEMP responses. Both the evaluations were carried out in acoustically treated single room suites with ambient noise levels meeting the requirements of ANSI standards [36].

Recording of Cervical Vestibular Evoked Myogenic Potentials. For the purpose of recording cVEMP, the participants were seated on a straight back chair. The recording of cVEMP was performed using the conventional electrode montage used previously [22, 37–40]. As per this, the noninverting electrode was placed over the middle part of the body of SCM muscle, inverting at the sternoclavicular junction and the ground on the forehead. During the recording of the responses, the participants were instructed to rotate their heads away from the ear of auditory stimulation in order to activate the sternocleidomastoid muscle. The muscle tension was maintained at a constant level within and between subjects by ensuring a constant target pointer on the shoulder resulting in about 60–70° head rotation from the midline in a direction opposite to the ear of acoustic stimulation. This method has been shown to produce similar values of variability to the use of an LED device for visual feedback and systems using electromyographic normalization [41]. It has also been shown to produce similar or better test-retest reliability than the use of an LED device for visual feedback [42, 43]. Using the etymotic ER-3A insert earphones of the Biologic Navigator Pro evoked potential system, alternating polarity 500 Hz tone-bursts were presented at an intensity of 125 dB SPL. The stimuli were grated using 2 ms rise/fall time and 1 ms plateau time as found optimum previously [39]. The stimuli were presented at a rate of 5.1 Hz. Responses from 200 stimuli were averaged to produce each waveform.

Recording of Cochlear Hydrops Analysis Masking Procedure. CHAMP was recorded with the participants seated in a comfortable position on a reclining chair. The recording of CHAMP involved placement of noninverting electrode on the vertex, inverting on the mastoid of the test ear and the ground electrode on the mastoid of the opposite ear (nontest ear), similar to those used in the previous studies [17, 32, 36]. The default settings of the Biologic Navigator Pro evoked potential system were used for recording CHAMP. Rarefaction polarity 60 dB nHL clicks were presented through a broadband insert 580-BINSER at a repetition rate of 45.5/s and averaged over 9200 stimuli. Responses were obtained for click alone and click with different ipsilaterally presented high-pass masking pink noises (81 dB SPL) with cut-off at octave frequencies from 8000 to 500 Hz (8000, 4000, 2000, 1000, and 500

Hz). An epoch of 16 ms was used in order to avoid un-ABR like responses that might arise beyond a latency of 16 ms. These responses were band-pass filtered between 0.1 Hz and 3000 Hz. A total of 6 responses were recorded: one for click alone stimulus condition and the remaining five corresponding to click along with each of the 5 high-pass masking noises. The responses were recorded twice for each stimulation condition in order to ensure reproducibility of the response.

Results

The present study compared cVEMP and CHAMP in order to arrive at the conclusion of a better test among the two for identifying Meniere's disease. In order to fulfill the objectives of the present study, 58 individuals with Meniere's disease were compared with an equal number of age and gender matched healthy individuals on cVEMP and CHAMP.

Cervical Vestibular Evoked Myogenic Potentials. Cervical VEMP were obtained from both ears of 58 individuals with Meniere's disease and same number of age and gender matched healthy individuals. The obtained waveforms were analyzed morphologically for peak-to-peak amplitude and asymmetry ratio. Figure 1 shows representative cVEMP waveforms recorded from an individual with unilateral definite Meniere's disease and an age and gender matched healthy individual.

Descriptive statistics was done to obtain mean and standard deviation of peak-to-peak amplitude and asymmetry ratio of cVEMP in individuals with Meniere's disease as well as healthy individuals. The lowest amplitudes were obtained in the affected ears with Meniere's disease followed by their unaffected ears. The individuals with Meniere's disease also portrayed larger asymmetry ratios than their healthy counterparts. The results of the descriptive statistics are shown in Table 1.

The statistical significance of the above observations for amplitude was evaluated using one-way repeated measures ANOVA for ears with group as the between subject factor (mixed ANOVA). The results demonstrated a significant main effect of ear [$F(1, 114) = 6.141, P < 0.05$] and group [$F(1, 114) = 22.035, P < 0.05$], but no significant interaction between ear and group [$F(1, 114) = 3.209, P > 0.05$]. Although the mixed ANOVA shows significant main effect of ear as well as group, it does not shed light on ear differences within each group and also group difference for each type of ear (Meniere's affected ears and unaffected ears). In order to evaluate the existence of difference between the ears within each group, separate paired t-tests were administered for each group and for identifying the presence of differences between the groups for each type of ear, independent samples t-test were done. Due to multiple t-tests, appropriate Bonferroni corrections were incorporated for the levels of significance. The results of paired t-test revealed significant difference between the ears in group of individuals with Meniere's disease [$t(57) = -3.106, P < 0.025$] but not in the groups of healthy individuals [$t(57) = 0.473, P > 0.025$]. The results of independent samples t-test revealed a significant difference between both, Meniere's affected ears and the matched ears of healthy individuals [$t(114) = -4.891, P < 0.025$] as well as the unaffected ears of individuals with Meniere's disease and matched ears of healthy individuals [$t(114) = -2.523, P < 0.025$]. These comparisons have been depicted in Figure 2 as box-plots. An independent samples t-test was also administered for asymmetry ratio comparison between the groups. The results revealed significant difference between the groups [$t(114) = 8.796, P < 0.05$]. Figure 2 also shows the box-plots of asymmetry ratio of cVEMP for both the groups. Thus, the results of cVEMP were suggestive of significantly smaller amplitude and larger asymmetry ratio in Meniere's disease compared to healthy individuals. Although the participants were unilaterally affected with Meniere's disease, the results revealed significantly smaller amplitude of cVEMP even in the unaff cted ears of individuals with Meniere's disease when compared to age and gender matched healthy individuals group.

Cochlear Hydrops Analysis Masking Procedure. CHAMP responses were obtained from all the 58 individuals with unilateral definite Meniere's as well as their healthy controls. Figure 3 shows CHAMP waveforms obtained for click alone and click with ipsilaterally presented high-pass masking pink noise with cut-off at 500 Hz.

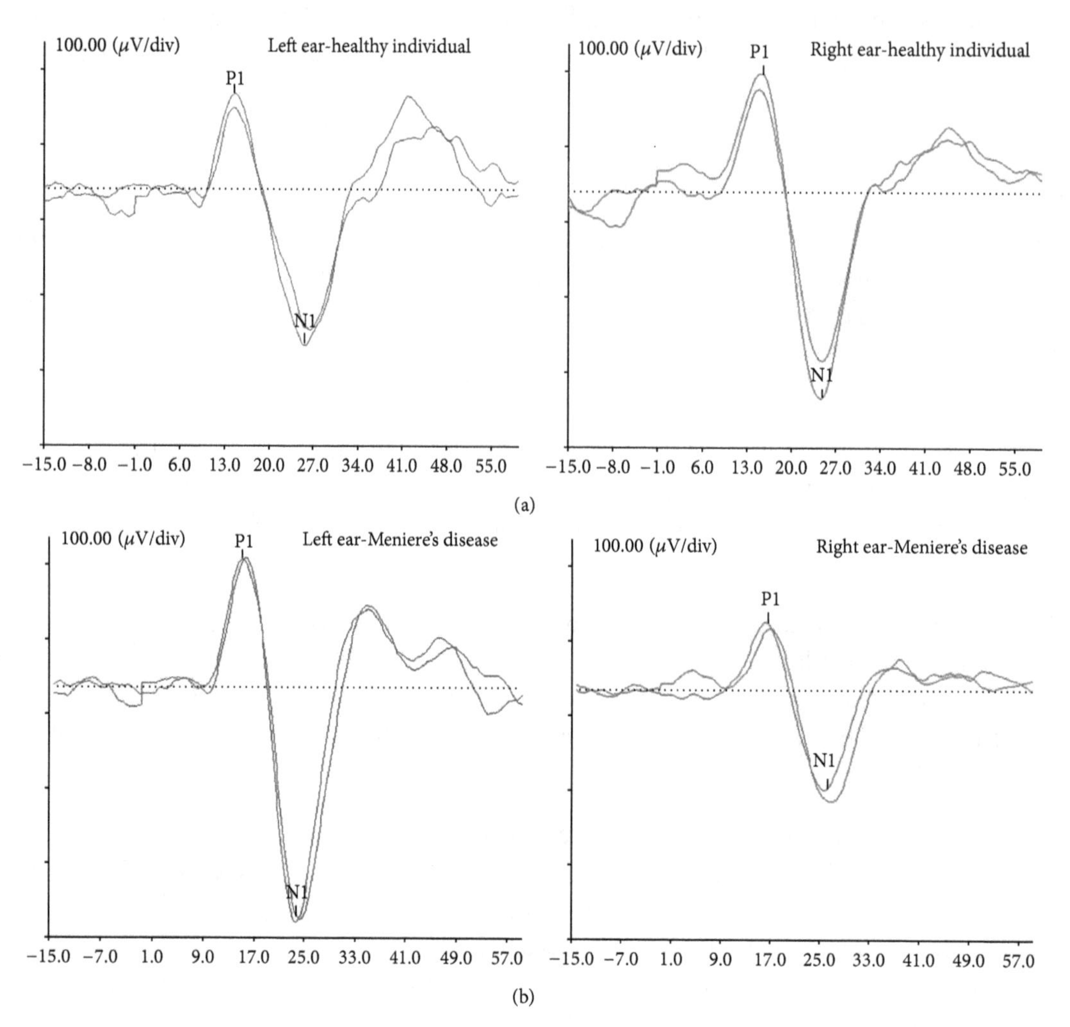

Figure 1: Representative cervical vestibular evoked myogenic potentials waveforms recorded from an individual with unilateral Meniere's disease (bottom panels) and an age and gender matched healthy individual (top panels). In this individual with Meniere's disease, right ear was the pathological ear. The positivity is indicated upwards.

Table 1: Mean and standard deviation for amplitude and asymmetry ratio of cervical vestibular evoked myogenic potentials and latency difference of wave V between click alone and click with 500 Hz high-pass masking pink noise in healthy individuals and individuals with Meniere's disease.

Population		cVEMP		CHAMP
		Amplitude (in μV)	Asymmetry ratio (in %)	Wave V latency difference (in ms)
Individuals with Meniere's disease	Affected ear	106.96 (74.00)	42.78 (22.48)	0.14 (0.10)
	Unaffected ear	124.92 (60.96)		0.89 (0.11)
Healthy individuals	Affected matched	151.31 (63.74)	16.19 (4.90)	0.96 (0.17)
	Unaffected matched	154.20 (63.99)		0.93 (0.15)

Note: "affected matched" and "unaffected matched" ears in healthy individuals are referred to the same side ears of the healthy individuals as that of individuals with Meniere's disease that were affected and not affected by the disease, respectively. The values within the brackets represent standard deviation.

Descriptive statistics was carried out in order to obtain mean and standard deviation values for latency difference between click alone condition and click along with ipsilaterally presented high-pass masking pink noise with cutoff at 500 Hz obtained from healthy individuals as well as individuals with Meniere's disease. Lowest mean difference was observed in the affected ears of individuals with Meniere's disease and largest difference between the stimulus conditions was obtained for ears of healthy individuals. The results of descriptive statistics are shown in Table 1.

The statistical significance of the above mentioned observation was evaluated using one-way repeated measures

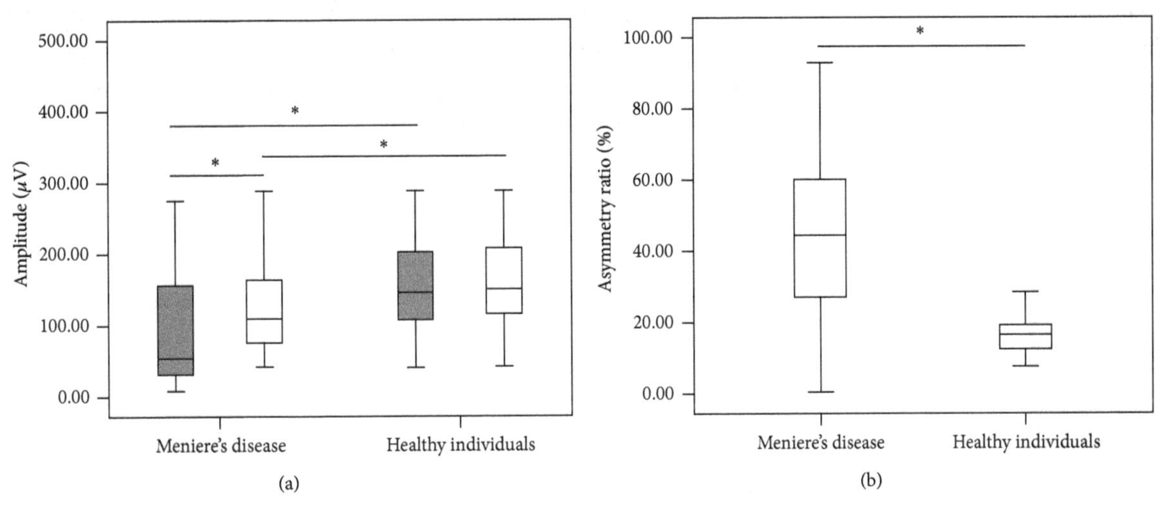

Figure 2: Box-plots for peak-to-peak amplitude (a) and asymmetry ratio (b) of cVEMP in healthy individuals and individuals with Meniere's disease; star marks above the horizontal lines represent statistically significant comparisons.

ANOVA for ears with group as the between subject factor for CHAMP. The results revealed a significant main effect of ear [$F(1, 114) = 360.724$, $P < 0.05$] and group [$F(1, 114) = 537.135$, $P < 0.05$]. There was also a significant interaction between ear and group [$F(1, 114) = 420.630$, $P < 0.05$]. This necessitated separate ear-wise analysis for groups and groupwise analysis for ears using one-way repeated measures ANOVA and MANOVA, respectively. One-way repeated measures ANOVA for ears demonstrated a significant main effect of ear in the group of individuals with Meniere's disease [$F(1, 57) = 1180.603$, $P < 0.05$]; however there was no significant main effect of ears in healthy individuals group [$F(1, 57) = 0.859$, $P > 0.05$]. MANOVA was done for groupwise analysis which revealed a significant main effect of group for comparison between aff cted ears of individuals with Meniere's disease and matched ears of healthy subjects [$F(1, 114) = 889.161$, $P < 0.05$] but not for unaffected ears of individuals with Meniere's disease and matched ears of healthy subjects [$F(1, 114) = 2.263$, $P > 0.05$].

Thus, CHAMP revealed significantly smaller latency difference of wave V between click alone and click with 500 Hz high-pass masking noise in affected ears of individual with Meniere's disease than their unaffected ears. The latency difference in affected ear with Meniere's disease was also significantly smaller than the ears of healthy individuals. There was no difference in the latency difference between the ears of healthy individuals. Figure 4 shows the box-plots for latency difference between the stimulus conditions (click alone and click with high-pass masking noise with cut-off frequency at 500 Hz) in individuals with Meniere's disease as well as healthy individuals.

Comparison between CHAMP and cVEMP. Receiver operating characteristic curves were obtained to examine sensitivity and specificity of CHAMP and cVEMP in identifying Meniere's disease (shown in Figure 5). Areas under the curve for cVEMP and CHAMP were 0.863 and 1.0, respectively. Asymmetry ratio of ≥31% is considered for abnormality in cVEMP [21] and ≤0.3 ms difference in wave V latency between click alone and click + 500 Hz high-pass masking noise is as established for diagnosis of Meniere's disease using CHAMP [17, 43]. Using these values, the sensitivity and specificity were found to be 65.5% and 100%, respectively, for cVEMP whereas they are 93.1% and 100%, respectively, for CHAMP. Present study's data revealed optimum criterion points of ≥29% asymmetry ratio of cVEMP and ≤0.48 for CHAMP for identifying Meniere's disease. The use of these values produced 70.7% and 100% sensitivity and specificity, respectively, for cVEMP against 100% sensitivity and specificity for CHAMP.

Discussion

Cervical VEMP and CHAMP were administered on all individuals of both the groups of the study. These two potentials have been investigated separately in several previous studies; nonetheless reports on the same group of individuals to facilitate the comparison of their relative efficiency in identifying Meniere's disease remained elusive until the present study. The present study is the first step in this direction.

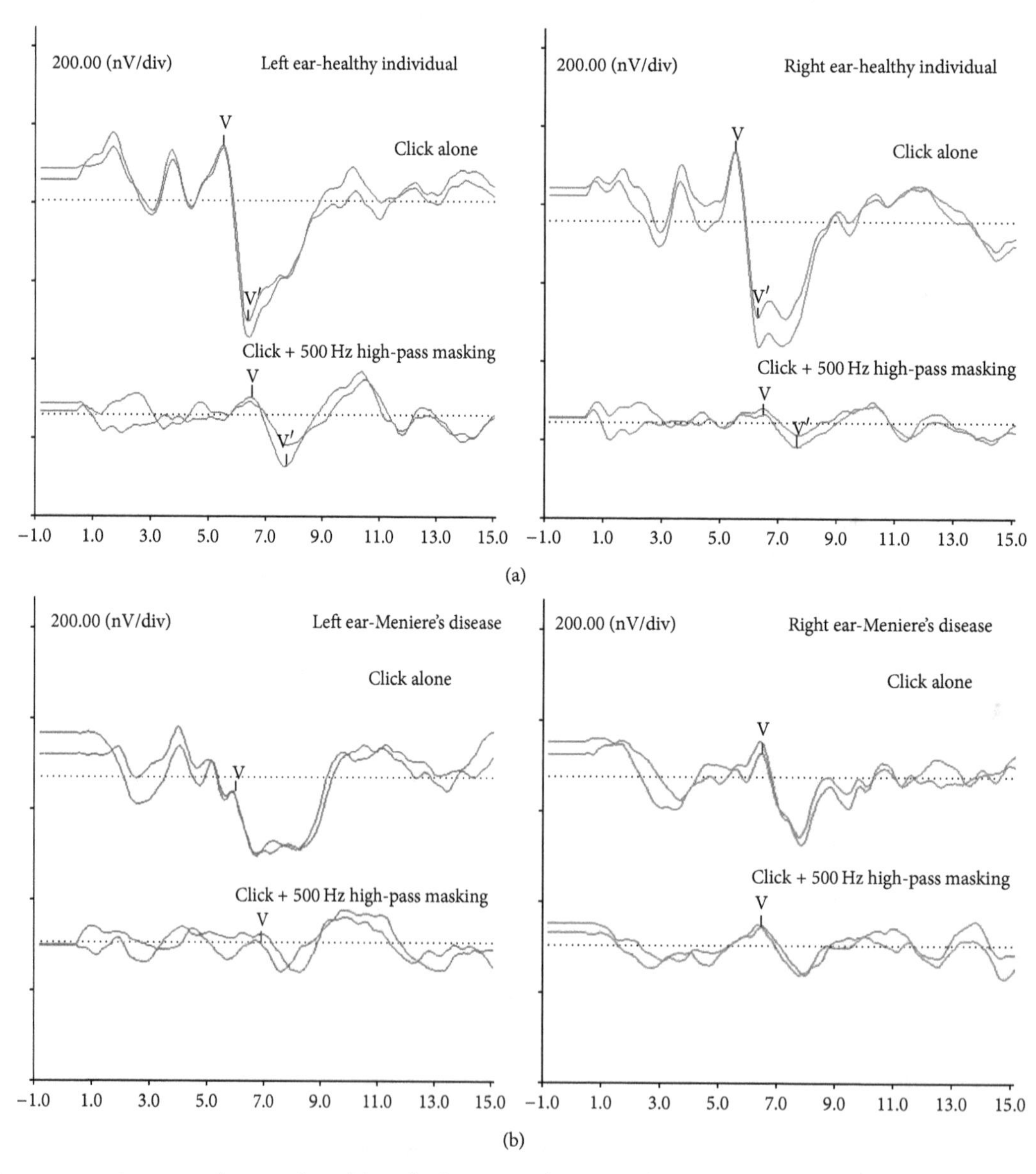

Figure 3: Representative waveforms of cochlear hydrops analysis masking procedure showing the responses for click alone and click with 500 Hz high-pass masking noise in an individual with Meniere's disease (bottom panels) and an age and gender matched healthy individual (top panels). In the individuals with Meniere's disease, right ear was the pathological ear.

Cervical Vestibular Evoked Myogenic Potentials in Meniere's Disease. The present study compared the findings of cVEMP between Meniere's disease and healthy individuals. The results revealed significantly smaller peak-to-peak amplitude of cVEMP in the Meniere's group compared to the healthy controls. This is in agreement with those reported previously in this regard [15, 16]. This might be attributed to the changes observed at the vestibular periphery, especially the saccule. The histopathological studies in individuals with Meniere's disease have revealed severe hydrops frequently resulting in the distortion of the saccule or even rupture of the saccular membrane [44–46]. This distorted or ruptured saccular membrane is likely to affect the mechanical energy transfer that vibrates the saccular macula and stimulates the saccular hair cells. This is therefore likely to result in reduced amplitude on the affected side of individuals with Meniere's disease.

The results of the present study further showed significantly smaller peak-to-peak amplitude of cVEMP in the unaffected (asymptomatic) ears of individuals with Meniere's disease than the ears of healthy controls. Affected cVEMP responses in the asymptomatic ears of individuals were also reported previously [47–49]. The postmortem studies on the temporal bones of individuals with Meniere's disease demonstrated the presence of saccular hydrops in nearly 35% of the asymptomatic ears [50], which further substantiates the findings of the present study. This was called the "occult saccular hydrops" in the previous reports [50]. This means that there is a likelihood of binaural involvement in these individuals with a later onset of the symptoms in the unaffected ears. This data (findings of present study and those reported in literature in asymptomatic ears) correlates well with the data on binaural involvement in Meniere's disease which suggests binaural involvement in nearly 30% of the individuals with Meniere's disease. Therefore, a possibility of binaural involvement with a later time of onset in the asymptomatic ears might explain the findings of the present study. However, this cannot be confirmed unless a longitudinal study on these individuals proves that occult saccular hydrops indeed was the reason for such a finding in the present study.

The results of comparison between the groups for asymmetry ratio of cVEMP revealed significantly higher value of asymmetry ratio in the group of individuals with Meniere's disease compared to the healthy individuals. This is in agreement with those reported previously [15, 16]. However, there is slight disagreement of these findings with Rauch et al. who reported no significant difference in asymmetry ratio between the group of Meniere's disease and healthy controls [25]. There was however an overall trend for greater asymmetry within Meniere's group compared to the controls in Rauch et al. [24]. Thus, the findings of the present study seem to be in agreement with those reported by Rauch et al. [25].

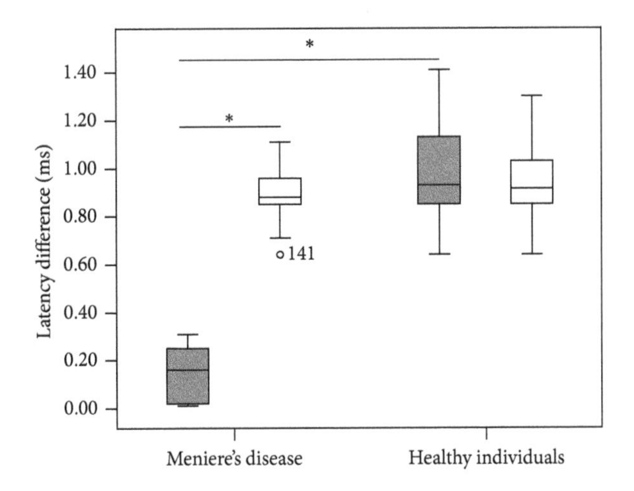

Figure 4: Box-plots for wave V latency difference between click alone and click + 500 Hz high-pass masking noise (CHAMP analysis) in healthy individuals and individuals with Meniere's disease. Grey shaded boxes represent affected ear of individuals with Meniere's disease and matched ear of healthy individuals. Unshaded boxes represent unaffected ears of individuals with Meniere's disease and matched ear of healthy individuals.

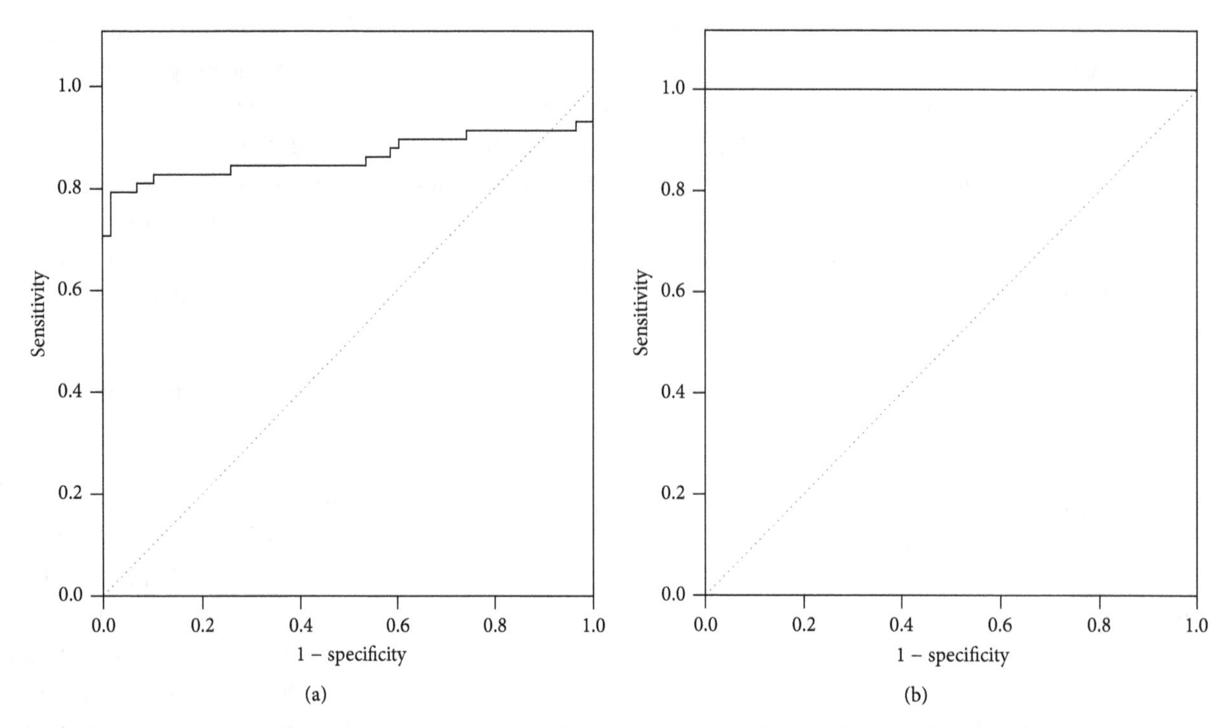

Figure 5: Receiver operating characteristic curves for sensitivity and specificity of cervical vestibular myogenic potential (a) and cochlear hydrops masking procedure (b) in identifying Meniere's disease.

The finding of larger asymmetry ratio of cVEMP in Meniere's disease might be attributed to the unilateral nature of the pathology. The previous research reports have shown Meniere's disease to be mostly a unilateral pathology [2, 6]. cVEMP, being an ipsilateral response with almost no contribution from the contralateral side [18, 21, 30, 51, 52], would therefore be affected on one side but not on the other side, thereby producing larger asymmetry between the sides in Meniere's disease compared to the healthy controls.

The saccule has been reported to be the second most frequent site of endolymphatic hydrops among the inner ear structures, possibly due to its close proximity to the endolymphatic duct [53]. The mechanism for this increase in volume of endolymph is relatively unknown; however it is hypothesized that osmotic or hydrostatic changes along with the changes in permeability of ion channels are responsible for the symptoms in Meniere's disease. These abnormalities could cause an irregular flow of ions across the labyrinthine membrane stimulating vestibular sensory cells. In addition it is likely that the enlargement of the saccular duct pushes the outer hair cell stereocilia into a less sensitive position, which could result in the deficits of mechanoelectrical transduction [6, 54]. While it is not certain how hydrops would mechanically affect the saccular macula, it is possible that the organ could be affected by one or more of the above pathological mechanisms. Overall, it is relatively clear that the abnormal cVEMP responses suggest an alteration in the normal physiology of the saccule in patients with Meniere's disease [26].

CHAMP in Meniere's Disease. The results of CHAMP revealed significantly smaller difference in latency of wave V between click alone and click with 500 Hz high-pass masking pink noise in Meniere's disease compared to healthy controls. This is in agreement with some of the previous reports [17, 27, 55] but in not in agreement with others [32, 36]. The dissimilarity in findings might be attributed to the use of different population between the two sets of studies. The present study utilized only "definite Meniere's disease" as opposed to no such criteria chosen for participants' selection in these studies [32, 36].

Smaller difference between unmasked and masked condition in Meniere's disease compared to healthy controls could be attributed to reduced efficiency of the masker as a result of changes in the stiffness characteristics of the basilar membrane precipitated by Meniere's disease [17, 55]. One of the major characteristic changes induced by the presence of Meniere's disease is an increase in the travelling wave velocity [56]. The increased velocity of the travelling wave would aff ct the properties of the basilar membrane but cannot aff ct the tonotopic organization along the basilar membrane. The increased velocity of the travelling wave is more likely to impact the low frequencies as they are represented towards the apical end on the basilar membrane (further away from generation point). When ABR latencies are obtained by presenting clicks along with the high-pass masking noise in individuals with Meniere's disease, the altered motion mechanics of the basilar membrane limits the ability of low frequency noise to mask the activity in high frequency [56]. Hence in individuals with Meniere's disease, we can observe the phenomenon of undermasking in highpass responses, whereas the undermasking phenomenon is not seen in normal individuals. This would in turn result in lesser latency difference between click alone and click with 500 Hz high-pass masking noise condition in ears with Meniere's disease than unaffected or normal ears.

Comparison between cVEMP and CHAMP in Identifying Meniere's Disease. The present study revealed higher sensitivity of CHAMP than cVEMP in identifying Meniere's disease. To the best of our knowledge, this is the first attempt at comparison between these two tests. The finding of better sensitivity of CHAMP than cVEMP in identifying Meniere's disease might be attributed to the extent of damage existing among different inner ear structures by the endolymphatic hydrops. The cochlea has been reported to be the most commonly involved site followed by the saccule and the utricle [53]. Since CHAMP is primarily a cochlea modulated auditory nerve response [17, 27, 55] and cVEMP a saccular response [18], lower sensitivity of cVEMP in comparison with CHAMP is justifiable. When a criterion of ≤0.48 for difference between click alone and click with 500 Hz highpass masking noise was used for identification of Meniere's disease, the results revealed 100% sensitivity and specificity, similar to those reported previously, although for slightly different criteria [17, 55].

The above comparison of sensitivity and specificity of cVEMP and CHAMP appears to suggest that CHAMP is a better test for evaluating inner ear functioning in Meniere's disease. However, an inherent constraint in the recording of CHAMP arises from the use of only 60 dB nHL for click intensity. It is well known that the nHL thresholds obtained using the auditory brainstem response to clicks are 10 to 20 dB higher than the behavioral auditory thresholds in HL [47, 57]. This would mean that for losses exceeding moderate degree, an auditory brainstem response to 60 dB nHL clicks would be absent since ABR thresholds for clicks have been reported to be 10–20 dB higher than the actual behavioral threshold. Thus CHAMP would appear to be useful only up to a moderate degree of hearing loss. On the contrary, the degree of sensorineural hearing loss does not impact the VEMP responses in anyway [47]. Therefore, it would be useful for evaluating patients of Meniere's disease with any degree of hearing loss. In the present study, all the participants had moderate or lesser degrees of hearing losses (although it was not planned to select participants with only such degrees of hearing losses), and hence the results show a higher sensitivity for CHAMP than cVEMP. This might not be the case, if the degree of hearing loss in some subjects exceeded moderate degree.

The results of the present study demonstrated significantly impaired cVEMP responses in the unaffected ears of individuals with Meniere's disease. However, such an occurrence was not observed for CHAMP which revealed no significant difference between the unaffected ears of Meniere's disease group and the ears of healthy controls. The postmortem studies on the temporal bones of individuals with Meniere's disease have previously revealed saccular involvement in the largest proportion of individuals followed by cochlea, utricle, and the semicircular canals [45]. This probably indicates that a saccular involvement without cochlear function compromise could be an early sign of onset of Meniere's disease in the asymptomatic ears. Since cVEMP is mainly a saccule mediated response while CHAMP is a cochlear mediated response, the lack of significantly altered CHAMP results in presence of significantly altered cVEMP responses in the asymptomatic ears could be understood. This further indicates that cVEMP could be a better tool to identify presymptomatic saccular hydrops and possibly predict the onset of binaural involvement of Meniere's disease in those who already have a unilateral pathology.

Conclusion

Both cVEMP and CHAMP showed statistically significant differences between individuals with Meniere's disease and healthy individuals and therefore both the tests are sensitive in identifying Meniere's disease induced changes in the inner ear. The receiver operating curves revealed 100% sensitivity and specificity for CHAMP as against 70.7% and 100% for cVEMP which appears to indicate that CHAMP is better test for evaluation of Meniere's disease than cVEMP. However, CHAMP can only be recorded for losses not exceeding moderate degree, which limits its use to identifying Meniere's disease with lesser degree of hearing losses only. No such limitations are imposed by the degree of hearing loss on cVEMP. Thus CHAMP could be the test of choice for hearing losses not exceeding moderate degree and cVEMP could be used for all degrees of hearing losses, although with slight constraint on sensitivity. Further, cVEMP could also prove useful in identifying the occult Meniere's disease in the asymptomatic ears of individuals with unilateral Meniere's disease.

References

[1] L. B. Minor, D. A. Schessel, and J. P. Carey, "Me´nie`re's disease," *Current Opinion in Neurology*, vol. 17, no. 1, pp. 9–16, 2004.

[2] H. F. Schuknecht, "Pathophysiology of Meniere's disease," *Otolaryngologic Clinics of North America*, vol. 8, no. 2, pp. 507–514, 1975.

[3] K. Yamakawa, "About the pathological alteration in a Meniere's patients," *Otorhinolaryngology Society Japan*, vol. 4, pp. 2310– 2312, 1938.

[4] M. M. Paparella and F. Mancini, "Trauma and Meniere's syndrome," *Laryngoscope*, vol. 93, no. 8, pp. 1004–1012, 1983.

[5] R. R. Gacek and M. R. Gacek, "Menie`re's disease as a manifestation of vestibular ganglionitis," *The American Journal of Otolaryngology-Head and Neck Medicine and Surgery*, vol. 22, no. 4, pp. 241–250, 2001.

[6] M. M. Paparella and H. R. Djalilian, "Etiology, pathophysiology of symptoms, and pathogenesis of Meniere's disease," *Otolaryngologic Clinics of North America*, vol. 35, no. 3, pp. 529–545, 2002.

[7] H. Masutani, H. Takahashi, I. Sando, and H. Sato, "Vestibular aqueduct in Meniere's disease and non-Meniere's disease with endolymphatic eyedrops: a computer aided volumetric study," *Auris Nasus Larynx*, vol. 18, no. 4, pp. 351–357, 1991.

[8] M. J. Ruckenstein, "Immunologic aspects of Meniere's disease," *The American Journal of Otolaryngology—Head and Neck Medicine and Surgery*, vol. 20, no. 3, pp. 161–165, 1999.

[9] C. S. Hallpike and H. Cairns, "Observations on the pathology of Meniere's syndrome," *Proceedings of the Royal Society of Medicine*, vol. 31, pp. 1317–1336, 1938.

[10] K. C. Horner, "Old theme and new reflections: hearing impairment associated with endolymphatic hydrops," *Hearing Research*, vol. 52, no. 1, pp. 147–156, 1991.

[11] D. T. Ries, M. Rickert, and R. S. Schlauch, "The peaked audiometric configuration in Meniere's disease: disease related?" *Journal of Speech, Language, and Hearing Research*, vol. 42, no. 4, pp. 829–843, 1999.

[12] R. W. Baloh and V. Honrubia, *Clinical Neurophysiology of Vestibular System*, Oxford University Press, New York, NY, USA, 3rd edition, 2001.

[13] N. Egami, M. Ushio, T. Yamasoba, T. Yamaguchi, T. Murofushi, and S. Iwasaki, "The diagnostic value of vestibular evoked myogenic potentials in patients with Meniere's disease," *Journal of Vestibular Research: Equilibrium and Orientation*, vol. 23, no. 4-5, pp. 249–257, 2013.

[14] D. Zack-Williams, R. M. Angelo, and Q. Yue, "A comparison of electrocochleography and high-pass noise masking of auditory brainstem response for diagnosis of Meniere's disease," *International Journal of Audiology*, vol. 51, no. 10, pp. 783–787, 2012.

[15] G. Magliulo, G. Cuiuli, M. Gagliardi, G. Ciniglio-Appiani, and R. D'Amico, "Vestibular evoked myogenic potentials and glycerol testing," *Laryngoscope*, vol. 114, no. 2, pp. 338–343, 2004.

[16] M.-Y. Lin, F. C. A. Timmer, B. S. Oriel et al., "Vestibular evoked myogenic potentials (VEMP) can detect asymptomatic saccular hydrops," *The Laryngoscope*, vol. 116, no. 6, pp. 987–992, 2006.

[17] M. Don, B. Kwong, and C. Tanaka, "A diagnostic test for Me´nie`re's disease and cochlear hydrops: impaired high-pass noise masking of auditory brainstem responses," *Otology and Neurotology*, vol. 26, no. 4, pp. 711–722, 2005.

[18] J. G. Colebatch, G. M. Halmagyi, and N. F. Skuse, "Myogenic potentials generated by a click-evoked vestibulocollic reflex," *Journal of Neurology Neurosurgery and Psychiatry*, vol. 57, no. 2, pp. 190–197, 1994.

[19] G. Zhou and L. C. Cox, "Vestibular evoked myogenic potentials: history and overview," *The American Journal of Audiology*, vol. 13, no. 2, pp. 135–143, 2004.

[20] D. Basta, I. Todt, A. Eisenschenk, and A. Ernst, "Vestibular evoked myogenic potentials induced by intraoperative electrical stimulation of the human inferior vestibular nerve," *Hearing Research*, vol. 204, no. 1-2, pp. 111–114, 2005.

[21] T. Murofushi, A. Ochiai, H. Ozeki, and S. Iwasaki, "Laterality of vestibular evoked myogenic potentials," *International Journal of Audiology*, vol. 43, no. 2, pp. 66–68, 2004.

[22] M. S. Welgampola and J. G. Colebatch, "Vestibulocollic reflexes: normal values and the effect of age," *Clinical Neurophysiology*, vol. 112, no. 11, pp. 1971–1979, 2001.

[23] M. Ohki, M. Matsuzaki, K. Sugasawa, and T. Murofushi, "Vestibular evoked myogenic potentials in ipsilateral delayed endolymphatic hydrops," *Oto-Rhino-Laryngology and Its Related Specialties*, vol. 64, no. 6, pp. 424–428, 2002.

[24] S. D. Rauch, M. B. Silveira, G. Zhou et al., "Vestibular evoked myogenic potentials versus vestibular test battery in patients with Me´nie`re's disease," *Otology and Neurotology*, vol. 25, no. 6, pp. 981–986, 2004.

[25] S. D. Rauch, G. Zhou, S. G. Kujawa, J. J. Guinan, and B. S. Herrmann, "Vestibular evoked myogenic potentials show altered tuning in patients with Meniere's disease," *Otology and Neurotology*, vol. 25, no. 3, pp. 333–338, 2004.

[26] G. Akkuzu, B. Akkuzu, and L. N. Ozluoglu, "Vestibular evoked myogenic potentials in benign paroxysmal positional vertigo and Meniere's disease," *European Archives of Oto-Rhino-Laryngology*, vol. 263, no. 6, pp. 510–517, 2006.

[27] S. K. Lee, C. I. Cha, T. S. Jung, D. C. Park, and S. G. Yeo, "Agerelated differences in parameters of vestibular evoked myogenic potentials," *Acta Oto-Laryngologica*, vol. 128, no. 1, pp. 66–72, 2008.

[28] Y.-H. Young, C.-C. Wu, and C.-H. Wu, "Augmentation of vestibular evoked myogenic potentials: an indication for distended saccular hydrops," *Laryngoscope*, vol. 112, no. 3, pp. 509–512, 2002.

[29] J. Tonnodorf, "The mechanism of hearing loss in early cases of endolymphatichydrops," *Annals of Otology, Rhinology and Laryngology*, vol. 66, pp. 766–784, 1957.

[30] G. Flottorp, "Cochlear nonlinearity in Meniere's syndrome," *Hearing Research*, vol. 2, no. 3-4, pp. 407–409, 1980.

[31] M. W. Li, D. Houlden, and R. D. Tomlinson, "Click evoked EMG responses in sternocleidomastoid muscles: characteristics in normal subjects," *Journal of Vestibular Research: Equilibrium and Orientation*, vol. 9, no. 5, pp. 327–334, 1999.

[32] C. F. J. de Valck, G. M. E. Claes, F. L. Wuyts, and P. H. van de Heyning, "Lack of diagnostic value of high-pass noise masking of auditory brainstem responses in Me´nie`re's disease," *Otology and Neurotology*, vol. 28, no. 5, pp. 700–707, 2007.

[33] Declaration of Helsinki (1964), 2013, http://irb.wayne.edu/policies/2-3 declaration of helsinki.pdf.

[34] "Committee on hearing and equilibrium guidelines for the diagnosis and evaluation of therapy in Meniere's disease," *Otolaryngology—Head and Neck Surgery*, vol. 113, no. 3, pp. 181–185, 1995.

[35] American National Standards Institute, *American National Standards for Maximum Permissible Ambient Noise Levels for Audiometric Test Rooms*, ANSI S3.1, American National Standards Institute, New York, NY, USA, 1999.

[36] C. M. Kingma and H. P. Wit, "Cochlear hydrops analysis masking procedure results in patients with unilateral Me´nie`re's disease," *Otology and Neurotology*, vol. 31, no. 6, pp. 1004–1008, 2010.

[37] N. K. Singh, L. Supreetha, R. S. Kashyap, and V. Sahana, "Characterization of age-related changes in sacculocolic response parameters assessed by cervical vestibular evoked myogenic potentials," *European Archives of Oto-Rhino-Laryngology*, vol. 271, no. 7, pp. 1869–1877, 2014.

[38] N. K. Singh, S. K. Sinha, R. Govindaswamy, and A. Kumari, "Are cervical vestibular evoked myogenic potentials sensitive to changes in the vestibular system associated with benign paroxysmal positional vertigo?" *Hearing, Balance and Communication*, vol. 12, no. 1, pp. 20–26, 2014.

[39] N. K. Singh, P. Kumar, T. H. Aparna, and A. Barman, "Rise/fall and plateau time optimization for cervical vestibular-evoked myogenic potential elicited by short tone bursts of 500 Hz," *International Journal of Audiology*, vol. 53, no. 7, pp. 490–496, 2014.

[40] N. K. Singh and K. Apeksha, "The effect of rise/fall time of 500 Hz short tone bursts on cervical vestibular evoked myogenic potential," *Vestibular Research*, vol. 24, pp. 25–31, 2014.

[41] D. L. McCaslin, G. P. Jacobson, K. Hatton, A. P. Fowler, and A. P. DeLong, "The effects of amplitude normalization and EMG targets on cVEMP interaural amplitude asymmetry," *Ear and Hearing*, vol. 34, no. 4, pp. 482–490, 2013.

[42] S. Isaradisaikul, D. A. Strong, J. M. Moushey, S. A. Gabbard, S. R. Ackley, and H. A. Jenkins, "Reliability of vestibular evoked myogenic potentials in healthy subjects," *Otology and Neurotology*, vol. 29, no. 4, pp. 542–544, 2008.

[43] B. J. Anoop and K. N. Singh, "Test-retest reliability of vestibular evoked myogenic potentials parameters," in *Student Research at AIISH (Articles Based on Dissertations Done at AIISH)*, vol. 9, pp. 51-60, 2011.

[44] J. R. Lindsay, R. I. Kohut, and P. A. Sciarra, "Menie`re's disease: pathology and manifestations.," *Annals of Otology, Rhinology and Laryngology*, vol. 76, no. 1, pp. 5–22, 1967.

[45] T. Okuno and I. Sando, "Localization, frequency, and severity of endolymphatic hydrops and the pathology of the labyrinthine membrane in meniere's disease," *Annals of Otology, Rhinology and Laryngology*, vol. 96, no. 4, pp. 438–445, 1987.

[46] F. Salvinelli, M. Greco, F. H. Trivelli, and J. R. Linthicum, "Meniere's disease. Histopathological changes: a post mortem study on temporal bones," *European Review for Medical and Pharmacological Sciences*, vol. 3, no. 4, pp. 189–193, 1999.

[47] S. Ribeiro, R. K. De Almeida, H. H. Caovilla, and M. M. Gananc¸a, "Vestibular evoked myogenic potentials in the affected and asymptomatic ears in the unilateral Me´nie`re's Disease," *Revista Brasileira de Otorrinolaringologia*, vol. 71, no. 1, pp. 60–66, 2005.

[48] M. Y. Lin, F. C. A. Timmer, B. S. Oriel et al., "Vestibular evoked myogenic potentials (VEMP) can detect asymptomatic saccular hydrops," *Laryngoscope*, vol. 116, no. 6, pp. 987–992, 2006.

[49] H. Fouly, M. E. Minawi, and T. E. Dessouki, "Value of VEMP in detecting saccular affection in the asymptomatic ear in the patients with meniere's disease ," *Medical Journal of Cario University*, vol. 80, no. 1, pp. 397–403, 2012.

[50] K. Tsuji, L. Velazquez-Villasenor, S. D. Rauch, R. J. Glynn, C. Wall, and S. N. Merchant, "Temporal bone studies of the human peripheral vestibular system. Meniere's disease," *Annals of Otology, Rhinology & Laryngology*, vol. 181, pp. 26–31, 2000.

[51] C. Ferber-Viart, R. Duclaux, B. Colleaux, and C. Dubreuil, "Myogenic vestibular-evoked potentials in normal subjects: a comparison between responses obtained from sternomastoid and trapezius muscles," *Acta Oto-Laryngologica*, vol. 117, no. 4, pp. 472–481, 1997.

[52] D. D. Robertson and D. J. Ireland, "Vestibular evoked myogenic potentials," *Acta Otolaryngologica*, vol. 24, no. 1, pp. 3–8, 1995.

[53] S. N. Merchant, J. C. Adams, and J. B. Nadol Jr., "Pathophysiology of Me´nie`re's syndrome: are symptoms caused by endolymphatic hydrops?" *Otology & Neurotology*, vol. 26, no. 1, pp. 74–81, 2005.

[54] A. N. Salt, "Acute endolymphatic hydrops generated by exposure of the ear to nontraumatic low-frequency tones," *Journal of the Association for Research in Otolaryngology*, vol. 5, no. 2, pp. 203–214, 2004.

[55] M. Don, B. Kwong, and C. Tanaka, "An alternative diagnostic test for active Me´nie`re's disease and cochlear hydrops using high-pass noise masked responses: the complex amplitude ratio," *Audiology and Neurotology*, vol. 12, no. 6, pp. 359–370, 2007.

[56] G. S. Donaldson and R. A. Ruth, "Derived-band auditory brainstem response estimates of traveling wave velocity in humans: II. Subjects with noise-induced hearing loss and Meniere's disease," *Journal of Speech, Language, and Hearing Research*, vol. 39, no. 3, pp. 534–545, 1996.

[57] Y.-H. Young, T.-W. Huang, and P.-W. Cheng, "Vestibular evoked myogenic potentials in delayed endolymphatic hydrops," *Laryngoscope*, vol. 112, no. 9, pp. 1623–1626, 2002.

5

The Treatment of Meniere's Disease by the Intratympanic Therapy

Maria Stella A. Amaral[1], Henrique F. Pauna[1], Ana Claudia M.B. Reis[2] and Miguel A. Hyppolito[1]*

[1]Department of Ophthalmology, Otorhinolaryngology and Head and Neck Surgery, Ribeirão Preto Medical School—University of São Paulo, Ribeirão Preto, São Paulo, Brazil

[2]Department of Health Sciences, Ribeirão Preto Medical School—University of São Paulo, Riberão Preto, São Paulo, Brazil

*Address all correspondence to: mahyppo@fmrp.usp.br

ABSTRACT

Meniere's disease represents one of the most frequent vestibulopathy, with prevalence of 46–200 cases per 100,000, without difference between genders and manifests in fourth decade of life. Features include dizziness/vertigo, hearing loss, tinnitus, and ear fullness. Individuals with Meniere's disease have poor quality of life due to dizziness, regarding physical, functional, and emotional aspects. The therapeutic measures are proposed, depending on the stage of the disease. About 95% of the patients are well controlled with conservative clinical treatment. The remaining 5% have incapacitating symptoms. These patients are candidates for surgical treatments classics, decompression of the endolymphatic sac, vestibular neurectomy, or labyrinthectomy. Intratympanic gentamicin injections emerged as an alternative to surgical treatments, whose risk and benefit ratio has been shown to be much more satisfactory. Aminoglycosides, such as gentamicin have been used since the decade of 1950 for the vestibular chemical ablation in cases of intractable vertigo. The drawback is that gentamicin causes irreversible destruction to cochlear hair cells with hearing loss. The selective vestibulotoxicity in the treatment of Meniere's disease can be used in the treatment of the vertigo promoting a chemical labyrinthectomy.

Keywords: Meniere's disease, vestibulopathy, vertigo treatment, chemical labyrinthectomy, vestibulotoxicity

INTRODUCTION

Meniere's disease (MD) is a clinical entity characterized by episodic vertigo, fluctuant sensorineural hearing loss (SNHL), tinnitus, and a pressure sensation of the ear. It can happen unior bilaterally, and diagnosis is made clinically, according to the classification of the American Academy of Otolaryngology—Head and Neck Surgery, updated in 2015 (**Table 1**) [1, 2]. MD is a chronic condition affecting about 190/100,000 patients in US, a general incidence about 50–200/100,000 per year, and a lower incidence of 17/100,000 per year in Japan [3].

The diagnosis of MD remains eminently clinical and its manifestations are widely variable. Many patients have audiological symptoms, some have mainly vestibular complaints and few patients have a combination of auditory and vestibular symptoms. The bilateral involvement can be observed in 10–50% of the patients, which leads to a condition difficult to treat and with unfavorable prognosis [4].

Definite	Two or more episodes of vertigo* plus audiometrically confirmed lowto medium-frequency SNHL in one ear on at least one occasion before, during, or after one of the episodes of vertigo; fluctuating aural symptoms** in the affected ear; not better accounted for by another vestibular diagnosis
Probable	Two or more episodes of vertigo or dizziness, each lasting 20 min to 24 h; fluctuating aural symptoms** in the affected ear; other causes excluded

Defined as spontaneous, rotational vertigo lasting 20 min to 12 h.

***Hearing, tinnitus, or fullness.*

Table 1. *Criteria of diagnosis of MD.*

Otopathology

Prosper Meniere, who worked as a director of the first school for the deaf-mute in Paris, described in 1861, a combination of vertigo, imbalance, and hearing impairment reflecting an inner ear disease [1]. But, only in 1937, with the discovery of endolymphatic hydrops (EH) in human temporal bones by Yamakawa and Hallpike and Cairns, the pathologic displacement of Reissner's membrane into the scala vestibuli—and so with the dilation of the scala media of the cochlea—was first stablished (**Figure 1**) [5].

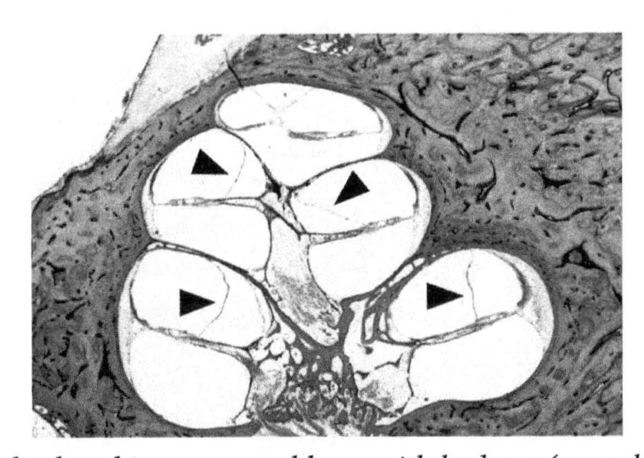

Figure 1. *Reissner's membrane displaced in a temporal bone with hydrops (arrowheads).*

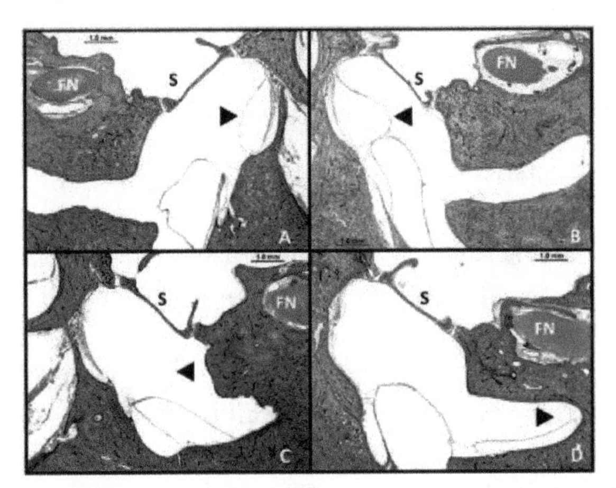

Figure 2. *Membranous structures displaced in MD. The arrowhead points the membranous structure called saccule, in different stages of hydrops (A, normal; B, slight; C, moderate; and D, severe). FN-facial nerve; S-stapes.*

Many other disorders can be related with hydrops, as aforementioned: temporal bone fracture, otosclerosis, diabetes mellitus, syphilis, hormonal disorders, migraine, and others. Diseases that can cause MD are as follows: food allergy, dyslipidemia, and autoimmune diseases [3, 6]. These disorders can also affect inner ear composition and displace in various degrees other membranous structures, including saccule, utricle, and the ampullae of the semicircular canals (**Figure 2**) [5].

Audiological findings

Several tests and evaluation methods have been employed for the diagnosis of MD. These include audiological tests, vestibular, radiological, clinical, and biochemical parameters. However, the lack of a definitive diagnostic test makes the process of diagnosis sometimes longer or frustrating. For this reason, the professional should be well experienced in the decision of when and what test should be used for the diagnostic process and, especially, to know how to interpret the results [7].

Although MD is not a rare condition, there is a delay in the diagnosis. Probably this is due to factors such as the difficulty of the differential diagnosis between other inner ear diseases, mainly due to the occurrence of nonspecific symptoms in the early stages of the disease and the absence of specific tests, in addition to the floating characteristic of MD which hinders the interpretation of the tests [8].

Patients with hearing loss and balance disorders are commonly diagnosed as having MD, which sometimes characterizes a diagnostic error, due to the lack of specific diagnostic tests [7, 8].

The main objective of early diagnosis is the early intervention, aiming to reduce the frequency and intensity of the crisis of vertigo and, at the same time, to preserve the hearing and vestibular functions [7]. Nonetheless, it is common among patients with MD, psychological suffering and loss in quality of life due to the crisis of vertigo [9, 10].

Some procedures significantly collaborate for the diagnosis of MD; however, it is important to emphasize the correlation of clinical history and symptoms with the results of the behavioral evaluation and testing goals for the conclusion of the case. In MD, a progressive hearing loss occurs with disappearance of vertigo in 70% of cases.

In addition, the audiological evaluation is important in monitoring treatment, as in the case of chemistry labyrinthectomy with gentamicin.

Tonal threshold audiometry is the basic examination used in the process of diagnosis and follow-up of MD and has a decisive role in treatment decisions. The progressive sensorineural hearing loss, with impairment of low frequencies and the fluctuations, is typical result observed in MD.

The degree of hearing loss seems to be related to the stage of the disease and has a relationship with the symptomatic period. It is common for MD patients a sensorineural hearing loss to moderate to severe before or on the first diagnosis. The settings of the hearing loss may vary; the most common is the ascendant or inverted "U." The flat configuration appears in more advanced stages of the disease. However, different audiometric results can be found and variations in the degree and configuration of hearing loss may be observed, depending on the stage of the disease. Although the low frequencies are generally more affected, hearing loss may be present in all frequencies when in an advanced state of the disease, configuring sometimes an audiogram with flat curve [11]. In this way, the diagnosis of MD should not be established in accordance with the configuration of the audiogram, because there is not a specific audiometric pattern [12]. There is no consensus in the literature that the auditory thresholds for pure tone should be investigated, including thresholds of air and bone conduction and, at least for the frequencies 250 Hz–8 kHz. A difference ≥10 dB is accepted as the float hearing for the MD. Relationship was found between the occurrence of fluctuation and the severity or progression of the hearing loss. Authors report that the hearing losses affecting the averages (between 500 and 2000 Hz) and high frequencies (between 3000 and 8000 Hz) suggest a worse prognosis than that one affects the low frequencies (between 125 and 500 Hz) [13]. The value of the results of the hearing evaluation by means of ATL has been shown to be significant, and the cochlear symptoms have been described in the literature as the most common initial sign of the disease and, many times, to appear before the vertigo.

The speech perception tests are also compromised. The percentage index of speech recognition (PISR) and the speech recognition threshold (SRT) are altered in MD [12, 13]. The average score of the PISR, when there is hearing loss can be around 56% or less if the MD is of long duration. In cases of unilateral hearing loss, percentages of PISR worst in relation to expected, considering the results of the auditory thresholds for pure tone. The speech in noise tests has helped in the intervention of the patients with MD; individuals with MD unilaterally submitted to simultaneous labyrinthectomy have improvement in sound localization and in speech understanding with and without competitive noise [13]. Acoustic immittance measures course with a type A configuration tympanometry, although in some patients with severe hearing loss of long term may present tympanometry curve characteristic of tubal dysfunction. The acoustic reflex threshold decreases in cochlear pathologies due to recruitment, the difference between the acoustic reflex thresholds of the frequencies of 500, 1000, and 2000 Hz and the tonal auditory thresholds obtained by air, the same frequencies of 60 dB or less, and outcome goal that suggests the presence of cochlear pathology (recruitment) [13]. It is worth mentioning that the acoustic immittance measures can be very useful in the diagnosis of MD, in cases of MD floating and nonfloating and with respect to the prediction of endolymphatic hydrops reversible and irreversible.

Electrocochleography (ECochG) can be used for MD diagnosis. The presence of endolymphatic hydrops is determined by the enlargement of the summation potential (SP) in relation to the action potential (AP), reflecting an increase in relation SP/AP. The SP enlargement is more evident when the patient presents fullness and mild hearing loss. In the initial stages of the MD, the increase in the endolymphatic volume alters the hydromechanical properties of cochlear stretching medium scale and changing SP. The specificity of the relationship SP/AP is larger than the sensitivity in MD. The increase of SP/AP relationship suggests the diagnosis of MD, but only in about 50% of the cases, the disease really exists [13].

Available treatments

The characteristics of the MD are well documented, as well as the treatments for this pathology. The available literature is focused to identify the etiology and how to clinically approach the symptomatic patient. The symptomatic treatment can be pharmacological and/or surgical.

The symptomatic treatment does not prevent the progression of the disease. This treatment may involve diet, vestibular therapy, and drug treatment [11]. In acute vertigo crisis, drugs that block the vestibular reflexes in the vestibule-cerebral shaft can be used. They are chlorpromazine, cinnarizine, promethazine, and diazepam [5, 14].

The endolymphatic hydrops found in MD is treated aiming to prevent its progression. In this way, there is a low sodium diet and use of diuretics, such as furosemide and hydrochlorothiazide [6].

Vasodilators are used for long-term treatment based on the fact that the hydrops can be caused by ischemia of the stria vascularis. Currently, the medical treatment of maintenance is betahistine with or without diuretic [6, 10].

Symptomatic chemical-surgical treatment

Studies have shown that the toxic effects of aminoglycosides in the sensorineural epithelium of the inner ear, particularly in the labyrinth, can be considered as a therapy for MD [6, 10].

In cases of MD with bilateral vestibular symptoms is difficult to control and with important hearing loss, has already been given in the past to ablation of the maze with systemic aminoglycosides because they control the vertigo. However, the cumulative doses of aminoglycosides increase the risk of ototoxicity with permanent cochlear damage and the possibility of causing ataxia and oscillopsia. Currently, with the possibility of injecting substances via transtympanic route, the indications for systemic use of aminoglycosides are limited [15].

Surgical treatment

In about 70% of the cases, MD evolves to progressive hearing loss with improvement to the vestibular symptoms. For the other 30% who do not present an improvement of vestibular symptoms, even with the clinical treatment, surgical treatment should be thought.

The decision to operate and the choice of procedure are often dictated by the understanding and experience of each surgeon [3]. Surgical treatment to be considered varies from conservative to destructive, depending on whether or not there is a hearing loss [3]. The surgery that is the most popular is the endolymphatic sac decompression, and it is known as a conservative surgical procedure and is widely accepted.

This surgery was first described by Portmann, in 1927, but the precise role by which the surgery works remains undefined [16]. Among the destructive surgical treatments, we have a vestibular neurectomy, the cochleo-sacculotomy, the transcanal labyrinthectomy, or postauricular labyrinthectomy [4].

Transtympanic treatment

The use of systemic aminoglycosides was replaced by intratympanic gentamycin instillations that are administered once a day by a limited number of days. The intratympanic administration of drugs for the treatment of the MD was primarily described by Schuknecht in 1957 [17]. The intratympanic injections of gentamicin provide a high rate of success in the control of vertigo with reduced number of side effects on hearing [18, 19].

The intratympanic injections of gentamicin were proposed by Stokroos. After anesthesia of the tympanic membrane, gentamicin is administered in the middle ear through a fine needle of lumbar puncture in a fixed dose of 30 mg/ml [20, 21].

One other substance that can be used is steroid, which may decrease the inflammatory reaction in the inner ear, thus decreasing the endolymphatic hydrops. It has been reported that the use of corticosteroids may help to control the inner ear dysfunction, thereby decreasing vestibular symptoms up to 91% of MD patients (with 1–4 injections of dexamethasone at a concentration of 12 mg/ml) [22, 23].

Another substance to be injected is methylprednisolone, with higher concentrations and with the possibility to last longer in the perilymph. However, many authors described data suggesting same effectiveness of both steroids [24, 25].

Both gentamicin and steroids are absorbed by perilymph through the round window membrane (which is semipermeable), the annular ligament of the oval window, and by the small lacunar mesh that surrounds the inner ear [25].

A randomized, double-blind controlled study compared the use of transtympanic gentamicin (40 mg/ml) and corticosteroids (methylprednisolone [62.5 mg/ml]), and no difference was observed regarding the effectiveness of both groups of treatments [26].

Injection protocols

1. Patient positioned at supine position;
2. Head is positioned in a slightly hyper-extension with 30° contralateral rotation;
3. Instillation 2% lidocaine in ear canal, removing completely after 15 min;
4. Under microscopic examination, tympanic membrane is anesthetized with 80–90% phenol solution at inferior and posterior tympanic membrane quadrant;
5. In few minutes, the transtympanic access could be performed using a spinal needle and a flexible catheter mounted on an insulin syringe;
6. Slow instillations of 1 ml of 26–40 mg/ml, not buffered with bicarbonate sodium in two 0.5 ml injection with 30 min apart;
7. Patient remained motionless for 30 min.

This protocol can be repeated each week or monthly for six times.

To maintain auditory function, patients must be evaluated with tone pure audiometry on every 2 weeks or before beginning each section. The treatment must be stopped in case of hearing thresholds becoming higher than 10 dB or in a case of decreasing in speech audiometry of more than 15%. A supportive drug treatment may be necessary until the vertigo control. A pretreatment auditory test is very important. The bone conduction pure tone thresholds average (0.5, 1.0, 2.0, and 3.0 kHz) is considered and repeated every 2 weeks and 2 weeks after treatment. The final audiometric exam is performed up to 12 months after transtympanic protocol initiation.

The success rate in transtympanic injection of gentamicin is about 87% in vertigo control, being a simple and safe procedure with few risks to hearing loss and tympanic membrane perforation [24, 27].

Acknowledgements

The authors wish to thank FAEPA and CAPES.

Conflict of interest

No conflict of interest.

References

[1] Gürkov R, Pyykö I, Zou J, Kentala E. What is Menière disease? A contemporary re-evaluation of endolymphatic hydrops. Journal of Neurology. 2016;**263**:71-81

[2] Lopez-Escamez JA, Carey J, Chung W-H, et al. Diagnostic criteria for Mennière's disease. Journal of Vestibular Research. 2015;**25**:1-7

[3] Wright T. Menière's disease. BMJ Clinical Evidence. 2015;**11**:505

[4] Saeed SR. Fortnightly review. Diagnosis and treatment of Ménière's disease. British Medical Journal. 1998;**316**(7128):368-372

[5] Salt AN, Plontke SK. Endolymphatic hydrops: Pathophysiology and experimental models. Otolaryngologic Clinics of North America. 2010;**43**(5):971-983

[6] Soderman AC, Bagger-Sjoback D, Bergenius J, Langius A. Factors influencing quality of life in patients with Meniere's disease, identified by a multidimensional approach. Otology & Neurotology. 2002;**23**(6):941-948

[7] Brookes GB. The pharmacological treatment of Menière's disease. Clinical Otolaryngology and Allied Sciences. 1996;**21**(1):3-11. Review

[8] Maudonnet EN, de Oliveira JA, Rossato M, Hyppolito MA. Gentamicin attenuates gentamicin-induced ototoxicity—Self-protection. Drug and Chemical Toxicology. 2008;**31**(1):11-25

[9] Strose A, Hyppolito MA, Colombari GC, Rossato M, Oliveira JA. Lack of protection against gentamicin ototoxicity by auditory conditioning with noise. Brazilian Journal of Otorhinolaryngology. 2014;**80**(5):390-396

[10] Hellström S, Ödkvist L. Pharmacological labyrinthectomy. Otolaryngologic Clinics of North America. 1994;**27**:307-315

[11] Güneri EA, Çakır A, Mutlu B. Validity and reliability of the diagnostic tests for Ménière's disease. Turkish Archives of Otorhinolaryngology. 2016;**54**:124-130

[12] Hoa M, Friedman RA, Fisher LM, Derebery MJ. Prognostic implications of and audiometric evidence for hearing fluctuation in Meniere's disease. The Laryngoscope. 2015;**125**(12):S1-S12

[13] Carey JP. Ménière's disease. Handbook of Clinical Neurophysiology. Elsevier; Baltimore, United States: 2010. pp. 371-381. DOI: 10.1016/S1567-4231(10)09028-3

[14] Santos PM, Hall RA, Snyder JM, Hughes LF, Dobie RA. Diuretic and diet effect on Menière's disease evaluated by the 1985 Committee on Hearing and Equilibrium guidelines. Otolaryngology and Head and Neck Surgery. 1993;**109**(4):680-689

[15] Nedzelski JM, Schessel DA, Bryce GE, Pheiderer AG. Chemical labyrinthectomy local application of gentamicin for the treatment of unilateral Ménière's disease. The American Journal of Otology. 1992;**13**:18-22

[16] Portmann G. Vertigo: Surgical treatment by opening the saccus endolymphaticus. Archives of Otolaryngology. 1927;**83**:316-319

[17] Beck C. Intratympanic application of gentamicin for treatment of Menière's disease. The Keio Journal of Medicine. 1986;**35**(1):36-41

[18] Cohen-Kerem R, Kisilevsky V, Einarson TR, et al. Intratympanic gentamicin for Ménière's disease: A meta-analysis. The Laryngoscope. 2004;**114**:2085-2091

[19] Diamond C, O'Connell DA, Hornig JD, et al. Systematic review of intratympanic gentamicin in Ménière's disease. The Journal of Otolaryngology. 2003;**32**:351-361

[20] Stokroos R, Kingma H. Selective vestibular ablation by intratympanic gentamicin in patients with unilateral active Meniere's disease: A prospective, double-blind, placebocontrolled, randomized clinical trial. Acta Oto-Laryngologica. 2004;**124**(2):172-175

[21] Sam G, Chung DW, van der Hoeven R, Verweij S, Becker M. The effect of intratympanic gentamicin for treatment of Ménière's disease on lower frequency hearing. International Journal of Clinical Pharmacy. 2016;**38**(4):780-783. DOI: 10.1007/s11096-016-0295-4

[22] Trune DR, Kempton JB, Kessi M. Aldosterone (mineralocorticoid) equivalent to prednisolone (glucocorticoid) in reversing hearing loss in MRL/MpJ-Fas1pr autoimmune mice. The Laryngoscope. 2000;**110**:1902-1906

[23] Boleas-Aguirre MS, Lin FR, Della Santina CC, Minor LB, Carey JP. Longitudinal results with intratympanic dexamethasone in the treatment of Ménière's disease. Otology & Neurotology. 2008;**29**(1):33-38. DOI: 10.1097/mao.0b013e31815dbafc

[24] Parnes LS, Sun AH, Freeman DJ. Corticosteroid pharmacokinetics in the inner ear fluids: An animal study followed by clinical application. The Laryngoscope. 1999;**109**(7 Pt 2):1-17

[25] Patel M. Intratympanic corticosteroids in Ménière's disease: A mini-review. The Journal of Otolaryngology. 2017;**12**(3):117-124. DOI: 10.1016/j.joto.2017.06.002

[26] Patel M, Agarwal K, Arshad Q , et al. Intratympanic methylprednisolone versus gentamicin in patients with unilateral Meniere's disease: A randomized, double-blind, comparative effectiveness trial. Lancet. 2016;**388**(10061):2753-2762

[27] Chia SH, Gamst AC, Anderson JP, et al. Intratympanic gentamicin therapy for Ménière's disease: A metaanalysis. Otology & Neurotology. 2004;**25**:544-552

6

The Intimate Relationship between Vestibular Migraine and Meniere Disease: A Review of Pathogenesis and Presentation

Yuan F. Liu and Helen Xu

Department of Otolaryngology, Head and Neck Surgery, Loma Linda University Medical Center, Loma Linda, CA, USA

Correspondence should be addressed to Yuan F. Liu; yfangl09@gmail.com

Academic Editor: Kadriye Agan

ABSTRACT

Vestibular migraine (VM) has only recently been recognized as a distinct disease entity. One reason is that its symptoms overlap greatly with those of other vestibular disorders, especially Meniere disease (MD). The pathophysiology of neither VM nor MD is entirely elucidated. However, there are many theories linking migraine to both disorders. We reviewed the current understanding of migraine, VM, and MD and described how VM and MD are similar or different from each other in terms of pathophysiology and presentation, including hypotheses that the two share a common etiology and/or are variants of the same disease.

INTRODUCTION

Vestibular migraine (VM) as a distinct disease entity came into the hesitant eye of the medical community no earlier than the advent of the new millennia [1]. Although monikers fitting of the disorder, migrainous vertigo, migraine-associated dizziness, benign recurrent vertigo, and others, have circulated for some 50 years, it was not until Neuhauser's landmark work in 2001 founding the first set of reliable criteria for what is now known as vestibular migraine that the disease began creeping into the physician's diagnostic repertoire [2, 3]. Even as late as 2010, skeptics voiced their denial of its existence [4]. Nevertheless, VM is now widely recognized as a distinct diagnostic entity by both the Barany Society and the International Headache Society (IHS), which jointly formulated the revised diagnostic criteria for VM in 2012 [5].

With an estimated lifetime prevalence of 1% and 1-year prevalence of 5% in women between the ages of 40 and 54, VM is likely the most common vestibular disorder [6–8]. It afflicts predominantly females, with a 5-fold increased risk, and has a mean age of onset of 38 in women and 42 in men [3]. VM accounts for about 10% of patients seen for migraine and about 10% of patients (although anecdotally up to 50% in the senior author's experience) seen for dizziness [9]. Episodes of vertigo, imbalance, dizziness, and/or disequilibrium seen in VM last from seconds to days and may or may not be temporally associated with migraine headaches, with or without aura [3, 5, 10]. The temporal association between VM and migraine headaches can also be inconsistent between patients and in the same patient [10, 11]. Often, vestibular symptoms in VM do not begin until several years after the onset of typical migraines, and, in some, there may be a headache-free interval of years before the onset of VM [10, 12, 13]. Despite VM's prevalence and new diagnostic criteria, its pathophysiology is unclear, its management is mostly anecdotal, and it remains a diagnosis of exclusion based only on history, without pathognomonic physical exam, laboratory, or imaging findings.

One of the reasons that physicians were so reluctant to accept VM as a distinct disease entity was that it produced so many symptoms overlapping with various well-established vestibular disorders such as Meniere disease (MD), benign paroxysmal positional vertigo (BPPV), and neurologic conditions that can elicit dizziness such as basilar migraine [5, 10, 13–17]. In some cases, VM may be indistinguishable from MD based on history and symptoms [1]. Furthermore, VM may be comorbid with MD, further confounding the diagnosis [15].

Meniere disease is characterized by vertigo associated with tinnitus, aural fullness, and/or hearing loss [18]. Its prevalence is 5 to 10 times lower than that of VM and has a lower female to male preponderance of 1.3 : 1 [12, 19]. Patients are affected usually in their 4th to 7th decades of life, often presenting with episodic vertigo with or without low-frequency hearing loss, though the disease course may be quite variable [18]. Like VM, the diagnosis of MD is based mainly on history, especially when audiological tests are normal; and its pathophysiology is also uncertain [19, 20].

One study found that of patients diagnosed with VM or MD in a tertiary dizziness clinic, about a quarter had symptoms which could have met criteria for either. Of the patients with VM alone, 38% presented with subjective hearing loss, aural pressure, and tinnitus during episodes of dizziness and headaches; and of the patients with MD alone, 49% presented with migrainous features such as photophobia and headache with vomiting or first degree relative to migraine [15]. MD patients have been found to be twice as likely to have migraine compared to those without MD [21]. And, interestingly, those with migraine are more likely to have earlier onset and bilateral hearing loss from MD [22, 23].

Clearly, the relationship between VM and MD is beyond that of chance alone. In this review, we explored the pathophysiology of these disorders and sought to clarify how the two disease processes are linked and why their presentations are so much alike.

Review

Current Theory of Migraine. Migraine is the common thread connecting VM and MD. Thus, the pathophysiology of migraine is crucial to the understanding of VM and MD. A brief discussion of the general concepts of migraine, especially aspects potentially important to the pathophysiology of VM and MD, is offered in lieu of a complete analysis of its mechanisms, as this study cannot do justice to the full scope of contemporary migraine theory.

The most widely accepted model of migraine resolves around the trigeminovascular system (TVS) [24, 25]. The TVS consists of the trigeminal nuclei, the trigeminal ganglion and nerve, and the meningeal vasculature which it innervates [24, 26]. More specifically, the ophthalmic division (V1) of the trigeminal nerve innervates dural and pial blood vessel nociceptors that, when activated, cause a release of vasoactive neuropeptides such as substance P, calcitonin gene-related peptide, and neurokinin A which in turn cause increased cerebral blood flow, release of proinflammatory factors, and a reaction called neurogenic inflammation [27]. The nociceptive afferent neurons project to what is called the trigeminocervical complex (TCC), consisting of the trigeminal nucleus caudalis in the brainstem and the spinal cord dorsal horns of C1 and C2. The TCC connects to the ventroposteromedial (VPM) and posterior nuclei of the thalamus, which relay information to the cerebral cortex, including the somatosensory cortex, the insular cortex, and the anterior cingulate cortex [24]. The TCC also has reciprocal connections with other parts of the brainstem, including the ventromedial medulla (VMM) and the ventrolateral periaqueductal gray (VLPAG), and hypothalamic areas. These areas are involved in nociceptive processing, and they also receive modulation from the cerebral cortex through descending pathways [24]. The activation of the TVS is how headaches are believed to occur in migraine.

What activates the TVS is uncertain. One hypothesis involves another popular but controversial theory, cortical spreading depression (CSD). CSD is a massive wave-like, slowly propagating depolarization of the brain that typically starts in the occipital cortex and leads to prolonged suppression of cortical activity [25]. CSD is triggered when the local concentration of certain ions reaches a threshold and activates NMDA receptors through release of glutamate from cortical pyramidal cells [28]. CSD is believed to be the cause of auras, which occur at a progression rate of a few minutes, similar to that of CSD, and include symptoms such as scotomas, hemianopsia, visual patterns, flashing lights, paresthesias, and hallucinations [24]. CSD disrupts transmembrane ionic gradients and increases extracellular concentrations of molecules that can activate meningeal nociceptors of the TVS as well as trigeminal nuclei of the TCC [29–31].

Another theory is that the TVS can be directly activated by the dysfunction and dysregulation of brainstem nociceptive nuclei, such as the VMM and VLPAG mentioned previously. Thereby, migraine headaches are triggered by direct activation of the TVS instead of through a sequential pathway starting from the meningeal nociceptors [24]. In summary, migraine can be seen as a pathological brain disease other than vascular or pain disorder, in which numerous pathways within the brain are activated and the central nervous system is oversensitized, making different systems, such as the vestibular system and the multisensory integrative routes it is involved in, prone to dysfunction [32].

How Migraine Produces Vestibular Symptoms. It has been postulated that the vestibular symptoms of VM are types of aura in migraines caused by the spread of CSD to the vestibular nuclei or cortices [13]. However, the vestibular symptoms in VM last from seconds to days, which do not fit the typical profile of auras. Also, it does not explain the unilateral vestibular canal paresis seen in some patients. When vertigo does occur like an aura, it is often associated with dysarthria, diplopia, ataxia, and altered consciousness, which is more diagnostic of basilar migraine [25].

Perhaps a better way to justify the relationship between VM and migraine is through vascular theories directly involving the TVS. It has been shown that the trigeminal nerve directly affects inner ear blow flow through the innervation of cochlear vasculature. Vass et al. demonstrated in Guinea pigs that the cochlea and the vestibular labyrinth receive trigeminal innervation from the ophthalmic branch, which provides parasympathetic innervation to the basilar and anterior inferior cerebellar arteries. Stimulation of the nerve led to increased vascular permeability and plasma protein extravasation [33–35]. Furthermore, Shore et al. showed that the trigeminal nerve also innervates the cochlear nucleus and the superior olivary complex [36]. A study in humans validated these results by showing that painful stimulation of the trigeminal nerve (through electrodes applied to the supraorbital point) elicited nystagmus or changes in preexisting nystagmus [37]. This provides a mechanism in which activation of the TVS, as in migraines, can cause peripheral vestibular dysfunction.

Central vestibular symptoms such as nystagmus during VM attacks and between attacks cannot simply be explained by ischemic events affecting the peripheral vestibular organs [16, 38]. A dysfunction of central processing of vestibular inputs along with other sensory information may be responsible for central vestibular findings in VM [24]. A specific vestibular cortex has yet to be discovered in humans [25]. However, vestibular information travels through and is processed in many areas including the ventroposterolateral (VPL) and VPM thalamus which are relay stations for visual and proprioceptive along with vestibular inputs. Activation of the thalamus shown through positron emission tomography (PET) and functional magnetic resonance imaging (fMRI) during migraine attacks suggests that the vestibular symptoms in VM are a result of faulty sensory integration [25, 29].

There are reciprocal connections between vestibular nuclei and nociceptive centers (e.g., VLPAG) and between vestibular nuclei and trigeminal nuclei (e.g., trigeminal nucleus caudalis), which can also explain vestibular symptoms in migraine patients [25, 39]. Other connections between vestibular nuclei and brainstem structures such as the parabrachial nucleus, raphe nuclei, and locus coeruleus may be responsible for sensitization of the TVS and nociceptive pathways during VM episodes [39–41]. The sensitization of thalamic pathways may be the cause of motion-sickness susceptibility in VM patients [42, 43]. Moreover, the degree of thalamic activation shown on fMRI during vestibular stimulation correlates with the frequency of migraine attacks in VM patients [25]. The reciprocity between the vestibular system and brain centers implicated in migraine is further demonstrated in another study, where rotational and caloric vestibular testing triggered migraines more in those with a history of migraine than in those without (49% versus 5%, resp.) [44]. Interesting, caloric stimulation has been reported to trigger migraine even in those without migraine history [45]. This shows that the peripheral vestibular system may have the ability to modulate migraines just as migraines may trigger vestibular dysfunction.

Anecdotally, the senior author has treated dizzy patients who presented with typical VM symptoms but have had histories typical of vestibular neuritis at the onset of their disease. These patients usually recount several days of severe, debilitating vertigo which resolves gradually but is never fully compensated and sometimes evolves into chronic dizziness/imbalance, along with migraine features like photophobia and phonophobia. Furthermore, in a yet unpublished study, we found that while examining the effects of intratympanic gentamycin injection on MD patient with or without migraine, migraines and vestibular migraines were triggered after chemical ablation of the vestibular system with gentamycin injections in several patients with migraine history but not in those without. Thus, our experience appears to be consistent with the previous studies, suggesting that insult to the peripheral vestibular system may be projected centrally.

Further evidence that VM is a disease of multisensory integration in the central nervous system was seen in a study of tilt perception in VM, migraine, and normal patients. When the 3 groups of patients sat in a centrifuge and an interaural centrifugal force was generated, the development of the perception of tilt in the roll plane was slower in the VM group compared to the other 2, but eye movement responses such as rotational axis shift were the same in all groups [46]. In other roll-type experiments, VM patients were found to have decreased motion perception thresholds when canal and otolith signals were presented simultaneously, but perception of tilt was slower when the signals were conflicting [47]. This may be a potential origin for motion sensitivity in VM patients. The authors believe that these results suggest VM is, at least in part, a result of dysfunctional vestibular signal integration and abnormal sensitization possibly of cerebellar origin [46, 47].

Pathophysiology of Meniere Disease. Similar to VM, although with a more extensive history of recognition and research, the pathophysiology of MD has yet to be fully elaborated [48]. The most well-known aspect of MD is the presence of endolymphatic hydrops (ELH), a hallmark of the disease which can be confirmed by pathology postmortem [20, 49]. However, even though ELH was found in all patients with MD in a study of temporal bones (28 patients), only 51 of 79 patients (65%) found to have ELH had MD [50]. Furthermore, ELH can be found in autoimmune inner ear disease, posttraumatic ears, otosyphilis, otosclerosis, endolymphatic sac tumors, and other disorders [20]. This brings about the question whether ELH is the cause of MD or if it is a byproduct of another process which causes both MD and ELH. It would seem that ELH is necessary but not sufficient for the development of MD.

Endolymphatic hydrops is a consequence of a disturbance in the homeostasis of endolymph. Some believe that MD is a result of a "fragile" ear in which certain factors make the inner ear more prone to dysregulation of homeostasis and more susceptible to changes in the body or the environment [48]. These changes may include stress, sleep deprivation, diet change, hormonal alterations, allergies, barometric pressure changes, or any of the diseases listed previously to be associated with ELH [20, 48]. The factors that actually make the ear vulnerable, however, are unclear.

Older theories of ELH postulated that obstructions to the flow of endolymph, from its production by the stria vascularis, passing through the endolymphatic duct (ELD), to its resorption in the endolymphatic sac (ELS), lead to the development of ELH [49]. This is supported by the observation of ELH in patients with ELD obstruction or ELD hypoplasia [20]. However, these conditions are not necessary for the presence of ELH, and the ionic homeostasis of endolymph does not seem to be significantly affected by this flow pathway [51]. Therefore, the theory of radial flow, wherein endolymph is both produced and absorbed in the cochlear duct, arose [20]. In this theory, molecules and channels such as aquaporins and gated ionic channels regulate the composition and volume of endolymph [52]. This may be why diuretics have shown some evidence of effectiveness in treating MD, though the effect has not been proven to be great [53].

Damage to the spiral ganglion by chronic excitotoxicity has been theorized to be the cause of gradual hearing loss in MD [20]. In this model, ELH in the cochlea results in the release of excitatory mediators such as glutamate and other amino acids, which can eventually lead to neuronal toxicity and death [54]. This process involves the apoptosis cascade, in which reactive oxygen species (ROS) are produced and a caspase-dependent pathway is activated, followed by cell death [54]. More specifically, in hydropic conditions, elevated levels of a glutamate aspartate transporter (GLAST) in the cochlea increase glutamate presence, which activates Nmethyl-D-aspartate (NMDA) receptors and subsequently activate nitric oxide synthase (NOS) [55, 56]. Nitric oxide produced by NOS combines with superoxide to create peroxynitrate, which is a potent ROS capable of cytotoxic neuronal apoptosis [54, 57]. In Guinea pig models, surgically induced hydrops reduced 8th cranial nerve diameter and caused differential nerve damage in that neuronal loss was greater than inner hair loss at the apex, consistent with typical low-frequency hearing loss in MD. However, the degree of hydrops did not correlate with the degree of reduction in 8th nerve diameter, and when aminoguanidine (an inhibitor of NOS) was used, there was no evidence of neuronal protection [58, 59]. Furthermore, the true relationship between ELH and neuronal damage is yet to be proven and can only be extrapolated to humans.

Comparing and Contrasting Vestibular Migraine and Meniere Disease. Prosper Meniere suggested a link between migraine and MD as early as 1861, but a definitive association has yet to be established [21]. Radtke et al. found the lifetime prevalence of migraine to be 56% in MD patients, compared to 25% in controls [21]. However, Gopen et al. found the incidence of migraine in MD to be 4.5%, which was not significantly different from those without MD (3.8%) [60]. Studies have supported both sides of the argument [61–64]. Nevertheless, there is an unequivocal overlap between many symptoms of VM and MD. Ghavami et al. found that, in 37 patients with definite MD, 95% had one or more features of migraine, 51% had migraine headaches, and 48% met the IHS criteria for diagnosis of VM [61].

MD patients typically have fluctuating aural symptoms of hearing loss, tinnitus, and aural fullness [18]. However, aural pressure may resemble headache and patients with migraine may also have tinnitus and hearing loss [65]. Phonophobia is a prominent symptom in VM but can commonly occur in MD [65]. The vestibular symptoms of VM are broadly defined to be vertigo, dizziness, or other imbalances lasting from 5 minutes to 72 hours, which can easily describe the type of vertigo seen in MD patients [5]. In fact, vertigo or dizziness occurs in migraine patients 25–35% of the time, with many episodes closely resembling MD attacks [2].

Based on the diagnostic criteria of both VM and MD, hearing loss stands out as a potential differentiating factor between the two disorders [5, 18]. Patients with definite MD must have audiograms showing low-frequency to mediumfrequency hearing loss [18]. However, hearing loss is not a requirement in probable MD, and many normal-hearing patients may develop hearing loss over time to be later diagnosed with definite MD [66]. Moreover, hearing loss can occur in VM. The mechanism can be explained by the previously mentioned animal studies demonstrating the trigeminovascular control of inner ear blood flow, which could involve cochlear perfusion as well as vestibular endorgan perfusion [34, 67]. Accordingly, reports have shown that fluctuating hearing loss or progressive sensorineural hearing loss can occur in up to 25% of migraine patients [68, 69].

As seen in the previous discussion on the pathophysiology of VM and MD, MD is a disorder of the peripheral vestibular end-organs, while VM is one of both central and vestibular dysfunctions originating from a central occurrence. How can the two be related? One study found that cervical and ocular vestibular-evoked myogenic potential (VEMP) responses from VM and MD patients were found to resemble each other and that no one test could differentiate between the two disorders [70]. Furthermore, caloric testing and motion-sensitivity questionnaires have been shown to be unsuccessful in distinguishing between VM and MD [43]. It has been suggested that the inability to discriminate between the two diseases by clinical testing is evidence of a common origin [61]. Some have hypothesized that ELH may result from end-organ damage to the inner ear caused by VM and that VM and MD in fact share the same etiology [70]. Other authors have found that family history is frequently positive for both VM and MD; and they believe that a heritable syndrome with variable expression of both VM and MD features exists [22]. It appears that the triggers suggested for ELH as mentioned previously (stress, sleep deprivation, diet change, etc.) are similar to those for migraine [48]. This could be another mechanism in which VM and MD are linked.

One common origin for VM and MD has been thought to be related to chronic underperfusion leading to end-organ damage [61]. Decreased perfusion of the spiral modiolar artery, which primarily supplies the middle and apical turns of the cochlea, has been thought to cause low-frequency hearing loss, as in that of typical MD [71]. One hypothesis is that chronic recurrent damage from vasospasm of the spiral modiolar artery causes the ELH found in MD [61]. By this proposed pathway, the TVS in migraine patients causes perfusion deficits in the inner ear, and based on individual anastomotic patterns, different parts of the inner ear are affected [61]. For example, involvement of the spiral modiolar artery would lead to the historically described "cochlear" MD with low-frequency hearing loss; additional involvement of the vestibular arteries would lead to typical MD findings with vertigo and hearing loss; and involvement of the cochlear artery (found to primarily perfuse the basal cochlea) would result in atypical high-frequency hearing loss in MD [61, 71]. The different types of hearing loss have been seen in representative audiograms that can be peaked or flat [68, 72]. Thereby, the different hearing loss and vertigo variations seen in MD represent phenotypes derived from differential injury to the inner ear based on development of its vasculature. Although this suggested mechanism for migraine being the predecessor of both VM and MD is unproven, based on their experience, the authors recommend treating patients who have both MD and migraine but do not fulfill the criteria for VM with migraine prophylactic agents before intratympanic or more invasive surgical therapy [61]. In fact, our unpublished data showed that, after intratympanic gentamycin injection, the quality of life in MD patients with migraine is much poorer than that in those without migraine, although the controls of major vertigo attack are similar in both groups of patients.

One way to discover whether VM and MD share a common etiology is by examining the evolution in symptomatology and findings over time to see where they deviate or converge. In VM, hearing loss may be present but is typically bilateral [73]. In MD, however, bilateral hearing loss is rare at its onset [74]. Cochlear symptoms of tinnitus, aural fullness, and hearing loss have been found to become more prevalent (from 15% to 49%) in a study of VM patients over an average of 9 years [75]. However, hearing levels in MD patients decrease to a mean of 50–60 decibels in 5–10 years, while hearing loss remains mild in VM patients and decreases much slower than that of MD patients [75]. The majority of VM patients still suffer from vertigo in the long run, while MD patients seem to experience fewer vertigo episodes. In one study, 87% of VM patients had recurrent vertigo after an average of 9 years with frequency reduced in 56%, increased in 29%, and unchanged in 16% [75]. In a study of 119 MD patients after at least 14 years, vertigo completely resolved in 50% and somewhat resolved in 28% [76]. In a review of retrospective studies totaling nearly 8000 MD patients, the overall frequency of vertigo attacks seemed to decrease [74]. There were some reports of patients who did not fare as well, however, and suffered from increasing severity or frequency of vertigo. In general, vertigo attacks in MD patients seemed to vary widely in terms of frequency and severity [74]. In VM, deterioration of vestibular function over time has been reported, evidenced by increased vestibular abnormalities such as central oculomotor dysfunction between episodes in about half of patients over nearly a decade [75, 77]. In MD, caloric tests have shown a general increase in hyporesponsiveness over time [74]. But, again, there was great variation in caloric results in patients with disease progression [74].

The reason VM and MD look so much alike in some cases, yet quite dissimilar in others, is that we do not yet truly understand the pathophysiology of either disease. And thus we use diagnostic criteria which are purposefully modest in specificity to encompass a broad spectrum of presentations. The arguments for a common etiology for VM and MD are provocative and feed our desire for an all-encompassing solution, but there is evidence that aspects of VM and MD can be very different from one another. As of yet, it is unclear if migraine or another trigger is the initiator of both VM and MD, if VM causes MD, if MD causes VM, or if the two simply occur in parallel due to an indirect cause with many degrees of separation. It could very well be, as we learn more about the vestibular disorders, that different subtypes of VM and MD will be parsed out.

While performing research on either disorder, we must keep in mind that previous work was performed when VM was not fully recognized and that it was (and is) often difficult to distinguish between VM and MD such that patients may have been mislabeled and conclusions were drawn based on historical diagnostic criteria. It may be that we will not be able to make significant strides in understanding either disease until new technology allows for novel pathways of experimentation, but we have taken important steps in recent years such as the use of new MRI protocols to image migraine and ELH in MD [78–80]. We do not wish to dishearten physicians who treat patients with dizziness by suggesting that VM and MD are far too difficult currently to distinguish and properly diagnose. In fact, we believe that the diagnostic criteria for *definite* VM and *definite* MD are clear and useful and that patients often can be appropriately classified into either category [5, 18]. The difficulty lies within the *probable* categories, which leave much to be desired in achieving specificity in differentiating between VM and MD. Redefined criteria, which will take more research to develop, are clinically imperative for the future. Our need to assign diagnoses even to patients with uncertain ailments and our need to categorize illnesses for the sake of satisfying patients' desires for therapy have put us in a position of both authority and skepticism.

Conclusion

The pathophysiology of vestibular migraine and Meniere disease has yet to be completely defined. As such, there is a great deal of overlap between the two disorders in terms of presentation and diagnostic criteria. Migraine is believed to be the cause of vestibular migraine through effects on the inner ear from the trigeminovascular system and through direct central activation of vestibular centers. While endolymphatic hydrops is still thought to be the cause of Meniere disease, this theory has been challenged and migraine has been implicated as a common etiology between vestibular migraine and Meniere disease. There is not enough evidence to definitively link vestibular migraine and Meniere disease in a mechanistic way, but awareness of the blurred lines between the two disorders may assist in clinical diagnosis and treatment.

Competing Interests

The authors have no competing interests.

References

[1] J. M. Furman and C. D. Balaban, "Vestibular migraine," *Annals of the New York Academy of Sciences*, vol. 1343, no. 1, pp. 90–96, 2015.

[2] A. Kayan and J. D. Hood, "Neuro-otological manifestations of migraine," *Brain*, vol. 107, part 4, pp. 1123–1142, 1984.

[3] H. Neuhauser, M. Leopold, M. von Brevern, G. Arnold, and T. Lempert, “The interrelations of migraine, vertigo, and migrainous vertigo,” *Neurology*, vol. 56, no. 4, pp. 436–441, 2001.

[4] J. Phillips, N. Longridge, A. Mallinson, and G. Robinson, “Migraine and vertigo: a marriage of convenience?” *Headache*, vol. 50, no. 8, pp. 1362–1365, 2010.

[5] T. Lempert, J. Olesen, J. Furman et al., “Vestibular migraine: diagnostic criteria,” *Journal of Vestibular Research*, vol. 22, no. 4, pp. 167–172, 2012.

[6] M. Cherchi and T. C. Hain, “Migraine-associated vertigo,” *Otolaryngologic Clinics of North America*, vol. 44, no. 2, pp. 367– 375, 2011.

[7] L.-C. Hsu, S.-J. Wang, and J.-L. Fuh, “Prevalence and impact of migrainous vertigo in mid-life women: a community-based study,” *Cephalalgia*, vol. 31, no. 1, pp. 77–83, 2011.

[8] H. K. Neuhauser, A. Radtke, M. von Brevern et al., “Migrainous vertigo: prevalence and impact on quality of life,” *Neurology*, vol. 67, no. 6, pp. 1028–1033, 2006.

[9] H. Neuhauser and T. Lempert, “Vertigo and dizziness related to migraine: a diagnostic challenge,” *Cephalalgia*, vol. 24, no. 2, pp. 83–91, 2004.

[10] J. M. Furman, D. A. Marcus, and C. D. Balaban, “Vestibular migraine: clinical aspects and pathophysiology,” *The Lancet Neurology*, vol. 12, no. 7, pp. 706–715, 2013.

[11] Y.-H. Cha, H. Lee, L. S. Santell, and R. W. Baloh, “Association of benign recurrent vertigo and migraine in 208 patients,” *Cephalalgia*, vol. 29, no. 5, pp. 550–555, 2009.

[12] H. K. Neuhauser and T. Lempert, “Vertigo: epidemiologic aspects,” *Seminars in Neurology*, vol. 29, no. 5, pp. 473–481, 2009.

[13] M. Dieterich and T. Brandt, “Episodic vertigo related to migraine (90 cases): vestibular migraine?” *Journal of Neurology*, vol. 246, no. 10, pp. 883–892, 1999.

[14] K. Brantberg and R. W. Baloh, “Similarity of vertigo attacks due to Meniere’s disease and benign recurrent vertigo, both with and without migraine,” *Acta Oto-Laryngologica*, vol. 131, no. 7, pp. 722–727, 2011.

[15] B. A. Neff, J. P. Staab, S. D. Eggers et al., “Auditory and vestibular symptoms and chronic subjective dizziness in patients with Me´nie`re’s disease, vestibular migraine, and Me´nie`re’s disease with concomitant vestibular migraine,” *Otology & Neurotology*, vol. 33, no. 7, pp. 1235–1244, 2012.

[16] M. von Brevern, A. Radtke, A. H. Clarke, and T. Lempert, “Migrainous vertigo presenting as episodic positional vertigo,” *Neurology*, vol. 62, no. 3, pp. 469–472, 2004.

[17] S. P. Cass, J. K. P. Ankerstjerne, S. Yetiser, J. M. Furman, C. Balaban, and B. Aydogan, “Migraine-related vestibulopathy,” *Annals of Otology, Rhinology and Laryngology*, vol. 106, no. 3, pp. 182–189, 1997.

[18] J. A. Lopez-Escamez, J. Carey, W.-H. Chung et al., “Diagnostic criteria for Menie`re’s disease: consensus document of the Ba´ra´ny Society, the Japan Society for Equilibrium Research, the European Academy of Otology and Neurotology (EAONO), the American Academy of Otolaryngology-Head and Neck Surgery (AAO-HNS) and the Korean Balance Society,” *Acta Otorrinolaringologica Espanola*, vol. 67, no. 1, pp. 1–7, 2016.

[19] S. S. da Costa, L. C. A. de Sousa, and M. R. D. T. Piza, “Meniere’s disease: overview, epidemiology, and natural history,” *Otolaryngologic Clinics of North America*, vol. 35, no. 3, pp. 455–495, 2002.

[20] M. T. Semaan and C. A. Megerian, “Contemporary perspectives on the pathophysiology of Meniere’s disease: implications for treatment,” *Current Opinion in Otolaryngology and Head and Neck Surgery*, vol. 18, no. 5, pp. 392–398, 2010.

[21] A. Radtke, T. Lempert, M. A. Gresty, G. B. Brookes, A. M. Bronstein, and H. Neuhauser, "Migraine and Me´nie`re's disease: is there a link?" *Neurology*, vol. 59, no. 11, pp. 1700–1704, 2002.

[22] Y. H. Cha, M. J. Kane, and R. W. Baloh, "Familial clustering of migraine, episodic vertigo, and Me´nie`re's disease," *Otology & Neurotology*, vol. 29, no. 1, pp. 93–96, 2008.

[23] N. T. Shepard, "Differentiation of Me´nie`re's disease and migraine-associated dizziness: a review," *Journal of the American Academy of Audiology*, vol. 17, no. 1, pp. 69–80, 2006.

[24] S. Akerman, P. R. Holland, and P. J. Goadsby, "Diencephalic and brainstem mechanisms in migraine," *Nature Reviews Neuroscience*, vol. 12, no. 10, pp. 570–584, 2011.

[25] J. M. Espinosa-Sanchez and J. A. Lopez-Escamez, "New insights into pathophysiology of vestibular migraine," *Frontiers in Neurology*, vol. 6, article 12, 2015.

[26] P. J. Goadsby, A. R. Charbit, A. P. Andreou, S. Akerman, and P. R. Holland, "Neurobiology of migraine," *Neuroscience*, vol. 161, no. 2, pp. 327–341, 2009.

[27] D. Pietrobon and M. A. Moskowitz, "Pathophysiology of migraine," *Annual Review of Physiology*, vol. 75, pp. 365–391, 2013.

[28] D. Pietrobon and M. A. Moskowitz, "Chaos and commotion in the wake of cortical spreading depression and spreading depolarizations," *Nature Reviews Neuroscience*, vol. 15, no. 6, pp. 379–393, 2014.

[29] H. Karatas, S. E. Erdener, Y. Gursoy-Ozdemir et al., "Spreading depression triggers headache by activating neuronal Panx1 channels," *Science*, vol. 339, no. 6123, pp. 1092–1095, 2013.

[30] X. Zhang, D. Levy, V. Kainz, R. Noseda, M. Jakubowski, and R. Burstein, "Activation of central trigeminovascular neurons by cortical spreading depression," *Annals of Neurology*, vol. 69, no. 5, pp. 855–865, 2011.

[31] X. Zhang, D. Levy, R. Noseda, V. Kainz, M. Jakubowski, and R. Burstein, "Activation of meningeal nociceptors by cortical spreading depression: implications for migraine with aura," *The Journal of Neuroscience*, vol. 30, no. 26, pp. 8807–8814, 2010.

[32] T. J. Schwedt, C. D. Chong, C. C. Chiang, L. Baxter, B. L. Schlaggar, and D. W. Dodick, "Enhanced pain-induced activity of pain-processing regions in a case-control study of episodic migraine," *Cephalalgia*, vol. 34, no. 12, pp. 947–958, 2014.

[33] Z. Vass, C. F. Dai, P. S. Steyger, G. Jancso´, D. R. Trune, and A. L. Nuttall, "Co-localization of the vanilloid capsaicin receptor and substance P in sensory nerve fibers innervating cochlear and vertebro-basilar arteries," *Neuroscience*, vol. 124, no. 4, pp. 919–927, 2004.

[34] Z. Vass, S. E. Shore, A. L. Nuttall, and J. M. Miller, "Direct evidence of trigeminal innervation of the cochlear blood vessels," *Neuroscience*, vol. 84, no. 2, pp. 559–567, 1998.

[35] Z. Vass, P. S. Steyger, A. J. Hordichok, D. R. Trune, G. Jancso´, and A. L. Nuttall, "Capsaicin stimulation of the cochlea and electric stimulation of the trigeminal ganglion mediate vascular permeability in cochlear and vertebro-basilar arteries: a potential cause of inner ear dysfunction in headache," *Neuroscience*, vol. 103, no. 1, pp. 189–201, 2001.

[36] S. E. Shore, Z. Vass, N. L. Wys, and R. A. Altschuler, "Trigeminal ganglion innervates the auditory brainstem," *Journal of Comparative Neurology*, vol. 419, no. 3, pp. 271–285, 2000.

[37] E. Marano, V. Marcelli, E. Di Stasio et al., "Trigeminal stimulation elicits a peripheral vestibular imbalance in migraine patients," *Headache*, vol. 45, no. 4, pp. 325–331, 2005.

[38] M. von Brevern, D. Zeise, H. Neuhauser, A. H. Clarke, and T. Lempert, "Acute migrainous vertigo: clinical and oculographic findings," *Brain*, vol. 128, no. 2, pp. 365–374, 2005.

[39] C. D. Balaban, "Migraine, vertigo and migrainous vertigo: links between vestibular and pain mechanisms," *Journal of Vestibular Research: Equilibrium and Orientation*, vol. 21, no. 6, pp. 315–321, 2011.

[40] A. L. Halberstadt and C. D. Balaban, "Organization of projections from the raphe nuclei to the vestibular nuclei in rats," *Neuroscience*, vol. 120, no. 2, pp. 573–594, 2003.

[41] A. L. Halberstadt and C. D. Balaban, "Anterograde tracing of projections from the dorsal raphe nucleus to the vestibular nuclei," *Neuroscience*, vol. 143, no. 2, pp. 641–654, 2006.

[42] L. Murdin, F. Chamberlain, S. Cheema et al., "Motion sickness in migraine and vestibular disorders," *Journal of Neurology, Neurosurgery and Psychiatry*, vol. 86, no. 5, pp. 585–587, 2015.

[43] J. D. Sharon and T. E. Hullar, "Motion sensitivity and caloric responsiveness in vestibular migraine and Meniere's disease," *Laryngoscope*, vol. 124, no. 4, pp. 969–973, 2014.

[44] L. Murdin, R. A. Davies, and A. M. Bronstein, "Vertigo as a migraine trigger," *Neurology*, vol. 73, no. 8, pp. 638–642, 2009.

[45] B. Seemungal, P. Rudge, R. Davies, M. Gresty, and A. Bronstein, "Three patients with migraine following caloric-induced vestibular stimulation," *Journal of Neurology*, vol. 253, no. 8, pp. 1000–1001, 2006.

[46] J. Wang and R. F. Lewis, "Abnormal tilt perception during centrifugation in patients with vestibular migraine," *Journal of the Association for Research in Otolaryngology*, vol. 17, no. 3, pp. 253–258, 2016.

[47] S. King, J. Wang, A. J. Priesol, and R. F. Lewis, "Central integration of canal and otolith signals is abnormal in vestibular migraine," *Frontiers in Neurology*, vol. 5, article 233, 2014.

[48] S. D. Rauch, "Clinical hints and precipitating factors in patients suffering from Meniere's disease," *Otolaryngologic Clinics of North America*, vol. 43, no. 5, pp. 1011–1017, 2010.

[49] M. M. Paparella and H. R. Djalilian, "Etiology, pathophysiology of symptoms, and pathogenesis of Meniere's disease," *Otolaryngologic Clinics of North America*, vol. 35, no. 3, pp. 529–545, 2002.

[50] S. N. Merchant, J. C. Adams, and J. B. Nadol Jr., "Pathophysiology of Me´nie`re's syndrome: are symptoms caused by endolymphatic hydrops?" *Otology & Neurotology*, vol. 26, no. 1, pp. 74–81, 2005.

[51] A. N. Salt, "Regulation of endolymphatic fluid volume," *Annals of the New York Academy of Sciences*, vol. 942, pp. 306–312, 2001.

[52] E. Beitz, H.-P. Zenner, and J. E. Schultz, "Aquaporin-mediated fluid regulation in the inner ear," *Cellular and Molecular Neurobiology*, vol. 23, no. 3, pp. 315–329, 2003.

[53] A. S. Thirlwall and S. Kundu, "Diuretics for Me´nie`re's disease or syndrome," *Cochrane Database of Systematic Reviews*, no. 3, Article ID CD003599, 2006.

[54] T. R. Van De Water, F. Lallemend, A. A. Eshraghi et al., "Caspases, the enemy within, and their role in oxidative stressinduced apoptosis of inner ear sensory cells," *Otology & Neurotology*, vol. 25, no. 4, pp. 627–632, 2004.

[55] D. N. Furness, J. A. Hulme, D. M. Lawton, and C. M. Hackney, "Distribution of the glutamate/aspartate transporter GLAST in relation to the afferent synapses of outer hair cells in the guinea pig cochlea," *Journal of the Association for Research in Otolaryngology*, vol. 3, no. 3, pp. 234–247, 2002.

[56] K. Matsuda, Y. Ueda, T. Doi et al., "Increase in glutamateaspartate transporter (GLAST) mRNA during kanamycininduced cochlear insult in rats," *Hearing Research*, vol. 133, no. 1-2, pp. 10–16, 1999.

[57] M. Urushitani, T. Nakamizo, R. Inoue et al., "N-methyl-Daspartate receptor-mediated mitochondrial Ca(2+) overload in acute excitotoxic motor neuron death: a mechanism distinct from chronic neurotoxicity after Ca(2+) influx," *Journal of Neuroscience Research*, vol. 63, no. 5, pp. 377–387, 2001.

[58] C. A. Megerian, "Diameter of the cochlear nerve in endolymphatic hydrops: implications for the etiology of hearing loss in Me´nie`re's disease," *The Laryngoscope*, vol. 115, no. 9, pp. 1525– 1535, 2005.

[59] S. R. Momin, S. J. Melki, K. N. Alagramam, and C. A. Megerian, "Spiral ganglion loss outpaces inner hair cell loss in endolymphatic hydrops," *Laryngoscope*, vol. 120, no. 1, pp. 159–165, 2010.

[60] Q. Gopen, E. Viirre, and J. Anderson, "Epidemiologic study to explore links between Me´nie`re syndrome and migraine headache," *Ear, Nose and Throat Journal*, vol. 88, no. 11, pp. 1200– 1204, 2009.

[61] Y. Ghavami, H. Mahboubi, A. Y. Yau, M. Maducdoc, and H. R. Djalilian, "Migraine features in patients with Meniere's disease," *Laryngoscope*, vol. 126, no. 1, pp. 163–168, 2016.

[62] W. Parker, "Meniere's disease: etiologic considerations," *Archives of Otolaryngology—Head and Neck Surgery*, vol. 121, no. 4, pp. 377–382, 1995.

[63] C. H. Rassekh and L. A. Harker, "The prevalence of migraine in Menie`re's disease," *Laryngoscope*, vol. 102, no. 2, pp. 135–138, 1992.

[64] P. Wladislavosky-Waserman, G. W. Facer, B. Mokri, and L. T. Kurland, "Meniere's disease: a 30-year epidemiologic and clinical study in Rochester, MN, 1951–1980," *The Laryngoscope*, vol. 94, no. 8, pp. 1098–1102, 1984.

[65] R. Gu¨rkov, C. Kantner, M. Strupp, W. Flatz, E. Krause, and B. Ertl-Wagner, "Endolymphatic hydrops in patients with vestibular migraine and auditory symptoms," *European Archives of OtoRhino-Laryngology*, vol. 271, no. 10, pp. 2661–2667, 2014.

[66] R. A. Battista, "Audiometric findings of patients with migraineassociated dizziness," *Otology and Neurotology*, vol. 25, no. 6, pp. 987–992, 2004.

[67] Z. Vass, S. E. Shore, A. L. Nuttall, G. Jancso´, P. B. Brechtelsbauer, and J. M. Miller, "Trigeminal ganglion innervation of the cochlea—a retrograde transport study," *Neuroscience*, vol. 79, no. 2, pp. 605–615, 1997.

[68] C.-S. Lee, M. M. Paparella, R. H. Margolis, and C. Le, "Audiological profiles and Meniere's disease," *Ear, Nose and Throat Journal*, vol. 74, no. 8, pp. 527–530, 1995.

[69] E. S. Viirre and R. W. Baloh, "Migraine as a cause of sudden hearing loss," *Headache*, vol. 36, no. 1, pp. 24–28, 1996.

[70] M. G. Zuniga, K. L. Janky, M. C. Schubert, and J. P. Carey, "Can vestibular-evoked myogenic potentials help differentiate Me´nie`re disease from vestibular migraine?" *Otolaryngology— Head and Neck Surgery*, vol. 146, no. 5, pp. 788–796, 2012.

[71] R. A. Tange, "Vascular inner ear partition: a concept for some forms of sensorineural hearing loss and vertigo," *ORL-Journal for Otorhinolaryngology and Its Related Specialties*, vol. 60, no. 2, pp. 78–84, 1998.

[72] M. M. Paparella, J. C. McDermott, and L. C. A. de Sousa, "Meniere's disease and the peak audiogram," *Archives of Otolaryngology*, vol. 108, no. 9, pp. 555–559, 1982.

[73] A. Radtke, H. Neuhauser, M. von Brevern, T. Hottenrott, and T. Lempert, "Vestibular migraine—validity of clinical diagnostic criteria," *Cephalalgia*, vol. 31, no. 8, pp. 906–913, 2011.

[74] D. Huppert, M. Strupp, and T. Brandt, "Long-term course of Menie`re's disease revisited," *Acta Oto-Laryngologica*, vol. 130, no. 6, pp. 644–651, 2010.

[75] A. Radtke, M. von Brevern, H. Neuhauser, T. Hottenrott, and T. Lempert, "Vestibular migraine: long-term follow-up of clinical symptoms and vestibulo-cochlear findings," *Neurology*, vol. 79, no. 15, pp. 1607–1614, 2012.

[76] J. D. Green Jr., D. J. Blum, and S. G. Harner, "Longitudinal followup of patients with Menie`re's disease," *Otolaryngology—Head and Neck Surgery*, vol. 104, no. 6, pp. 783–788, 1991.

[77] J. M. Furman and D. A. Marcus, "Migraine and motion sensitivity," *CONTINUUM: Lifelong Learning in Neurology*, vol. 18, no. 5, pp. 1102–1117, 2012.

[78] M. Dieterich, M. Obermann, and N. Celebisoy, "Vestibular migraine: the most frequent entity of episodic vertigo," *Journal of Neurology*, vol. 263, supplement 1, pp. 82–89, 2016.

[79] J. Hornibrook, E. Flook, S. Greig et al., "MRI inner ear imaging and tone burst electrocochleography in the diagnosis of Me´nie`re's disease," *Otology & Neurotology*, vol. 36, no. 6, pp. 1109–1114, 2015.

[80] G. Tedeschi, A. Russo, F. Conte, M. Laura, and A. Tessitore, "Vestibular migraine pathophysiology: insights from structural and functional neuroimaging," *Neurological Sciences*, vol. 36, supplement 1, pp. 37–40, 2015.

7

Altered Chromogranin A Circulating Levels in Meniere's Disease

Roberto Teggi,[1] Barbara Colombo,[2] Matteo Trimarchi,[1] Mimma Bianco,[2] Angelo Manfredi,[3] Mario Bussi,[1] and Angelo Corti[2]

[1]ENT Division, San Raffaele Scientific Institute, Milan, Italy

[2]Division of Experimental Oncology, San Raffaele Scientific Institute, Milan, Italy

[3]Department of Internal Medicine and Division of Regenerative Medicine, Stem Cells & Gene Therapy, San Raffaele Scientific Institute, Universita` Vita-Salute San Raffaele, Milan, Italy

Correspondence should be addressed to Roberto Teggi; teggi.roberto@hsr.it

Academic Editor: Benoit Dugue

ABSTRACT

Objectives. Meniere's disease (MD) is an inner ear disorder characterized by episodic vertigo, ear fullness, and hearing loss; usually vertigo attacks cluster in specific period. We studied in MD patients the circulating levels of chromogranin A (CgA) and vasostatin1 (VS-1), secreted by the neuroendocrine system and involved in the regulation of the endothelial barrier function. Methods. Serum levels were assessed in 37 MD patients and 36 controls. The ratio between VS-1 and CgA was calculated. Results. CgA was increased in patients compared to controls (1.46 versus 0.67 nM, $p = 0.01$) while no difference was detected for VS-1 (0.41 versus 0.39, resp.). CgA levels in patients positively correlated with the frequency of vertigo spells in the previous four weeks ($p = 0.008$) and negatively with the time in days from the last vertigo attack ($p = 0.018$). Furthermore, the VS-1/CgA ratio negatively correlated with the frequency of vertigo spells ($p = 0.029$) and positively correlated with the time from the last attack ($p = 0.003$). Conclusion. The results indicate that variations of CgA levels, but not of VS-1, occur in the blood of patients with active MD, depending on the frequency of vertigo spells and the time from the last crisis.

INTRODUCTION

Meniere's disease (MD) is an inner ear disorder characterized by episodic vertigo associated with low-frequency sensorineural hearing loss, tinnitus, and aural fullness. Commonly accepted pathophysiology includes increased endolymphatic pressure (hydrops). Histopathologic findings in temporal bones support this hypothesis [1], although the relationship between hydrops and MD symptoms remains unproven. Furthermore, according to some authors, hydrops might be an epiphenomenon of MD that arises in end stage as a consequence of a variety of damaging processes of the inner ear [2, 3]. Most MD cases are sporadic and are thought to arise from the interplay of genetic and environmental factors. Normally MD attacks cluster in defined periods, followed by periods of quiescence [4, 5]. Among nongenetic factors, different possibilities might contribute to incite MD relapses, including viruses [6,

7], allergy [8], autoimmunity [9–11], and factors related to fluid and ionic homeostasis [12, 13]. Since MD patients present a higher rate of migraine, some common pathophysiological mechanisms between the two disorders have been postulated [14]. Finally, patients with MD also present a higher rate of psychiatric disorders, above all depression and anxiety [15].

Chromogranin A (CgA) is a 439-residue long protein originally discovered as a major secretory protein of chromaffin cells of the adrenal medulla and was found later to be stored in the secretory granules of many other neuroendocrine cells and neurons [16, 17]. This protein is exocytotically released in circulation, together with the coresident hormone, upon appropriate cell stimulation. Abnormal levels of immunoreactive CgA have been detected in the blood of patients with neuroendocrine tumors or with heart failure, with important diagnostic and prognostic implications [18]. Increased levels have been detected in several other pathological conditions, including renal failure, rheumatoid arthritis, atrophic gastritis, inflammatory bowel disease, and sepsis, or in subjects treated with proton pump inhibitors (a class of drugs commonly used to treat acid peptic disorders) [17–19]. This protein plays an intracellular function in secretory granules biogenesis and hormone condensation and an extracellular function, upon secretion, as a precursor of a variety of bioactive peptides and fragments [16, 17].

CgA may undergo various posttranslational modifications, including glycosylation, sulfation, phosphorylation, and proteolytic processing [17, 20]. A growing body of evidence suggests that CgA fragments exert different and even contrasting biological effects. For example, a peptide corresponding to residues 352–372, called catestatin, acts as a potent inhibitor of nicotinic-cholinergic stimulated catecholamine secretion, induces vasodilation in humans, exerts proangiogenic effects, and plays a cardioregulatory role [16, 21, 22]. A fragment corresponding to the N-terminal region 1–76, named vasostatin-1 (VS-1), inhibits vasoconstriction in isolated blood vessels, is neurotoxic in neuronal/ microglial cell cultures, exerts antibacterial effects, regulates cell adhesion, depresses myocardial contractility/ relaxation, counteracts the β-adrenergic-induced positive inotropism, and modulates coronary tone [17, 23]. In addition, VS-1 is a potent inhibitor of endothelial cell activation caused by cytokines, enhances the endothelial barrier function, protects vessels from TNF-induced vascular leakage, and exerts antiangiogenic effects in various in vitro and in vivo assays [23–26]. CgA has been demonstrated to be expressed in different portions of inner ear of guinea pig, including organ of Corti, utricle, and saccule [27]. Moreover, other investigators showed the presence of catestatin in the auditory and vestibular pathways, suggesting its possible role as a neuromodulatory peptide [28].

Based on the notions that CgA and VS-1 can play important roles in the endothelial barrier function and vascular homeostasis and that altered fluid homeostasis might represent a pathogenetic event in MD, we investigated the circulating levels of these polypeptides in MD patients. We found that the relative levels of VS-1 and CgA change in MD depending on the frequency of vertigo spells and the time from the last attack.

Materials and Methods

Study Population. The study population included 37 consecutive MD patients (24 females, mean age 45.3±10.8 years), recruited at the Outpatients Clinic of the Vestibular Disorders Unit at San Raffaele Hospital, Milan, Italy. All patients fulfilled all AAO-NHSF criteria for definite MD according to AAO-HNS guidelines [29] and were selected when referring at least with one attack of vertigo in the last 30 days. The study was approved by the Ethics Committee of the San Raffaele Scientific Institute and all subjects signed informed consent. Exclusion criteria were clinical history of therapies with proton pump inhibitors or serotonin selective reuptake inhibitors in the month before recruitment and a clinical history of heart, hepatic, or renal failure.

The following clinical data were recorded for each MD patient: (a) history of hypertension or migraine and first attack of migrainous headache; (b) familial history of episodic vertigo of any kind; (c) positivity for one of the following autoantibodies: nucleus, smooth muscle, mitochondria, thyroid, cardiolipin, beta 2 glycoprotein, lupus-like anticoagulant, and rheumatoid factor; (d) time from the last attack of vertigo (in days) and number of attacks in the last 30 days; and (e) age at the first vertigo attack.

Table 1: Demographic data (sex and age) and body mass index (BMI) of normal subjects and MD patients.

Subjects	(n)	Sex	Age	BMI
Controls	36	22 females	43.9 ± 12.6	24.98 ± 3.63
MD patients	37	24 females	45.3 ± 10.8	24.26 ± 2.76
(p value)		*ns*	*ns*	*ns*

Control subjects ($n = 36$) referred with a negative clinical history for vertigo and no clinical conditions were known to be associated with increased levels of CgA. They were selected with gender distribution and mean age overlapped with patients (mean age 43.9 ± 12.6 years; 22 were females). Exclusion criteria included treatment with proton pump inhibitors or serotonin selective reuptake inhibitors in the 30 days before blood collection.

In subjects of both groups a body mass index has been calculated; sex, age, and body mass index (BMI) of control subjects and MD patients are reported in Table 1.

CgAand VS-1-ELISAs. Blood samples from control subjects and patients were collected into tubes without anticoagulants (Becton Dickinson, France), immersed in ice, and immediately transported to the laboratory for processing. Blood was allowed to clot for 30 min, centrifuged (3000 ×g, 10 min), and stored at −20°C.

CgA-ELISA. Serum levels of CgA were detected using a sandwich ELISA, previously described, based on the use, in the capture step, of monoclonal antibody (mAb) B4E11 against an epitope located within CgA residues 68–71 and, in the detection step, of a rabbit anti-recombinant CgA polyclonal antibody against epitopes located in central region of CgA (immunodominant epitopes 90–133, 163–187, 222–256, and 315–338). This assay recognizes full-length CgA1-439 and fragments containing the N-terminal and part or all central regions (e.g., CgA1-436, CgA1-409, CgA1-400, and CgA1373), but not CgA1-76 (VS-1) [25]. This ELISA has been previously used for CgA detection in the blood of patients with cancer, heart failure, renal failure, rheumatoid arthritis, or other diseases [19, 26].

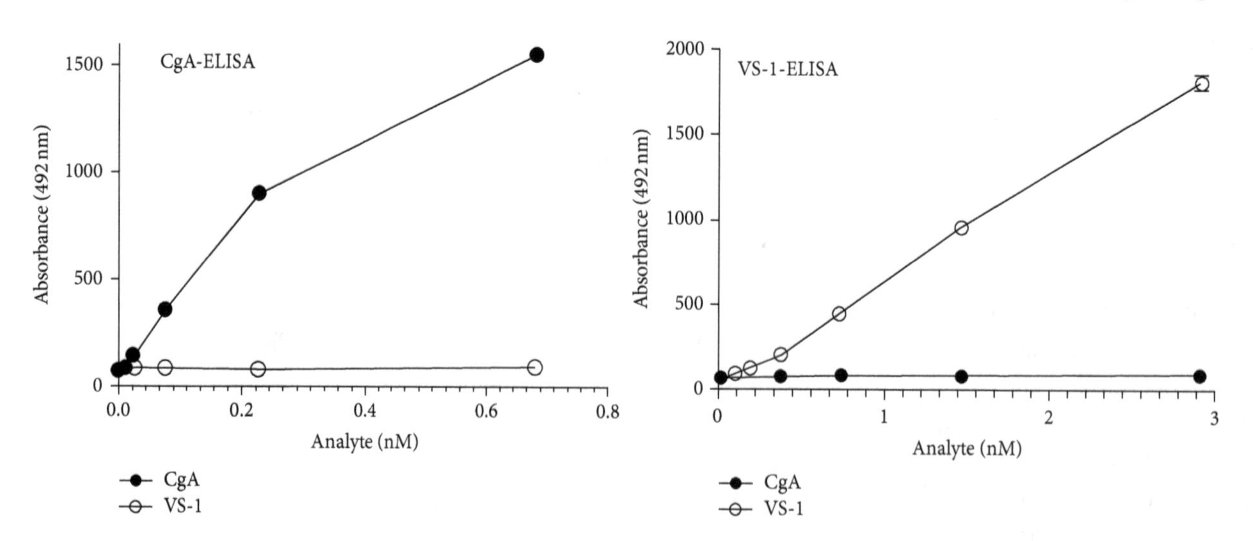

Figure 1: Dose-response curve of CgA-ELISA and VS-1-ELISA to recombinant human CgA and VS-1.

VS-1-ELISA. Serum levels of VS-1 were detected using a sandwich ELISA, previously described, based on the use of mAb 5A8 (against an epitope located within residues 53–57 of CgA) in the capture step and a rabbit polyclonal antibody raised against the peptide KERAHQQ (with a free carboxyl group) coupled to Keyhole Limpet Hemocyanin in the detection step [25]. This antibody, which is against a peptide that corresponds to the C-terminal sequence of CgA1-76 (VS1), can recognize VS-1, but not the full-length CgA precursors. Consequently, the VS-1-ELISA can detect VS-1, but not larger fragments or full-length CgA. The use of this combination of antibodies in a sandwich ELISA has been previously reported for the detection for VS-1 in the sera of patients with sepsis [26]. The dose-response curves of CgA-ELISA and VS-1ELISA showing the assay specificity and dynamic ranges for these analytes are shown in Figure 1.

Statistical Analyses. Continuous variables are described as mean and standard deviation. The significance of difference between groups was evaluated by *t*-test for independent samples. A Mann-Whitney test was performed when data did not present a normal distribution. A Spearman test was performed to investigate the association between CgA, VS-1, and ratio values and migraine, hypertension, familial history of vertigo, positivity for autoantibodies, frequency of vertigo spells in the last month, and time (in days) from the last attack of vertigo; finally, a general linear model was performed to assess the independent role of age, BMI, and frequency of vertigo spells in CgA levels.

Results

Five out of 37 MD patients presented arterial hypertension (14%), 16 had a diagnosis of migraine (43%), 11 were positive for at least one of the autoantibodies tested (30%), and 9 referred with a familial history of episodic vertigo (24%). The age of the first attack of vertigo was 41.2 ± 9.8 years. The mean value of time from the last attack of vertigo was 15.6±8.6 days; the mean value of number of spells in the last 30 days from blood collection was 3 ± 1.9.

The circulating levels of CgA, VS-1, and the VS-1/CgA ratio in patients and controls are reported in Table 2 and Figure 2. MD patients presented higher serum levels of CgA, while no significant difference was observed for VS-1. Notably, some patients had abnormally elevated levels of circulating CgA.

Since CgA values in patients did not show a normal distribution, a Spearman test was performed to assess the correlation of CgA with other clinical variables. Serum levels of CgA positively correlated with the vertigo frequency occurring within 30 days before blood collection (rs stat 0.43; $p = 0.008$) and negatively correlated with the time in days from the last vertigo attack (rs stat −0.39; $p = 0.018$) (Figure 3). Notably, subjects with values greater than the median CgA value (0.75 nM) had a higher number of vertigo spells in the last month (4 ± 2.4 versus 2.3 ± 0.8, $p = 0.011$) (Figure 3). No correlation was observed between CgA levels and migraine, hypertension, positivity of at least one of autoantibodies, and familial cases of episodic vertigo. Moreover a general linear model test demonstrated no association between CgA levels and BMI ($p = 0.44$) or age ($p = 0.55$). Moreover, every increase of a single attack determined an increase of CgA value of 0.363 ($p = 0.363$; SD 0.101).

Subjects	(n)	ELISA assay CgA (nM)	VS-1 (nM)	VS-1/CgA (%)
Controls	*36*	0.67 ± 0.27	0.39 ± 0.18	54 ± 19
MD patients	*37*	1.46 ± 1.79	0.41 ± 0.19	52 ± 38
(p value)		*(0.01)*	*(0.5)*	*(0.6)*

Table 2: Circulating levels of immunoreactive CgA and VS-1 in normal subjects and MD patients.

No correlation was observed between VS-1 serum levels and number of crises in the last month and time from the last attack. Consequently we observed a negative correlation between the VS-1/CgA ratio and vertigo frequency in the last 30 days (Spearman; rs = −0.36; $p = 0.029$) and a positive correlation with the time in days from the last crisis (rs = 0.47; $p = 0.003$) (Figure 3). No correlation was observed between these clinical variables and clinical history of migraine, hypertension, familial cases, and positivity for at least one autoantibody.

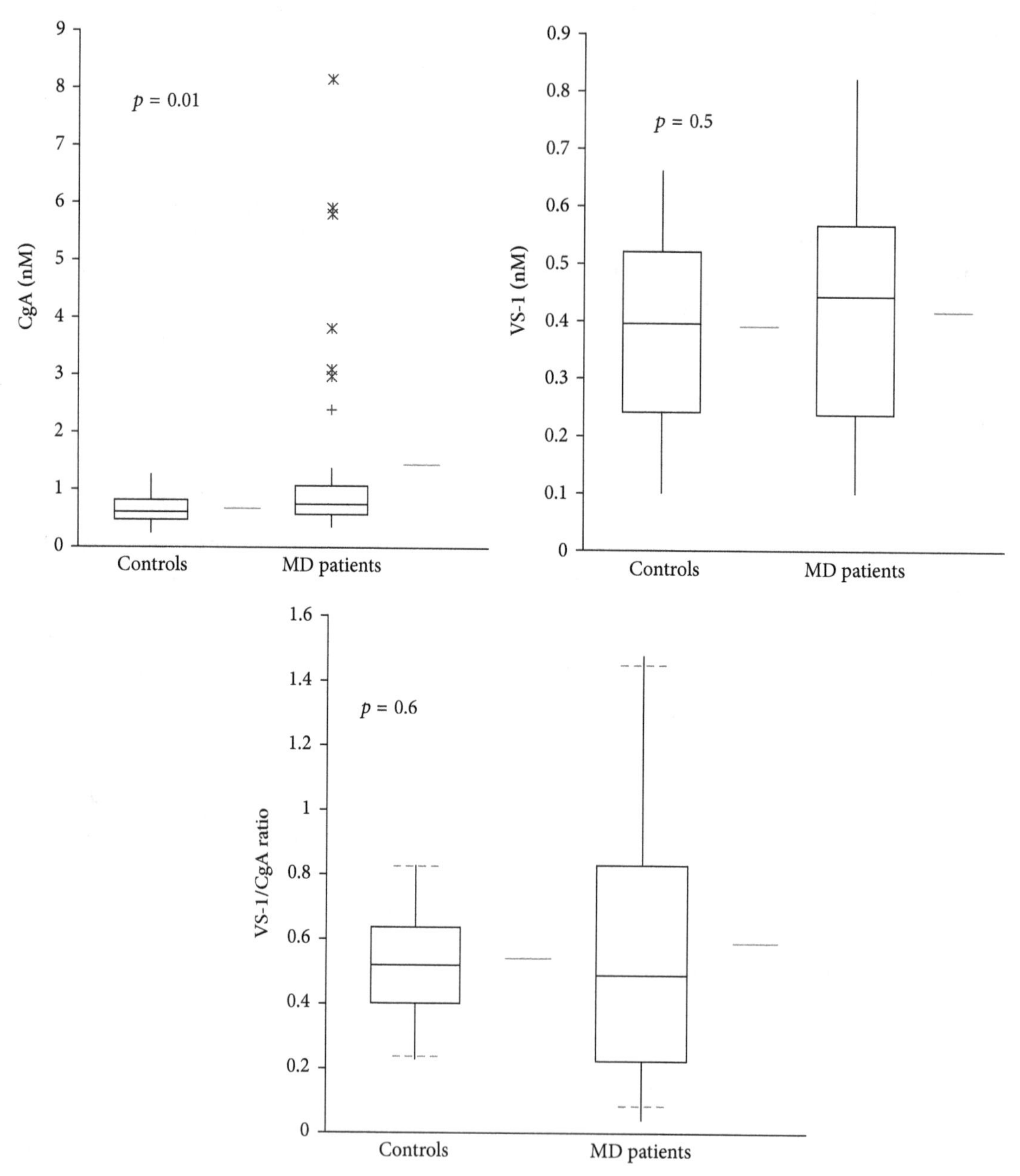

Figure 2: Serum levels of CgA, VS-1, and VS-1/CgA ratio in normal subjects ($n = 37$) and MD patients ($n = 37$).

Discussion

The results show that variations of CgA levels, but not of VS1, occur in the blood of patients with active MD, depending on the frequency of vertigo spells and the time from the last crisis. In particular, the results show that the serum levels of CgA, but not of VS-1, correlate with the number of crises in the last 30 days from blood collection and the time from the last vertigo attack, being higher in patients with a higher number of vertigo spells in the last month and in patients referring with more recent attacks. Considering that CgA is stored and coreleased with serotonin and other catecholamines by cells of the neuroendocrine system [30], the increased circulating levels of CgA observed in MD patients referring with a high number of vertigo spells in the last month may be related to activation of the autonomic system

(in which serotonin has been demonstrated to be an important neurotransmitter) consequent to vestibular overloading [31]. Furthermore, since serotonin is present in the inner ear and vestibular nuclei of the rat [32], we cannot exclude that repetitive vestibular stimulation and the possible consequent release of CgA in these brain areas might contribute to enhancing the circulating levels of this protein. At variance no difference has been detected in the VS-1 levels of controls and patients. As a consequence, a marked reduction of VS-1/CgA ratio occurs in MD patients with higher recurrence of vertigo spells. Furthermore the VS-1/CgA ratio positively correlates with the time from the last attack, pointing to a possible change in the proteolytic processing of CgA or to differential secretion or metabolism of these polypeptides in patients with increased clustering of vertigo. Given that VS-1 and CgA fragments can exert complex and even opposite effects in the homeostatic regulation of the endothelial lining of vessels [26], these findings may have important pathophysiological implications. For example, it is possible that CgA/VS-1dependent changes in the homeostatic mechanisms related to endothelial barrier may have a role in hydrops and, consequently, in vertigo clustering attack.

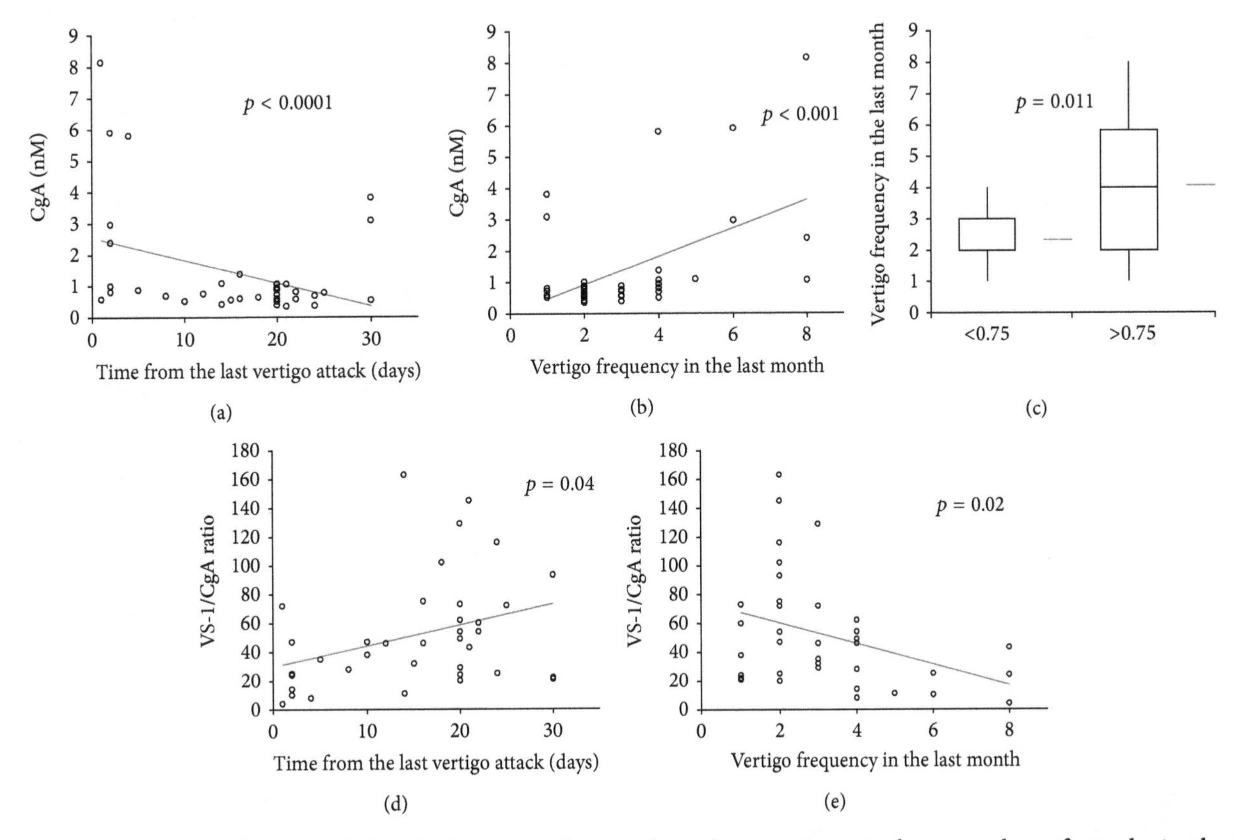

Figure 3: Correlation of CgA or VS-1/CgA ratio with time from last vertigo attack or number of attacks in the last month (a, b, d, and e). Number of vertigo attacks in MD patients with CgA < 0.75 nM or >0.75 (median value) (c).

Further studies are necessary to verify this hypothesis. Although this is a descriptive study performed on a small sample size and without serial samples (which represent important study limitations), our results may stimulate new studies on a larger cohort of MD patients aimed at assessing whether the detection of circulating CgA has a predictive value regarding vertigo recurrence.

References

[1] H. Sajjadi and M. M. Paparella, "Meniere's disease," *The Lancet*, vol. 372, no. 9636, pp. 406–414, 2008.

[2] S. N. Merchant, J. C. Adams, and J. B. Nadol Jr., "Pathophysiology of Me´nie`re's syndrome: are symptoms caused by endolymphatic hydrops?" *Otology and Neurotology*, vol. 26, no. 1, pp. 74–81, 2005.

[3] C. A. Foster and R. E. Breeze, "Endolymphatic hydrops in Me´nie`re's disease: cause, consequence, or epiphenomenon?" *Otology and Neurotology*, vol. 34, no. 7, pp. 1210–1214, 2013.

[4] J. T. Vrabec, "Genetic investigations of Meniere's diseasee," *Otolaryngologic Clinics of North America*, vol. 43, no. 5, pp. 1121– 1132, 2010.

[5] T. Requena, I. Gazquez, A. Moreno et al., "Allelic variants in TLR10 gene may influence bilateral affectation and clinical course of Meniere's disease," *Immunogenetics*, vol. 65, no. 5, pp. 345–355, 2013.

[6] J. T. Vrabec, "Herpes simplex virus and Meniere's disease," *Laryngoscope*, vol. 113, no. 9, pp. 1431–1438, 2003.

[7] R. R. Gacek, "Evidence for a viral neuropathy in recurrent vertigo," *ORL*, vol. 70, no. 1, pp. 6–14, 2008.

[8] M. J. Derebery, "Allergic and immunologic aspects of Meniere's disease," *Otolaryngology—Head and Neck Surgery*, vol. 114, no. 3, pp. 360–365, 1996.

[9] A. Greco, A. Gallo, M. Fusconi, C. Marinelli, G. F. Macri, and M. De Vincentiis, "Meniere's disease might be an autoimmune condition?" *Autoimmunity Reviews*, vol. 11, no. 10, pp. 731–738, 2012.

[10] I. Gazquez, A. Soto-Varela, I. Aran et al., "High prevalence of systemic autoimmune diseases in patients with menie`re's disease," *PLoS ONE*, vol. 6, no. 10, Article ID e26759, 2011.

[11] T. Requena, J. M. Espinosa-Sanchez, S. Cabrera et al., "Familial clustering and genetic heterogeneity in Meniere's disease," *Clinical Genetics*, vol. 85, no. 3, pp. 245–252, 2014.

[12] G. Ishiyama, I. A. Lo´pez, and A. Ishiyama, "Aquaporins and Meniere's disease," *Current Opinion in Otolaryngology and Head and Neck Surgery*, vol. 14, no. 5, pp. 332–336, 2006.

[13] R. Teggi, C. Lanzani, L. Zagato et al., "Gly460Trp α-adducin mutation as a possible mechanism leading to endolymphatic hydrops in Me´nie`re's syndrome," *Otology and Neurotology*, vol. 29, no. 6, pp. 824–828, 2008.

[14] A. Radtke, T. Lempert, M. A. Gresty, G. B. Brookes, A. M. Bronstein, and H. Neuhauser, "Migraine and Me´nie`re's disease: is there a link?" *Neurology*, vol. 59, no. 11, pp. 1700–1704, 2002.

[15] C. Best, A. Eckhardt-Henn, R. Tschan, and M. Dieterich, "Psychiatric morbidity and comorbidity in different vestibular vertigo syndromes: results of a prospective longitudinal study over one year," *Journal of Neurology*, vol. 256, no. 1, pp. 58–65, 2009.

[16] Y. P. Loh, Y. Cheng, S. K. Mahata, A. Corti, and B. Tota, "Chromogranin A and derived peptides in health and disease," *Journal of Molecular Neuroscience*, vol. 48, no. 2, pp. 347–356, 2012.

[17] K. B. Helle, A. Corti, M.-H. Metz-Boutigue, and B. Tota, "The endocrine role for chromogranin A: a prohormone for peptides with regulatory properties," *Cellular and Molecular Life Sciences*, vol. 64, no. 22, pp. 2863–2886, 2007.

[18] A. Corti, "Chromogranin A and the tumor microenvironment," *Cellular and Molecular Neurobiology*, vol. 30, no. 8, pp. 1163– 1170, 2010.

[19] C. Ceconi, R. Ferrari, T. Bachetti et al., "Chromogranin A in heart failure: a novel neurohumoral factor and a predictor for mortality," *European Heart Journal*, vol. 23, no. 12, pp. 967–974, 2002.

[20] S. K. Mahata, M. Mahata, M. M. Fung, and D. T. O'Connor, "Catestatin: a multifunctional peptide from chromogranin A," *Regulatory Peptides*, vol. 162, no. 1–3, pp. 33–43, 2010.

[21] M. Theurl, W. Schgoer, K. Albrecht et al., "The neuropeptide catestatin acts as a novel angiogenic cytokine via a basic fibroblast growth factor-dependent mechanism," *Circulation Research*, vol. 107, no. 11, pp. 1326–1335, 2010.

[22] B. Tota, T. Angelone, and M. C. Cerra, "The surging role of Chromogranin A in cardiovascular homeostasis," *Frontiers in Chemistry*, vol. 2, article e64, 2014.

[23] A. Corti and E. Ferrero, "Chromogranin A and the endothelial barrier function," *Current Medicinal Chemistry*, vol. 19, no. 24, pp. 4051–4058, 2012.

[24] G. Di Comite, C. M. Rossi, A. Marinosci et al., "Circulating chromogranin a reveals extra-articular involvement in patients with rheumatoid arthritis and curbs TNF-α-elicited endothelial activation," *Journal of Leukocyte Biology*, vol. 85, no. 1, pp. 81–87, 2009.

[25] L. Crippa, M. Bianco, B. Colombo et al., "A new chromogranin A-dependent angiogenic switch activated by thrombin," *Blood*, vol. 121, no. 2, pp. 392–402, 2013.

[26] K. B. Helle and A. Corti, "Chromogranin A: a paradoxical player in angiogenesis and vascular biology," *Cellular and Molecular Life Sciences*, vol. 72, no. 2, pp. 339–348, 2015.

[27] S. H. Yoo and D. J. Lim, "Ubiquitous presence of chromogranin A in the inner ear of guinea pig," *FEBS Letters*, vol. 317, no. 1-2, pp. 113–117, 1993.

[28] M. Bitsche, S. K. Mahata, J. Marksteiner, and A. Schrott-Fischer, "Distribution of catestatin-like immunoreactivity in the human auditory system," *Hearing Research*, vol. 184, no. 1-2, pp. 16–26, 2003.

[29] "Committee on hearing and equilibrium: guidelines for the diagnosis and evaluation of therapy in Meniere's disease," *Otolaryngology—Head and Neck Surgery*, vol. 113, no. 3, pp. 181– 185, 1995.

[30] L. X. Cubeddu, D. T. O'Connor, and R. J. Parmer, "Plasma chromogranin A: a marker of serotonin release and of emesis associated with cisplatin chemotherapy," *Journal of Clinical Oncology*, vol. 13, no. 3, pp. 681–687, 1995.

[31] C. D. Balaban and J. D. Porter, "Neuroanatomic substrates for vestibulo-autonomic interactions," *Journal of Vestibular Research: Equilibrium and Orientation*, vol. 8, no. 1, pp. 7–16, 1998.

[32] R. Khalmuratova, Y.-S. Hah, S.-K. Ahn, S.-Y. Jeon, J.-P. Kim, and C. D. Balaban, "Immunohistochemical and biomolecular identification of 5-HT7 receptor in rat vestibular nuclei," *Journal of Vestibular Research: Equilibrium and Orientation*, vol. 20, no. 6, pp. 401–406, 2010.

8

Surgical Procedures for Ménière's Disease

Ricardo Ferreira Bento and Paula Tardim Lopes*

Department of Otorhinolaryngology and Neurotology, Hospital das Clínicas— University of São Paulo, São Paulo, Brazil

*Address all correspondence to: paula.tardim@hc.fm.usp.br

ABSTRACT

The aim of this chapter is to present a literature review on some of the main articles describing different interventions for the treatment in patients with progressive intractable Ménière disease symptoms. Even though each paper presents good results in defending its techniques, there have been few well-designed clini cal studies, that is, studies involving control groups or long-term observation, in the efficacy of surgery with respect to vertigo control and hearing preservation. Focusing on presenting the different techniques established in the literature, we discuss the main indications and results obtained regarding the control of vertigo and the audiological outcomes after the procedure. Physicians should offer additional treatment strategies for Meniere's disease patients with a long history of limiting symptoms or associated hearing loss. The surgical options for such patients should be considered carefully because surgery can damage the ipsilateral ear and the hearing function of the contralateral ear is often suboptimal. Its importance is that alternatives for treatment can only be offered to a patient when doctor knows them.

Keywords: Ménière's disease, hearing loss, vertigo, endolymphatic sac, vestibular rehabilitation

INTRODUCTION

Ménière's disease is a clinical diagnosis based on the 1995 classification by the American Academy of Otolaryngology-Head and Neck Surgery (AAO-HNS) Committee on Hearing and Equilibrium [1]. The definitive diagnosis of Ménière's disease can be made with specific tests such as audiometry and electrocochleography in the exacerbated states of the disease. Recently, a study by Bernaerts [2] showed diagnostic evidences with the use of magnetic resonance imaging (MRI) scans, which showed an enlargement of the perilymphatic spaces in Ménière's disease.

The endolymphatic sac physiologically maintains the hydrostatic pressure and endolymph homeostasis in the inner ear, and its dysfunction may contribute to the pathophysiology of Ménière's disease. The classic tetrad of symptoms in endolymphatic hydrops includes recurrent attacks of vertigo lasting for hours, fluctuating hearing loss, auricular fullness, and tinnitus. Ménière's disease is idiopathic, as its aetiology remains unknown. Over the years, different surgical procedures for intractable vertigo secondary to Ménière's disease have been carried out, and although many authors consider these procedures effective, some argue that they only have a placebo effect. Usually, surgical procedures are indicated in about 20% of the patients when the possibilities of treatment with drugs for vestibular rehabilitation have already been exhausted [3–6].

The surgical technique for the treatment of vertigo depends on the diagnostic hypothesis, clinical condition, age, and hearing level of the patient.

Conservative procedures for Ménière's disease

This chapter describes the different surgical procedures performed for Ménière's disease. They can be divided into two types: non-destructive surgery, aimed at altering the disease expression and at reducing the frequency and intensity of vestibular drop attacks; and destructive surgery, aimed at controlling vertigo by stopping the vestibular function.

The most common procedures are the endolymphatic sac decompression with or without the endolymphatic duct opening and shunt in the endolymphatic sac, endolymphatic duct blockage, and intratympanic corticosteroid injection.

Endolymphatic sac decompression and shunt in the endolymphatic sac

Decompression of the endolymphatic sac involves reducing pressure in this space. It is considered a conservative procedure because of the low rate of hearing loss and the high success rate (around 80% or more) of vertigo control [7, 8].

The first surgical procedure for the treatment of Ménière's disease was described in 1927 by Portmann [9, 10], who first opened the endolymphatic sac to decrease the endolymphatic pressure. In 1938, Hallpike and Cairns [11] showed the pathological findings of endolymphatic hydrops in post-mortem temporal bones of patients who were also diagnosed with Ménière's disease. These bones showed signs of ischemia in the sensory terminal endings at the lateral walls of the membranous labyrinth, which could have been caused by the presence of hydrops.

In 1962, William House [12] showed that draining endolymphatic hydrops using a subarachnoid shunt had good outcomes. In 1967, Kimura [13] obliterated the endolymph duct and attenuated the endolymphatic hydrops in guinea pigs, following which surgeons innovated new techniques of mastoid shunts. In 1976, Paparella [14] described a technique that emphasised the need to make a wide incision in the dura mater of the posterior fossa to completely decompress the endolymphatic sac and duct, increasing its drainage through a valve created in this duct with the placement of a T-tube.

Paparella described that this surgical technique was a modification of the surgical technique of the endolymphatic sac described by Portmann and showed a 94% control rate for vertigo [15].

In a 2014 meta-analysis conducted by Sood et al. [16], the various endolymphatic surgical techniques were analysed, along with their efficacy in vertigo control and hearing maintenance. The study demonstrated that the decompression procedures of the endolymphatic sac both alone and associated with shunt placement in the mastoid were effective, without any statistical difference in the 75% control of vertigo symptoms in a short period of 12–24 months.

Bento et al. [17] conducted a retrospective study of endolymphatic sac decompression using the retrolabyrinthine approach in 95 patients with Ménière's disease who did not undergo long-term clinical treatment. In the group with unilateral disease, vertigo was controlled in 94.3%, cochlear function significantly improved in 14%, and hearing was preserved or improved in 88% of patients. In the group with bilateral disease, vertigo was controlled in 85.7%, cochlear function improved in 28%, and auditory function was preserved in 71% of patients. Considerable improvement in hearing was an improvement of more than 20 dB in the bone conduction threshold or improvement by more than 20% in the discrimination score (**Figures 1** and **2**).

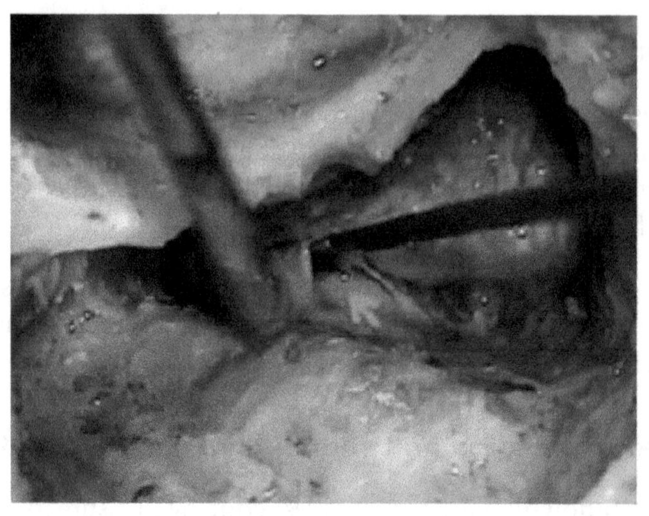

Figure 1. *The sac is opened (arrowhead).*

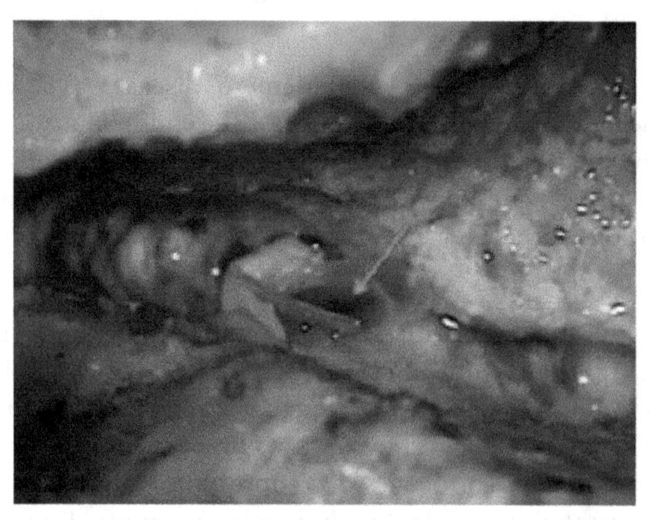

Figure 2. *A silastic sheet (arrow) is placed to keep the sac opened.*

The surgical method of endolymphatic sac decompression and drainage of the endolymphatic duct, as previously described by Paparella et al. [18–20], involves a broad exposure of the mastoid cortex, wall-up mastoidectomy, and extensive removal of the pre-sigmoidal and retrolabyrinthine cells.

A very thin skeletal bone should cover the sigmoid sinus, and a small bone island should be left over it to avoid damage from pressure and bleeding. With the Trautmann's triangle fully exposed, the overlying bone is removed with a curette or microdissector, and the sac is then identified as a dense white thickening in the dura mater pointing toward the lower portion of the posterior semicircular canal. Mostly, the sac is clearly differentiated from the adjacent dura mater by its greater thickness in the region and lack of blood vessels. After identifying the endolymphatic sac, a small aperture is created in it with a paracentesis blade or a scalpel, often below the bone border, by retracting the dura mater with a suction tip to expose the lumen. To keep the opening intact, a T-shaped silastic sheet is cut to about 0.127 mm thickness and positioned in the opening, or a T-tube is used. After the procedure, an absorbable gelatine haemostatic sponge is placed in the mastoid cavity, and the wound is closed.

Endolymphatic duct block

In this technique, the sac is not incised. The surgeon dissects the bone around the endolymphatic duct to expose it and blocks it with two small titanium clips. The endolymphatic sac gets isolated, so the production and absorption of endolymph in the inner ear balance. Saliba et al. [21] conducted a randomised controlled, non-blinded study comparing this technique with the endolymphatic sac decompression and showed that 96.5% of the patients in the endolymphatic block group achieved vertigo control compared to 37.5% of the patients in the endolymphatic sac decompression group, with no statistical differences between the groups in preand post-operative auditory thresholds.

In summary, endolymphatic duct blockade has potential as a surgical technique that results in good control of vertigo.

Corticosteroid therapy

In 1986, Brookes [22] showed the presence of high levels of circulating immunocomplexes in up to 54% of patients with Ménière's disease. Later, Alleman et al. [23] extracted the circulating immunocomplexes from patients with Ménière's disease and exposed them to endolymphatic sac tissue from other patients with the disease, showing that in only 10% of cases, there was a reaction between the immune complexes and tissues. Hence, it is suggested that although the levels of circulating immunocomplexes in these patients is high, they can represent an induction (viral, allergic, or traumatic) that is greater than an autoimmune phenomenon. Another pathophysiological analysis of Ménière's disease showed that the immune-mediated responses in the inner ear, endolymphatic sac, and vascular striae could be the main causative factors. In 1997, Shea et al. [24] showed that combined administration of systemic and intratympanic dexamethasone completely suppressed vertigo in 63.4% and significantly improved hearing in 35.4% of patients within 2 years after treatment. Later in 2001, Sennaroglu et al. [25] reported that intratympanic perfusion of dexamethasone completely suppressed vertigo in 42.0% and significantly improved hearing in 16% of patients within 2 years after treatment.

Destructive surgeries for Ménière's disease

These labyrinthine surgeries cure the patient of vertigo by destroying the final vestibular organ. The brain compensates for the loss of vestibular function on one side using the contralateral labyrinth, as long as it is functioning properly. Destructive labyrinthine procedures have a high risk of destroying the cochlea and should be avoided in patients with adequate hearing. Vestibulocochlear nerve neurectomy, chemical labyrinthectomy, surgical labyrinthectomy, and sacculotomy are common destructive surgeries.

Vestibulocochlear nerve neurectomy

The neurectomy of the vestibulocochlear nerve for the treatment of Ménière's disease was described in 1933 by Dandy [26]. It is a surgical technique involving a selective section of the vestibular nerve at its entrance to the brain to reduce vertigo but inevitably causing total hearing loss in the operated ear.

Several authors modified the original technique. In 1989, Silverstein [27] proposed the retrosigmoid approach for neurectomy and observed a substantial improvement in dizziness in 92% with a significant hearing loss in only 4% of patients.

House [28] introduced the middle fossa approach. Regardless of the access, the decompression technique had a success rate of up to 90% in the control of vertigo [29–33]. Colletti et al. [4] conducted a comparative study on 209 patients who underwent neurectomy, comparing a group of 24 patients who received intratympanic gentamicin (ITG), chemical labyrinthectomy neural ablation therapy. To perform a homogenous comparison of results in the present paper, it considered all the 24 ITG patients and the last 24 patients who underwent VN from 2000 to 2002 via the retrosigmoid approach.

Vertigo was controlled in 95.8% of neurectomy patients and in 75% of gentamicin patients. Speech discrimination in the neurectomy group was reduced from 85 to 82% and in the gentamicin group from 87% to 65%.

Chemical labyrinthectomy: intratympanic application of gentamicin in the middle ear

This technique was first used in 1978 by Beck [34, 35] and aims to perform a chemical ablation of the labyrinth to decrease the frequency and intensity of vertigo episodes but can result in hearing loss, as gentamicin is ototoxic and reduces labyrinthine activity. It can be injected directly into the tympanic cavity using a thin needle or applied daily through a Politzer ventilation tube first placed at the tympanic membrane for penetrating the round and oval windows. A study [36] showed 90% efficacy in the cessation of vertigo among 92 patients.

In the 2000 literature review by Blakley et al. [37], 18 articles were found on the techniques of intratympanic injection of gentamicin in the treatment of Ménière's disease. The articles reported high success rates in vertigo treatment, but the technique, dose, duration, and treatment philosophy varied considerably among them. Hearing loss was typically reported in about 30% of patients, and no technique had any significant medical advantage over the other. Until new controlled studies indicate otherwise, this therapy is an alternative treatment for patients with major comorbidities.

Surgical labyrinthectomy

This technique can decrease vertigo by the total destruction of the labyrinth but leads to total hearing loss in the operated ear.

Lake first described this procedure in 1904 [38], and in the mid-twentieth century, labyrinthectomy was established as a less-invasive alternative to neurectomy of the vestibular nerve [39, 40]. The surgical technique involves opening the semicircular canals up to the endolymphatic ducts in the opening of the vestibule with the complete destruction of neuroepithelium and Scarpa's ganglion [41, 42]. No technique was observed to be superior in vertigo control among labyrinthectomy, neurectomy, and a combination of both [43, 44].

Labyrinthectomy, in particular, is an alternative [45] (demonstrating approximately 100% success rate in vertigo treatment) for old patients, and in this case, the transmastoid technique presented a lower permanent imbalance rate after the procedure than the transcanal technique. Labyrinthectomy is the treatment of choice for patients over 60 years of age [46]. Surgical labyrinthectomy of the affected labyrinth always ends in total deafness. Therefore, it should be reserved for patients with non-functional hearing and should be one of the last therapeutic options (**Figure 3**).

Sacculotomy

In 1964, Fick [47, 48] described a procedure in which a fenestra is made in the stapes footplate or round window membrane, and therefore, a permanent shunt for draining of the saccule is created with the destruction of the cochlear function [49].

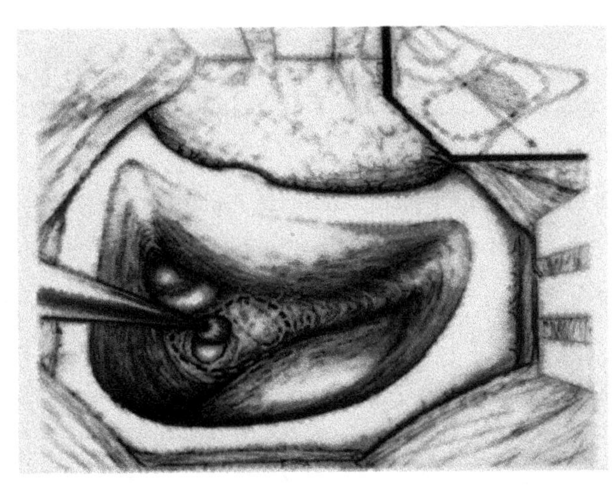

Figure 3. *Schematic drawing of Labyrinthectomy.*

Giddings et al. [50] reported hearing loss after cochleo-sacculotomy in 80% of the patients and recurrent vertigo episodes in a mean follow-up of 17 months in 4 of 11 patients so that a destructive intervention had to be carried out again. Kinney et al. [51] and Wielinga et al. [52] recommended cochleo-sacculotomy as a minimally invasive surgical method, especially for old patients, as an alternative to neurectomy because good results were obtained with regard to vertigo control, although with significant hearing loss in almost all patients.

In 2015, in a comparative study [53] between cochlear sacculotomy techniques and endolymphatic sac decompression, the control of vertigo was significantly better in patients after cochleo-sacculotomy but also with significant deterioration of hearing. The cochleo-sacculotomy procedure performed simultaneously with cochlear implant surgery in patients with deafness and persistent vertigo in Ménière's disease is an alternative already proposed by some authors [54–56], and they have reported good results.

Conclusion

The surgical procedures described in this chapter demonstrated satisfactory results in the control of incapacitating vertigo in patients diagnosed with endolymphatic hydrops refractory to clinical drug treatment, adequate diet, and vestibular rehabilitation. The choice of method would depend on the quality of residual hearing, contralateral hearing, and on the ability to develop compensatory mechanisms if surgical techniques destroyed vestibular function.

Conflict of interest

The authors have no conflict of interest.

References

[1] Committee on Hearing and Equilibrium. Committee on hearing and equilibrium guidelines for the diagnosis and evaluation of therapy in Meniere's disease. American Academy of Otolaryngology—Head and Neck Foundation, Inc. Otolaryngology and Head and Neck Surgery. 1995;**113**(3):181-185

[2] Bernaerts A, Vanspauwen R, Blaivie C, et al. The value of four stage vestibular hydrops grading and asymmetric perilymphatic enhancement in the diagnosis of Menière's disease on MRI. Neuroradiology. 2019;**61**(4):421-429. DOI: 10.1007/s00234-019-02155-7

[3] Liston SL, Nissen RL, Paparella MM, Da Costa SS. Surgical treatment of vertigo. In: Paparella MM, Shumrick DA, Gluckman JL, Meyerhoff WL, editors. Otolaryngology. Volume II. Philadelphia: WB Saunders Company; 1991. pp. 1715-1732

[4] Colletti V, Carner M, Colletti L. Auditory results after vestibular nerve section and intratympanic gentamicin for Ménière's disease. Otology & Neurotology. 2007;**28**(2):145-151. DOI: 10.1097/MAO.0b013e31802c7989

[5] Sajjadi H, Paparella MM. Ménière's disease. Lancet. 2008;**372**(9636): 406-414. DOI: 10.1016/ S0140-6736(08)61161-7

[6] Yokota Y, Kitahara T, Sakagami M, Ito T, Kimura T, Okayasu T, et al. Surgical results and psychological status in patients with intractable Ménière's disease. Auris, Nasus, Larynx. 2016;**43**(3):287-291. DOI: 10.1016/j.anl.2015.10.007

[7] Brinson GM, Chen DA, Arriaga MA. Endolymphatic mastoid shunt versus endolymphatic sac decompression for Ménière's disease. Otolaryngology and Head and Neck Surgery. 2007;**136**(3):415-421. DOI: 10.1016/j.otohns.2006.08.031

[8] Kitahara T, Horii A, Imai T, Ohta Y, Morihana T, Inohara H, et al. Effects of endolymphatic sac decompression surgery on vertigo and hearing in patients with bilateral Ménière's disease. Otology & Neurotology. 2014;**35**(10):1852-1857. DOI: 10.1097/ MAO.0000000000000469

[9] Portmann G. The saccus endolinphaticus and the operation for draining the same for relief of vertigo. The Journal of Laryngology and Otology. 1927;**42**:809-817

[10] Portamann G. Surgical treatment of vertigo by opening of the saccus endolymphaticus. Archives of Otolaryngology. 1969;**89**(6):809-815

[11] Hallpike CS, Cairns H. Observation on pathology of Ménière's syndrome. The Journal of Laryngology and Otology. 1938;**53**:624-654

[12] House WF. Subarachnoid shunt for drainage of endolymphatic hydrops. A preliminary report. Laryngoscope. 1962;**72**:713-729. DOI: 10.1288/00005537-196206000-00003

[13] Kimura RS. Experimental blockage of the endolymphatic duct and sac and its effects on the inner ear of the guinea pig. A study on endolymphatic hydrops. The Annals of Otology, Rhinology, and Laryngology. 1967;**76**(3):664-687. DOI: 10.1177/000348946707600311

[14] Paparella MM, Hanson DG. Endolymphatic sac drainage for intractable vertigo (method and experiences). The Laryngoscope. 1976;**86**(5):697-703. DOI: 10.1288/00005537-197605000-00010

[15] Paparella MM, Goycoolea M. Panel of Menière's disease. Endolymphatic sac enhancement surgery for Menière's disease: An extension of conservative therapy. The Annals of Otology, Rhinology, and Laryngology. 1981;**90**(6 Pt 1):610-615. DOI: 10.1177/000348948109000620

[16] Sood AJ, Lambert PR, Nguyen SA, Meyer TA. Endolymphatic sac surgery for Ménière's disease: A systematic review and meta-analysis. Otology & Neurotology. 2014;**35**(6):1033-1045. DOI: 10.1097/ MAO.0000000000000324

[17] Bento RF, Cisneros JC, De Oliveira Fonseca AC. Endolymphatic sac drainage for the treatment of Ménière's disease. The Journal of Laryngology and Otology. 2016;**131**(2):144-149. DOI: 10.1017/S0022215116009713

[18] Paparella MM, Goycoolea M. Panel of Ménière's disease. Endolymphatic sac enhancement surgery for Ménière's disease: An extension of conservative therapy. The Annals of Otology, Rhinology, and Laryngology. 1981;**90**(6 Pt 1):610-615. DOI: 10.1177/000348948109000620

[19] Paparella MM, Sajjadi H. Endolymphatic sac enhancement. Otolaryngologic Clinics of North America. 1994;**27**(2):381-402

[20] Paparella MM. Revision of endolymphatic sac surgery for recurrent Ménière's disease. Otolaryngologic Clinics of North America. 2002;**35**(3):607-619

[21] Saliba I, Gabra N, Alzahrani M, Berbiche D. Endolymphatic duct blockage: A randomized controlled trial of a novel surgical technique for Ménière's disease treatment. Otolaryngology and Head and Neck Surgery. 2015;**152**(1):122-129. DOI:10.1177/0194599814555840

[22] Brookes GB. Circulating immune complexes in Meniere's disease. Archives of Otolaryngology—Head & Neck Surgery. 1986;**112**(5):536-540

[23] Alleman AM, Dornhoffer JL, Arenberg IK, Walker PD. Demonstration of autoantibodies to the endolymphatic sac in Meniere's disease. The Laryngoscope. 1997;**107**(2):211-215

[24] Shea JJ Jr. The role of dexamethasone or streptomycin perfusion in the treatment of Meniere's disease. Otolaryngologic Clinics of North America. 1997;**30**(6):1051-1059

[25] Sennaroglu L, Sennaroglu G, Gursel B, Dini FM. Intratympanic dexamethasone, intratympanic gentamicin, and endolymphatic sac surgery for intractable vertigo in Meniere's disease. Otolaryngology and Head and Neck Surgery. 2001;**125**(5):537-543. DOI: 10.1067/ mhn.2001.119485

[26] Dandy WE. Treatment of Meniere's disease by section of only the vestibular portion of the acoustic nerve. Bulletin of the Johns Hopkins Hospital.1933;**53**:52-55

[27] Silverstein H, Jackson LE. Vestibular nerve section. Otolaryngologic Clinics of North America. 2002;**35**(3):655-673

[28] House WF. Surgical exposure of the internal auditory canal and its contents through the middle cranial fossa. The Laryngoscope. 1961;**71**:1363-1385. DOI: 10.1288/00005537-196111000-00004

[29] Reid CB, Eisenberg R, Halmagyi GM, Fagan PA. The outcome of vestibular nerve section for intractable vertigo: The patient's point of view. The Laryngoscope. 1996;**106** (12 Pt 1):1553-1556

[30] Pappas DG Jr, Pappas DG Sr. Vestibular nerve section: Long-term follow-up. The Laryngoscope. 1997;**107**(9):1203-1209

[31] De Diego JI, Prim MP, Melcon E, de Sarriá MJ, Gavilán J. Result of middle fossa vestibular neurectomy in Meniere's disease. Acta Otorrinolaringológica Española. 2001;**52**(4):283-286

[32] Nakahara H, Takemori S, Seki Y, Umezu H. Hearing changes and questionnaire responses in patients with paramedian suboccipital vestibular neurectomy. Acta Oto-Laryngologica. Supplementum. 2001;**545**:108-112

[33] Schlegel M, Vibert D, Ott SR, Häusler R, Caversaccio MD. Functional results and quality of life after retrosigmoid vestibular neurectomy in patients with Ménière's disease. Otology & Neurotology. 2012;**33**(8):1380-1385

[34] Beck C, Schmidt CL. 10 years of experience with intratympanally applied streptomycin (gentamycin) in the therapy of morbus Meniere. Archives of Oto-Rhino-Laryngology. 1978;**221**(2):149-152

[35] Beck C. Intratympanic application of gentamicin for treatment of Meniere's disease. The Keio Journal of Medicine. 1986;**35**(1):36-41

[36] Lange G. Gentamicin and other ototoxic antibiotics for the transtympanic treatment for Meniere's disease. Archives of Oto-RhinoLaryngology. 1989;**246**(5):269-270

[37] Blakley BW. Update on intratympanic gentamicin for Meniere's disease. The Laryngoscope. 2000;**110** (2 Pt 1):236-240

[38] Lake R. Removal of the semicircular canals in a case of unilateral aural vertigo. Lancet. 1904;**1**:1567-1568

[39] Cawthorne TE, Hallpike CS. Some recent work on the investigation and treatment of "Ménière's" disease. Proceedings of the Royal Society of Medicine. 1943;**36**(10):533-550

[40] Day KM. Surgical treatment of hydrops of the labyrinth; surgical destruction of the labyrinth for Ménière's disease. The Laryngoscope. 1952;**62**(6):547-555

[41] Jones R, Silverstein H, Smouha E. Long-term results of transmeatal cochleovestibular neurectomy: An analysis of 100 cases. Otolaryngology and Head and Neck Surgery. 1989;**100**(1):22-29

[42] Langman AW, Lindeman RC. Surgery for vertigo in the nonserviceable hearing ear: Transmastoid labyrinthectomy or translabyrinthine vestibular nerve section. The Laryngoscope. 1993;**103**(12):1321-1325

[43] Gacek RR, Gacek MR. Comparison of labyrinthectomy and vestibular neurectomy in the control of vertigo. The Laryngoscope. 1996;**106**(2 Pt 1): 225-230

[44] Eisenman DJ, Speers R, Telian SA. Labyrinthectomy versus vestibular neurectomy: Long-term physiologic and clinical outcomes. Otology & Neurotology. 2001;**22**(4):539-548

[45] Schwaber MK, Pensak ML, Reiber ME. Transmastoid labyrinthectomy in older patients. The Laryngoscope. 1995;**105**(11):1152-1154

[46] Langman AW, Lindeman RC. Surgical labyrinthectomy in the older patient. Otolaryngology and Head and Neck Surgery. 1998;**118**:739-742

[47] Fick IA. Decompression of the labyrinth: A new surgical procedure for Meniere's disease. Archives of Otolaryngology. 1964;**79**:447-458

[48] van Fick IA. Symposium: Management of Ménière's disease. VI. Sacculotomy for hydrops. The Laryngoscope. 1965;**75**(10):1539-1546

[49] Schuknecht HF. Cochleosacculotomy for Meniere's disease: Theory, technique and results. The Laryngoscope. 1982;**92**(8 Pt 1):853-858

[50] Giddings NA, Shelton C, O'Leary MJ, Brackmann DE. Cochleosacculotomy revisited: Long-term results poorer than expected. Archives of Otolaryngology—Head & Neck Surgery. 1991;**117**(10):1150-1152

[51] Kinney WC, Nalepa N, Hughes GB, Kinney SE. Cochleosacculotomy for the treatment of Menière's disease in the elderly patient. The Laryngoscope. 1995;**105**(9 Pt 1):934-937

[52] Wielinga EW, Smyth GD. Longterm results of sacculotomy in older patients. The Annals of Otology, Rhinology, and Laryngology. 1989;**98**(10):803-806

[53] Soheilipour S, Abtahi SH, Soltani M, Khodadadi HA. Comparison the results of two different vestibular system surgery in patients with persistent Meniere's disease. Advanced Biomedical Research. 2015;**4**:198. DOI: 10.4103/2277-9175.166134

[54] Mukherjee P, Eykamp K, Brown D, Curthoys I, Flanagan S, Biggs N, et al. Cochlear implantation in Ménière's disease with and without labyrinthectomy. Otology & Neurotology. 2017;**38**(2):192-198. DOI: 10.1097/MAO.0000000000001278

[55] Prenzler NK, Bültmann E, Giourgas A, Steffens M, Salcher RB, Stolle S, et al. Cochlear implantation in patients with definite Meniere's disease. European Archives of Oto-RhinoLaryngology. 2017;**274**(2):751-756. DOI: 10.1007/s00405-016-4356-z

[56] Heywood RL, Atlas MD. Simultaneous cochlear implantation and labyrinthectomy for advanced Ménière's disease. The Journal of Laryngology and Otology. 2016;**130**(2):204-206. DOI: 10.1017/S0022215115003345

9

Outcomes of Endolymphatic Sac Surgery for Meniere's Disease with and without Comorbid Migraine

Norman A. Orabi,[1] Brian M. Kellermeyer,[1] Christopher A. Roberts,[1] Stephen J. Wetmore,[1] and Adam M. Cassis[2]

[1]West Virginia University School of Medicine Department of Otolaryngology, P.O. Box 9200, Morgantown, WV 26506, USA

[2]Arizona Hearing & Balance Center, 225 S Dobson Rd#1, Chandler, AZ 85224, USA

Correspondence should be addressed to Brian M. Kellermeyer; bmkellermeyer@hsc.wvu.edu

Academic Editor: Gerd J. Ridder

ABSTRACT

Purpose. To explore outcomes of endolymphatic sac surgery for patients with Meniere's disease with and without the comorbid condition of migraine. Materials and Methods. A retrospective chart review of adult patients undergoing endolymphatic sac surgery at a single tertiary care center from 1987 to 2019 was performed. All adult patients who failed medical therapy and underwent primary endolymphatic sac surgery were included. The main outcome measures were vertigo control and functional level scale (FLS) score. Patient characteristics, comorbidities, and audiometric outcomes were tracked as well. Results. Patients with Meniere's disease and migraine had a stronger association with psychiatric comorbidities (64.29% vs. 25.80%, $p = 0.01$), shorter duration of vertigo episodes (143 vs. 393 min, $p = 0.02$), and younger age (36.6 vs. 50.8 yr, p = 0.005) at the time of endolymphatic sac surgery. Postoperative pure tone averages and word recognition scores were nearly identical to preoperative baselines. Class A vertigo control (47.92%) was most common, followed by class B vertigo control (31.25%). The FLS score improved from 4.2 to 2.8 ($p < 0.001$). Both patients with and without migraine had classes A-B vertigo control (66.67% vs. 80.95%) without any statistically significant difference ($p = 0.59$). Of the patients who required secondary treatment (10.42%), none had migraine. Conclusions. Endolymphatic sac surgery is an effective surgical intervention for Meniere's disease with and without migraine. Patients with comorbid migraine tend to be younger and present with psychiatric comorbidities.

INTRODUCTION

Meniere's disease is a rare condition with a prevalence of 190 per 100,000 but has detrimental effects on function and quality of life [1]. The condition is defined by (1) two or more spontaneous episodes of vertigo lasting 20 minutes to 12 hours, (2) at least one occasion of audiometrically documented low-to-medium frequency sensorineural hearing loss in the affected ear before, during, or after one of the episodes of vertigo, (3) fluctuating aural symptoms (hearing, tinnitus, or fullness) in the affected ear, and (4) another vestibular diagnosis not better accounted for [2].

Although the etiology is unclear, it has been associated with anatomical changes in the inner ear from increased endolymph, which is termed endolymphatic hydrops. The association with endolymphatic hydrops supports the theory that the episodic symptoms are due to endolymphatic duct distention leading to microtears in Reisner's membrane and influx of toxic levels of potassiumrich endolymph [2]. Individual patients often present with a unique constellation of symptoms. For example, two studies by Frejo et al. have used cluster analysis to identify 5 clinical subgroups of Meniere's disease, which includes the Type 4 subgroup that is characterized by comorbid migraine [3, 4]. Moreover, these symptoms overlap with other clinical entities making the diagnosis elusive. The American Academy of Otolaryngology (AAO) published several guidelines to assist in the diagnosis, evaluation, and treatment of Meniere's disease [2, 5].

Initial treatment consists of medical management with low salt diet, diuretics, and betahistine. Antiemetics, vestibular suppressants, and corticosteroids are reserved for symptomatic control during acute episodes. Unfortunately, more aggressive treatment may be necessary for those who continue to have disabling vertigo. Additional treatment consists of intratympanic injection of corticosteroids or gentamicin or surgical options including endolymphatic sac surgery (ESS), vestibular nerve section, and labyrinthectomy. Each treatment option carries its own risks and morbidity. For example, labyrinthectomy is the gold standard for vertigo control but is a destructive procedure resulting in a total loss of hearing [6]. ESS is effective with AAO classes A-B vertigo control of 64.5–77% and minimal risk to hearing [7–9].

Migraine affects about 15.3% of the general population and is characterized by head pain, nausea, vomiting, and sensitivity to environmental stimuli [10]. It is a common comorbidity with Meniere's disease, affecting about 43–56% of these patients [11, 12]. A subset of classical migraine patients develop vestibular migraine, which is often underdiagnosed due to overlapping symptoms with other vestibular disorders such as Meniere's disease [13, 14]. Vestibular migraine has only relatively recently been recognized as a cause of episodic vertigo and did not have a consensus definition by the Barany Society until 2012 [15]. Moreover, vestibular migraine can be accompanied by otologic symptoms (tinnitus, aural fullness, and hearing loss), and it is not uncommon for patients to have both Meniere's disease and vestibular migraine [2, 16]. Some authors have proposed that migraine and Meniere's disease may even be variants of one other and share a common pathophysiological origin through disorders of ionic regulation [17, 18]. When there is uncertainty in the diagnosis or concern for concurrent vestibular migraine, noninvasive medical therapy should be pursued prior to surgical intervention and can be quite effective [2, 14]. Despite the symptoms of migraine and potential to develop vestibular migraine, no studies exploring the effect of migraine on outcomes of ESS in patients with Meniere's disease have been reported. Given the variable outcomes of ESS, we aim to explore the outcomes of ESS in those with a preexisting diagnosis of migraine. We hypothesize that patients with preexisting migraine diagnosis may have a worse outcome with ESS compared to those without migraine.

Methods

Our study was approved by our university's Institutional Review Board. We conducted a retrospective chart review of all adult patients (≥18 years) with Meniere's disease who underwent ESS at a single tertiary care center from 1987 through 2019 after failing medical therapy. All included patients retrospectively fulfilled Barany Society diagnostic criteria for Meniere's disease. Patients were excluded if they did not undergo ESS or underwent ESS at an outside institution. All surgeries were ESS with mastoid shunt using an arrow-shaped piece of silastic inserted into the sac with the tail of the arrow extending into the mastoid cavity performed by three fellowship trained neurotologists. Seventy-six patients were identified and underwent chart review including paper and electronic medical records. A power analysis was deferred, given that we were able to review the entire available cohort of 76 patients.

Preoperative demographics, comorbidities, and baseline characteristics were collected for all patients. Due to the long time period of data collection extending well before the diagnosis of vestibular migraine, any form or variant of migraine was recorded as positive if present in the past medical history with diagnosis made by either surgeon, primary care provider, or neurologist. Migraine treatment history was not obtained due to the large number of included patients coming from a time period before the knowledge of vestibular migraine and was not routinely available in the records. Baseline functional level scale (FLS) score and Meniere's stage were assessed as per the 1995 AAO Guidelines for Meniere's disease. The FLS score was determined via self-assessment on a standard form or by patient history during clinic visits. Meniere's staging was based on the four-tone average of the pure tone thresholds at 0.5, 1, 2, and 3 kHz of the worst audiogram during the 6-month period before ESS.

Paired preoperative and postoperative pure tone averages (PTAs) and word recognition scores (WRSs) were compared to assess hearing outcomes. Most postoperative audiograms were from the 18–24-month period. If unavailable, we included the postoperative audiogram within 12–36 months that was closest to the preferred 18–24-month postoperative period. There were 42 paired preoperative and postoperative audiograms available for analysis.

Vertigo control grade was used to assess the efficacy of ESS. As per the 1995 AAO Guidelines for Meniere's disease, vertigo control grade classes are divided into classes A–F by dividing the number of definitive vertigo spells in the 6month period prior to treatment by the number of definitive vertigo spells in the 18–24-month posttreatment period. Classes are defined as $A = 0\%$, $B = 1–40\%$, $C = 41–80\%$, $D = 81–120\%$, and $F > 120\%$. Of the 76 patients, 28 patients were excluded due to inadequate data in the 18–24-month posttreatment period. Good and poor vertigo controls were defined as vertigo classes A-B and vertigo classes C–F, respectively.

Of note, our patient population had an overlap with a previous descriptive study on primary ESS for the treatment of MD [7]. Unlike the previous study, we focused on preoperative characteristics and postoperative outcomes for primary ESS with migraine as an independent variable. Moreover, our patient population was larger due to the addition of more recent patients since the prior study was completed.

Statistical analysis was performed using RStudio Version 1.4.1103 (© 2009–2021 RStudio, PBC). Descriptive statistics were used for patient demographics. Univariate analysis with a p value set at $p = 0.05$ was used to analyze the remainder of the data with a subset analysis based on the comorbidity of migraine as an independent variable. We used the two-sample t-test for continuous variables and Fisher's exact test for categorical variables.

Results

Demographics and baseline characteristics were analyzed for 76 patients based on the presence or absence of migraine as shown in Table 1. Meniere's disease with migraine was designated MD + M and Meniere's disease without migraine as MD − M. The average age at the time of surgery was lower at 36.6 years in MD + M compared to 50.8 years in the MD − M group ($P = 0.005$). There was a slight female predominance among all patients due to increased prevalence in MD + M patients. Psychiatric comorbidities were present in 64.29% of MD + M patients compared to 25.80% of MD − M patients ($P = 0.01$). Comorbidities were anxiety, depression, and panic attacks. The majority of patients in both groups were treated by diuretics, followed by diuretics with either oral or intratympanic steroids. In the MD − M group, there were four patients who received other forms of treatment: two patients received diuretics, intratympanic steroids, and betahistine; one patient received diuretics and used the Meniett device; and one patient received diuretics, oral and intratympanic steroids, and intratympanic gentamycin. Audiometric baselines were similar in MD + M and MD − M patients. Meniere's stage 3 comprised the majority of patients in both groups. The average FLS score was 4.0 and 4.3 in MD + M and MD − M patients, respectively ($p = 0.5$). The time from diagnosis to surgery was 47.43 and 52.00 months in the MD + M and MD − M patients, respectively ($p = 0.74$).

Analysis of the 42 paired audiograms demonstrated stable hearing outcomes without any significant difference (Table 2). Regarding vertigo control, there were 48 patients with appropriate follow-up in the postoperative 18–24-month period. Overall, ESS decreased the frequency of major vertigo episodes (16.0 vs. 2.4 episodes per month, $p < 0.001$) and FLS score (4.2 vs. 2.8, $p < 0.001$). Class A vertigo control (47.92%) was most common, followed by class B vertigo control (31.25%) (Table 2). Five patients required secondary treatment: two patients underwent revision ESS followed by labyrinthectomy, one vestibular nerve section, one revision ESS followed by vestibular nerve section, and one revision ESS. Decision for revision surgery was based on a relapse of vertigo symptoms after temporary improvement following the initial ESS.

Six of the 48 patients had MD + M as shown in Table 3. MD + M patients had a shorter duration of major vertigo episodes than MD – M patients (143 vs. 393.4 min, $P = 0.02$). Mean vertigo control percentage was similar in MD + M and MD – M patients ($p = 0.96$) (Figure 1). The MD + M group had 33.33% of MD + M with class A control and 33.33% with classes C–F control compared to 50.00% with class A control and 19.05% with classes C–F control in the MD – M group. Both groups had similar postoperative FLS scores and classes A-B vertigo control without any statistically significant differences ($p = 0.09$ and $p = 0.59$) (Table 3 and Figure 2). None of the patients who underwent a secondary procedure were in the MD + M group.

Discussion

Meniere's disease has detrimental effects on function and quality of life. Although most cases can be managed with medical therapy, a significant proportion of cases require surgical treatment. Migraine is a common comorbidity in these patients. Given the variable outcomes of ESS and possibility of coexisting vestibular migraine, presence of migraine could factor in when considering ESS. Our study is the first to assess the effect of migraine on preoperative characteristics and postoperative outcomes for ESS. We discovered several differences in preoperative characteristics and confirmed the relatively high efficacy of ESS in both MD + M and MD – M patients.

There were several key differences between MD + M patients and MD – M patients. In our study, MD + M patients were more than twice as likely to have psychiatric comorbidities than MD – M patients (Table 1). It is well known that there is a higher association of psychiatric disorders with both Meniere's disease and migraine compared to rates in the general population [19, 20]. Interestingly, vestibular migraine has higher rates of psychiatric comorbidity than Meniere's disease [21]. One explanation for the increased prevalence of psychiatric disorders would be that a subset of our MD + M patients was affected by vestibular migraine given their history of classical migraines, which often predate the vertiginous symptoms of vestibular migraine.

MD + M patients were about 14.2 years younger on average at the time of surgery. Meniere's disease has its highest prevalence in the 5th and 6th decades compared to 4th and 5th decades for migraine, which is consistent with our finding of younger average age for those patients with Meniere's disease and migraine [2, 10, 22]. Although both migraine and Meniere's disease have a female predominance, migraine has a greater association with females as seen in large-scale epidemiological studies [1, 19]. Prior studies on ESS do not consistently demonstrate a female predominance in their surgical candidates [7, 9, 23, 24]. There was a higher female prevalence in MD + M patients but not in MD – M patients. This finding was not statistically significant, but our data are limited by our small population sizes. Vestibular migraine patients are younger and more likely to be female compared with patients with Meniere's disease [2]. These observations in the MD + M group fit the typical demographics for what we now know is vestibular migraine which was not known at that time. There is a possibility that this migraine subset of patients had elements of vestibular migraine contributing to their dizziness.

For patients with Meniere's disease refractory to medical management, more invasive treatment strategies can be pursued including intratympanic injection of corticosteroids or gentamicin, ESS, vestibular nerve section, and labyrinthectomy. ESS is an attractive option because it avoids the total hearing loss and permanent vestibular dysfunction seen with labyrinthectomy. On the other hand, intratympanic gentamycin allows the patient to avoid the morbidity of a surgical procedure but has the potential to damage hearing and vestibular function [25]. Previous studies on ESS have demonstrated excellent vertigo control and improvements in FLS scores. Following ESS, classes A-B vertigo control ranged from 64.5 to 77% and FLS decreased by an average of 0.8–2.0 points [7, 9, 26, 27]. Moreover, a study by Gibson et al. demonstrated similar classes A-B vertigo control between patients receiving ESS and those receiving intratympanic gentamycin injections (73.1% vs. 66.8%, p = 0.76). However, chronic posttreatment unsteadiness was encountered more frequently in the patients receiving intratympanic gentamycin injections compared to patients receiving ESS (25.0% vs. 0%, p = 0.009) [25]. Overall, we had classes A-B vertigo control in 79.17% of patients and decreased FLS from 4.2 to 2.8. Our results demonstrated similar efficacy to other studies in the literature.

Table 1: All patient demographics stratified by migraine as a comorbidity.

Characteristic	MD+M[a] (N=14)	MD−M[b] (N=62)	P value [95% CI]
Age (yr)	36.6±15.5	50.8±11.6	0.005*S [4.8, 23.6]
Sex			
Male	3 (21.43%)	31 (50.00%)	0.07**
Female	11 (78.57%)	31 (50.00%)	
Psychiatric comorbidity	9 (64.29%)	16 (25.80%)	0.01**S [1.3, 22.2]
Pure tone average (dB)	49.5±18.6	49.4±15.1	0.99* [−11.4, 11.3]
Word recognition score (%)	69.8±37.2	65.7±32.7	0.70* [−27.0, 18.6]
Preoperative FLS Prior treatment	4.0±1.0	4.3±0.8	0.50* [−0.6, 1.2]
Diuretics	11 (78.57%)	49 (79.03%)	0.73**
Diuretics+steroids	3 (21.43%)	9 (14.52%)	
Other	0 (0%)	4 (6.45%)	
Meniere's stage		(N=56)[c]	0.35**
1: ≤25 dB	3 (21.43%)	4 (7.14%)	
2: 26–40 dB	2 (14.29%)	13 (23.21%)	
3: 41–70 dB	8 (57.14%)	36 (64.29%)	
4: >70 dB	1 (7.14%)	3 (5.36%)	0.74*
Diagnosis to surgery (months)	47.43±39.41	52.00±65.61	

[a]Meniere's disease with migraine. [b]Meniere's disease without migraine. [c]Population of 56 due to six missing values. *Two-sample t-test. **Fisher's exact test. [S]Significant at 5% level of significance.

Table 2: Overall outcomes for endolymphatic sac surgery.

Variable	Preoperative period	Postoperative period	*P* value [95% CI]
Pure tone average (*N* = 42)	50.1 ± 16.2	50.36 ± 21.4	0.91* [−5.2, 4.6]
Word recognition score (*N* = 42)	64.2 ± 34.2	63.2 ± 32.6	0.55* [−5.8, 10.7]
Frequency of major vertigo episodes (per month) (*N* = 48)	16.0 ± 18.5	2.4 ± 5.2	<0.001*S [8.1, 19.0]
Functional level scale (*N* = 48)	4.2 ± 0.8	2.8 ± 1.7	<0.001*S [0.7, 1.9]
1995 AAO vertigo control (*N* = 48)			
Class A		23 (47.92%)	
Class B		15 (31.25%)	
Class C		1 (2.08%)	
Class D		4 (8.33%)	
Class E		0 (0.00%)	
Class F		5 (10.42%)**	

*Paired two-sample *t*-test. **Secondary treatment procedures included the following: two patients underwent revision ESS followed by labyrinthectomy, one vestibular nerve section, one revision ESS followed by VNS, and one revision ESS. [S]Significant at 5% level of significance.

Table 3: Outcomes for endolymphatic sac surgery stratified by migraine as a comorbidity.

Variable	MD + M[a] (*N* = 6[c])	MD − M[b] (*N* = 42[c])	*P* value [95% CI]
Preoperative baseline			
Frequency of major vertigo episodes (per month)	11.2 ± 10.1	16.6 ± 16.7	0.30* [−16.7, 5.6],
Duration of major vertigo episodes (minutes)	143 ± 73.4	393.4 ± 600.7	0.02*S [−458.9, −42.0]
Functional level scale	1.8 ± 0.96	2.9 ± 1.83	0.09* [−2.6, 0.25]*
1995 AAO vertigo control			
Class A	2 (33.33%)	21 (50.00%)	
Class B	2 (33.33%)	13 (30.95%)	
Class C	0 (0.00%)	1 (2.38%)	
Class D	2 (33.33%)	2 (4.76%)	
Class E	0 (0.00%)	0 (0.00%)	
Class F	0 (0.00%)	5 (11.90%)	
Good control: classes A-B	4 (66.67%)	34 (80.95%)	0.59**
Poor control: classes C–F	2 (33.33%)	8 (19.05%)	
Mean vertigo control (%)	32.8 ± 48.9	34.0 ± 65.8	0.96* [−48.4, 51.2]

[a]Meniere's disease with migraine. [b]Meniere's disease without migraine. [c]Patients with available data in accordance with time intervals specified by 1995 AAO Guidelines. *Two-sample *t*-test. **Fisher's exact test. [S]Significant at 5% level of significance.

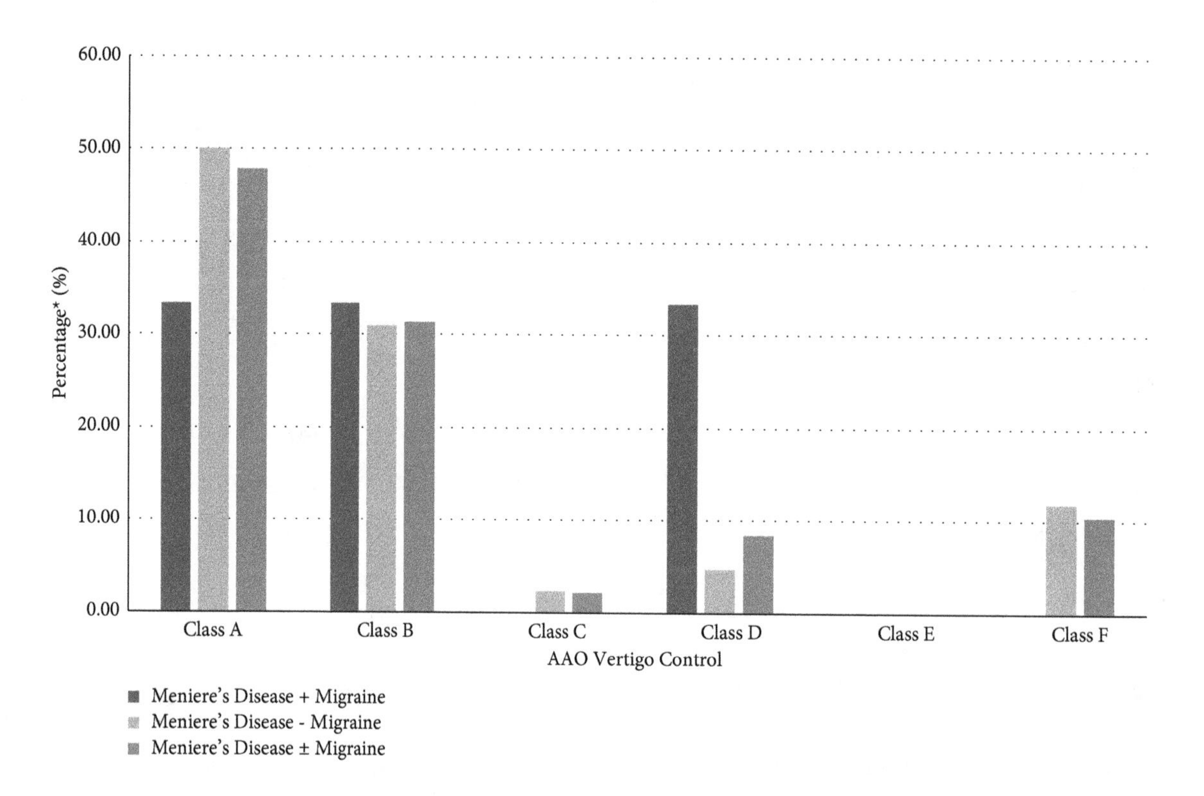

Figure 1: Vertigo outcomes following endolymphatic sac surgery. *Based on specific population sizes for each respective patient category. See Tables 2 and 3 for numerical representation of results.

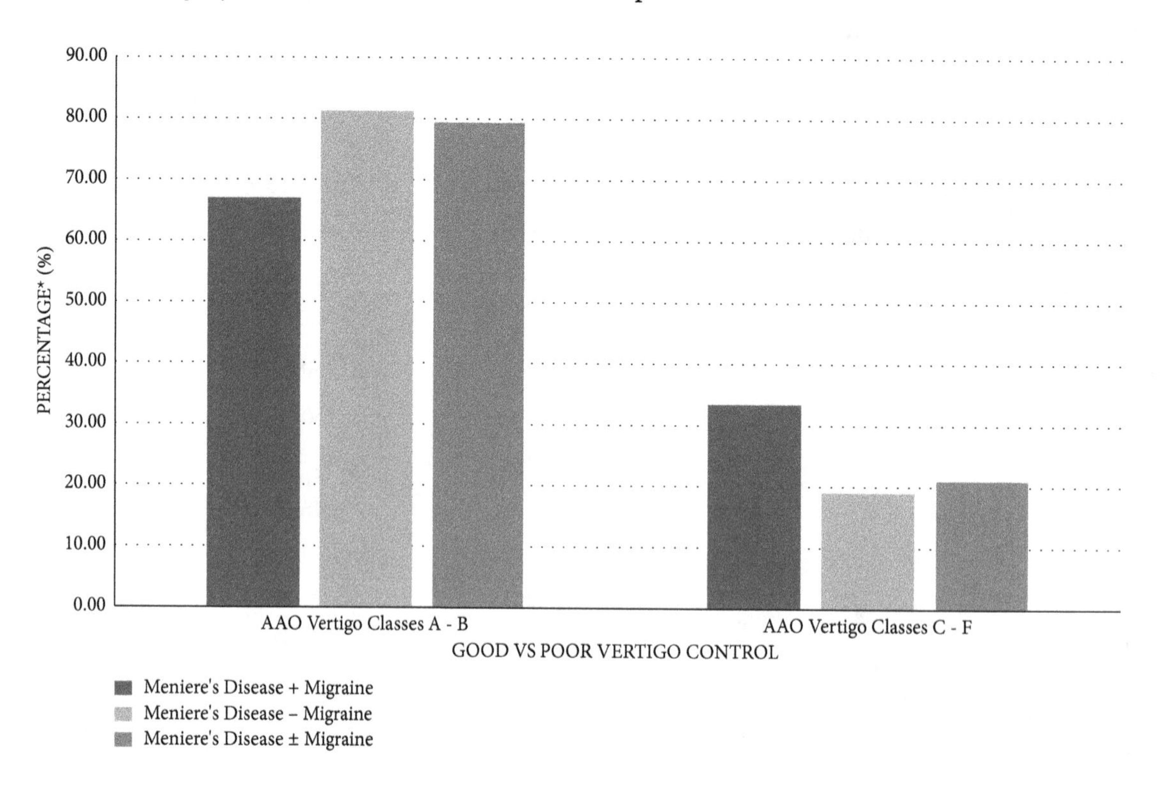

Figure 2: Vertigo control following endolymphatic sac surgery. Good control was defined as AAO classes A-B. Poor control was defined as AAO classes C–F. *Based on specific population sizes for each respective patient category. See Tables 2 and 3 for numerical representation of results.

Migraine is a common comorbidity with Meniere's disease and may confound the decision to pursue ESS. Yet, there are no studies of exploring the effect of comorbid migraine on ESS. Our study demonstrated that 66.67% of MD + M patients had classes A-B control, which is similar to MD – M patients (Table 3, Figure 2) and the aforementioned studies on ESS. Moreover, postoperative FLS scores did not show any statistically significant difference between the two groups ($p = 0.09$). These findings partially agree with a recent study by Liu et al. that demonstrated similar rates of vertigo control but with a trend of poorer FLS scores in MD + M than in MD – M patients following intratympanic gentamicin injection [28]. Therefore, MD + M patients can be treated with similar confidence as their MD – M counterpart when considering ESS for intractable vertigo.

Lastly, our MD + M patients had a shorter duration of major vertigo episodes than MD – M (Table 3). Our study is the first to report this interesting finding. Whether this finding represents a true observation or a Type I falsepositive error is unclear given our small and unequal patient population.

Our study had several limitations. It was a retrospective review conducted at a single institution. Over one-third of our initial patient population was excluded from postoperative analysis due to inadequate records. Unfortunately, regular follow-up is often difficult for many of our patients who reside in rural parts of the state and travel a long distance to receive care at our tertiary care center. There was also no control group to account for the natural history of Meniere's disease compared to effect of the intervention.

Another significant limitation was the small patient population. ESS is not a high-volume surgery, so obtaining a large patient population at a single institution is a difficult and common limitation of similar studies. Moreover, the number of migraine patients may be underreported given that the prevalence (18.42%) was similar to the general population, which would be less than expected in patients with Meniere's disease [11, 19].

In our study, migraine is referred to as any form or variant of migraine without a distinction for vestibular migraine. Vestibular migraine is an evolving diagnosis based on a history of migraine and vestibular symptoms, which did not have a consensus definition until 2012 and may occur concurrently with Meniere's disease [2, 15, 17]. If treated today, a subset of our patients may have been also diagnosed with vestibular migraine given that our patients spanned from 1987 to 2019. Hence, migraine treatment was not recorded or mentioned in documentation nor was it recommended by the neurotologist at the time for most of these patients. Ideally, vestibular migraine would have been screened for and treated prior to consideration of ESS, which could be addressed in future studies now that the 2020 Meniere's Disease Guideline recommend screening for it. Nonetheless, we are the first study to account for the migraine comorbidity in Meniere's disease patients undergoing ESS. Further studies are needed to investigate and elaborate on the differences and similarities we observed between the two groups.

Conclusion

In conclusion, Meniere's disease has a profound impact on patients due to severe vertigo and functional impairment. Migraine is a common comorbidity in those with Meniere's disease. MD + M patients are associated with more psychiatric comorbidities and younger age at the time of ESS than MD – M patients. Nonetheless, ESS appears to have a similarly high efficacy in Meniere's disease with and without migraine.

References

[1] J. P. Harris and T. H. Alexander, "Current-day prevalence of Meniere's syndrome," *Audiology and Neurotology*, vol. 15, no. 5, pp. 318–322, 2010.

[2] G. J. Basura, M. E. Adams, A. Monfared et al., "Clinical practice guideline: Meniere's disease," *Otolaryngology-Head and Neck Surgery*, vol. 162, no. 2_suppl, pp. S1–S55, 2020.

[3] L. Frejo, E. Martin-Sanz, R. Teggi et al., "Extended phenotype and clinical subgroups in unilateral Meniere disease: a crosssectional study with cluster analysis," *Clinical Otolaryngology*, vol. 42, no. 6, pp. 1172–1180, 2017.

[4] L. Frejo, A. Soto-Varela, S. Santos-Perez et al., "Clinical subgroups in bilateral Meniere disease," *Frontiers in Neurology*, vol. 7, p. 182, 2016.

[5] "Committee on hearing and equilibrium guidelines for the diagnosis and evaluation of therapy in Meniere's disease," *Otolaryngology-Head and Neck Surgery*, vol. 113, pp. 181–185, 1995.

[6] K. B. Teufert and J. Doherty, "Endolymphatic sac shunt, labyrinthectomy, and vestibular nerve section in Meniere's disease," *Otolaryngologic Clinics of North America*, vol. 43, no. 5, pp. 1091–1111, 2010.

[7] S. J. Wetmore, "Endolymphatic sac surgery for Meniere's disease," *Archives of Otolaryngology-Head and Neck Surgery*, vol. 134, no. 11, pp. 1144–1148, 2008.

[8] R. F. Bento, J. C. Cisneros, and A. C. De Oliveira Fonseca, "Endolymphatic sac drainage for the treatment of Me´nie`re's disease," *Journal of Laryngology & Otology*, vol. 131, no. 2, pp. 144–149, 2017.

[9] A. Hu and L. S. Parnes, "10-year review of endolymphatic sac surgery for intractable Meniere disease," *Journal of Otolaryngology-Head & Neck Surgery*, vol. 39, pp. 415–421, 2010.

[10] R. Burch, P. Rizzoli, and E. Loder, "The prevalence and impact of migraine and severe headache in the United States: figures and trends from government health studies," *Headache: The Journal of Head and Face Pain*, vol. 58, no. 4, pp. 496–505, 2018.

[11] A. Radtke, T. Lempert, M. A. Gresty, G. B. Brookes, M. Bronstein, and H. Neuhauser, "Migraine and Meniere's disease: is there a link?" *Neurology*, vol. 59, no. 11, pp. 1700–1704, 2002.

[12] R. Teggi, R. A. Battista, F. Di Berardino et al., "Evaluation of a large cohort of adult patients with Me´nie`re's disease: bedside and clinical history," *Acta Otorhinolaryngologica Italica*, vol. 40, no. 6, pp. 444–449, 2020.

[13] Y. F. Liu and H. Xu, "The intimate relationship between vestibular migraine and Meniere disease: a review of pathogenesis and presentation," *Behavioural Neurology*, vol. 2016, Article ID 3182735, 8 pages, 2016.

[14] A. Van Ombergen, V. Van Rompaey, P. Van de Heyning, and F. Wuyts, "Vestibular migraine in an Otolaryngology clinic," *Otology & Neurotology*, vol. 36, no. 1, pp. 133–138, 2015.

[15] T. Lempert, J. Olesen, J. Furman et al., "Vestibular migraine: diagnostic criteria," *Journal of Vestibular Research*, vol. 22, no. 4, pp. 167–172, 2012.

[16] R. Teggi, B. Colombo, R. Albera et al., "Clinical features, familial history, and migraine precursors in patients with definite vestibular migraine: the VM-phenotypes projects," *Headache: The Journal of Head and Face Pain*, vol. 58, no. 4, pp. 534–544, 2018.

[17] Y. Ghavami, H. Mahboubi, A. Y. Yau, M. Maducdoc, and H. R. Djalilian, "Migraine features in patients with Meniere's disease," *The Laryngoscope*, vol. 126, no. 1, pp. 163–168, 2016.

[18] R. Teggi, B. Colombo, L. Zagato, and M. Filippi, "Could ionic regulation disorders explain the overlap between Meniere's disease and migraine?" *Journal of Vestibular Research*, vol. 31, no. 4, pp. 297–301, 2021.

[19] R. C. Burch, D. C. Buse, and R. B. Lipton, "Migraine," *Neurologic Clinics*, vol. 37, no. 4, pp. 631–649, 2019.

[20] A. Eckhardt-Henn, C. Best, S. Bense et al., "Psychiatric comorbidity in different organic vertigo syndromes," *Journal of Neurology*, vol. 255, no. 3, pp. 420–428, 2008.

[21] C. Lahmann, P. Henningsen, T. Brandt et al., "Psychiatric comorbidity and psychosocial impairment among patients with vertigo and dizziness," *Journal of Neurology, Neurosurgery & Psychiatry*, vol. 86, no. 3, pp. 302–308, 2015.

[22] X. H. Hu, L. E. Markson, R. B. Lipton, W. F. Stewart, and M. L. Berger, "Burden of migraine in the United States," *Archives of Internal Medicine*, vol. 159, no. 8, pp. 813–818, 1999.

[23] T. Kitahara, A. Horii, T. Imai et al., "Effects of endolymphatic sac decompression surgery on vertigo and hearing in patients with bilateral Me´nie`re's disease," *Otology & Neurotology*, vol. 35, no. 10, pp. 1852–1857, 2014.

[24] M. J. Derebery, L. M. Fisher, K. Berliner, J. Chung, and K. Green, "Outcomes of endolymphatic shunt surgery for Me´nie`re's disease," *Otology & Neurotology*, vol. 31, no. 4, pp. 649–655, 2010.

[25] A. W. Gibson, I. J. Moon, J. S. Golub, and J. T. Rubinstein, "A comparison of endolymphatic shunt surgery and intratympanic gentamicin for Meniere's disease," *The Laryngoscope*, vol. 130, no. 10, pp. 2455–2460, 2020.

[26] G. M. Brinson, D. A. Chen, and M. A. Arriaga, "Endolymphatic mastoid shunt versus endolymphatic sac decompression for Me´nie`re's disease," *Otolaryngology-Head and Neck Surgery*, vol. 136, no. 3, pp. 415–421, 2007.

[27] V. Ostrowski and J. M. Kartush, "Endolymphatic sac-vein decompression for intractable Meniere's disease: long term treatment results," *Otolaryngology-Head and Neck Surgery*, vol. 128, no. 4, pp. 550–559, 2003.

[28] Y. F. Liu, E. Renk, S. D. Rauch, and H. X. Xu, "Efficacy of intratympanic gentamicin in Meni`ere's disease with and without migraine," *Otology & Neurotology*, vol. 38, no. 7, pp. 1005–1009, 2017.

10

Concomitant Obstructive Sleep Apnoea in Patients with Meniere's Disease

Wong Kein Low[1,2] and Esther Jiayi Lim[1]

[1]Novena Ent-Head & Neck Surgery Specialist Centre, 04-21/22/34, Mount Elizabeth Novena Medical Centre, 38 Irrawaddy Road, Singapore

[2]Duke-NUS Graduate Medical School, 8 College Road, Singapore

Correspondence should be addressed to Wong Kein Low; low.wong.kein@gmail.com

Academic Editor: Augusto Casani

ABSTRACT

Meniere's disease (MD) is a condition characterised by fluctuating and progressive hearing loss, aural fullness, tinnitus, and intermittent attacks of vertigo. The disabling vertigo symptoms can be controlled in most patients by lifestyle changes and medications such as diuretics. Should standard medical therapy fail, the patient may require surgery in order to control the disease, but such surgical procedures can be functionally destructive. Obstructive sleep apnoea syndrome (OSAS) is common, especially in people who are grossly overweight. Up to 15% of patients with MD may have concomitant OSA. Unless the OSA is well controlled, such patients may continue to experience MD symptoms despite receiving adequate standard medical therapy for MD. Moreover, MD patients may experience insomnia as a result of vertigo and/or tinnitus where sedatives are indicated. The use of sedatives with muscle relaxant properties may inadvertently further aggravate OSA resulting in a vicious cycle of symptoms. Symptoms suggestive of concomitant OSA must be proactively sought as these patients do not necessarily exhibit the obvious phenotypic features of OSA. This is especially so in Asians where OSAS is commonly observed in people who are not overly obese. We report a case of a female patient who presented with recalcitrant MD disease and was later found to have concomitant OSA. The relevant literature will be reviewed, and learning points will be discussed from the perspective of the otologist/neurotologist. The clinician must always be mindful of the existence of concomitant "silent" OSAS as this impacts the management of patients with MD.

INTRODUCTION

Meniere's disease (MD) is a condition characterised by fluctuating and progressive hearing loss, aural fullness, tinnitus, and intermittent attacks of vertigo. Although the aetiology of MD is largely unknown, the pathology is the result of hydropic distension of the endolymphatic system [1]. Various factors such as stress are known to trigger or contribute to MD [2, 3]. Obstructive sleep apnoea syndrome (OSAS) is a sleep-related breathing disorder where episodes of apnoea/ hypopnea occur during sleep due to a collapse of the upper airway. The direct consequences of the collapse are intermittent hypoxia and hypercapnia, recurrent arousals, and increase in respiratory efforts, leading to secondary sympathetic activation, oxidative stress, and systemic inflammation [4]. The cardiovascular complications of OSA are well documented [5], but the neurotological consequences have only been studied recently [6]. A mainstay of treatment for OSA is continuous positive airway pressure (CPAP), which corrects the hypoxia and associated body stresses.

In recent years, there have been some reports linking MD and OSA [6–10]. Up to 15% of patients with MD have been found to have concomitant OSAS [11]. It is important to identify this subset of patients because unless the OSA is well controlled, such patients may continue to experience MD symptoms despite receiving adequate standard medical treatment for MD. Moreover, MD patients may experience insomnia from the vertigo and/or tinnitus where sedatives are indicated. The use of sedatives with muscle relaxant properties may inadvertently further aggravate OSAS resulting in a vicious cycle of symptoms. It is noteworthy that identification of OSAS in patients with MD may not be forthcoming as these patients do not necessarily exhibit obvious phenotypic features such as gross obesity that characterise OSAS. This is, especially so in Asians [6].

We report a case to illustrate the relationship between MD and OSA and highlight some of the challenges encountered. Th relevant literature will be reviewed and discussed from the perspective of the otologist/neurotologist.

Case Report

A 53-year-old Chinese female was first seen by us in September 2016 with an 18-month history of recurrent episodes of vertigo associated with nausea and vomiting. Each of these vertiginous episodes typically lasted for 7-8 hours and appeared to be aggravated by stress. She also experienced fluctuating tinnitus, hearing loss, and aural fullness in the right ear. She had a history of rhinitis.

She also complained of headaches which were usually located at the back or the top of the head. Often occurring after sleep, they were described as dull in nature and not pulsatile. The headaches were mild to moderate in severity which did not interfere nor prohibit daily activities. They might be aggravated by stress but not by physical activities. She did not have photophobia, phonophobia, nor visual auras. The fluctuating aural symptoms (but not the headaches) occurred around the time of the vertiginous episodes.

The patient was anxious about her symptoms which were affecting her quality of life and work. She had difficulty sleeping, which she attributed to her MD symptoms. It was noteworthy that she did not offer at presentation a history of snoring, apneic episodes during sleep, or any history suggestive of OSAS.

With a body weight of 57 kg and a height of 157 cm, her body mass index (BMI) was 23.1 kg/m^2. She did not have any craniofacial features to suggest OSAS. Neurootological assessment was unremarkable. Audiogram showed sensorineural hearing loss in the right ear, especially in the lower frequencies (Figure 1). MRI scan of the brain was normal.

Based on the amended diagnostic criteria (2015) for MD by the American Academy of Otolaryngology-Head and Neck Surgery (AAO-HNS), a clinical diagnosis of MD was made [12]. This was further substantiated by audiometric documentation of fluctuating low-to-midfrequency hearing levels at different time points (Figure 1).

Lifestyle changes such as a low-sodium and low-caffeine diet were advised. A course of Apotriazide was prescribed for each episode of attacks with betahistine being used as maintenance. However, she continued to have recurrent vertiginous attacks and fluctuating right aural symptoms. She still experienced difficulty sleeping and was referred to a psychiatrist who prescribed clonazepam and Valdoxan. Th family sought a second opinion from an ear specialist in the USA who concurred with the diagnosis of MD.

After almost 1 year of standard medical therapy, her MD was still not adequately controlled with recurring bouts of vertigo. The patient had a supportive spouse who was keen to exclude any comorbidity that could have contributed to the disease. Having observed her sleeping patterns, he suspected that she might have OSAS. A sleep study was done in September 2017 which confirmed severe sleep apnoea with an apnoea-hypopnea index (AHI) of 35.6 events per hour. The results of the study suggested that the sleep apnoea was obstructive and not central in origin. Upon direct questioning, she admitted to having regular snoring with apneic episodes during sleep. Nasopharyngoscopy showed narrowing of the hypopharyngeal space. Hypertrophic inferior turbinates and deviated nasal septum were also observed. The tonsils were, however, not enlarged.

Upon diagnosis of OSA, she was started on continuous positive airway pressure (CPAP). Since then, she had complete resolution of vertigo as well as headaches over a followup period of 28 months. She had continued with betahistine (but not Apotriazide) as maintenance for about 15 months after starting CPAP and used only CPAP thereafter.

Discussion

The diagnosis of MD is a clinical one. The AAO-HNS issued a set of amended diagnostic criteria for MD in 2015 (Table 1), which were formulated together with the Classification Committee of the Barany Society, the Japan Society for Equilibrium Research, the European Academy of Otology and Neurotology, and the Korean Balance Society [12]. As shown in Table 1, our patient possessed the clinical features that defined definite MD. Our patient also had audiometric documentation of fluctuating hearing levels involving mainly the lowto midfrequencies which further supported the diagnosis of MD (Figure 1).

Episodes of vertigo developing in a patient with headaches raise the possibility of vestibular migraine as the cause. Table 2 outlines the diagnostic criteria of vestibular migraine issued by the Barany Society and the International Headache Society [13]. Based on this set of criteria, our patient clearly did not have vestibular migraine (Table 2). Instead, the headaches experienced by our patient were more likely a result of her OSA [14]. This was substantiated by the fact that her headaches completely resolved after CPAP treatment.

The prevalence of MD has been reported to be between 12 and 46 per 100,000, with a geographical variation [7]. The otologist/neurotologist routinely manages MD patients, and standard medical therapy includes lifestyle changes such as dietary salt restriction and medications such as diuretics, migraine prophylaxis, and steroid therapy [15]. Should adequate standard medical therapy fail to control frequent disabling vertigo, more effective but potentially functionally destructive treatment modalities such as gentamicin ablation, vestibular neurectomy, and labyrinthectomy may be indicated [1]. Such procedures will result in total loss of vestibular function in the operated ear, and if the opposite ear is subsequently affected by MD, the patient may end up with significant loss of vestibular function in both ears which can be functionally disabling. This is because the vestibular function in an ear affected by MD can possibly be lost as a result of the disease itself. In this respect, it is important to note that MD not uncommonly affects both ears over time. In one study, 14% of patients with unilateral MD became bilateral over an average follow-up period of 7.6 years (SD = 7.0 years) [16]. Hence, any comorbidity, which if treated can lead to better outcomes with conservative treatment, should be identified and managed. As illustrated by the present case report, concomitant OSA is potentially such a comorbidity that has often been underappreciated.

The prevalence of clinically significant OSAS in the general adult population has been reported to be at least 8.5% [7]. In a longitudinal study, the association between MD and OSA patients was studied based on a nationwide 9year longitudinal cohort database of 1,025,340 South Korean patients [9]. In this study, no overall association between OSA and MD was observed. However, in a subgroup analysis, female and middle-aged (45–64 years) patients with OSAS were independently associated with a two-fold higher incidence of subsequent MD compared to those without

OSA. These findings are consistent with the profile of our patient in the present case report. Among patients with MD, the prevalence of concomitant OSA has been reported to be up to 15% [11].

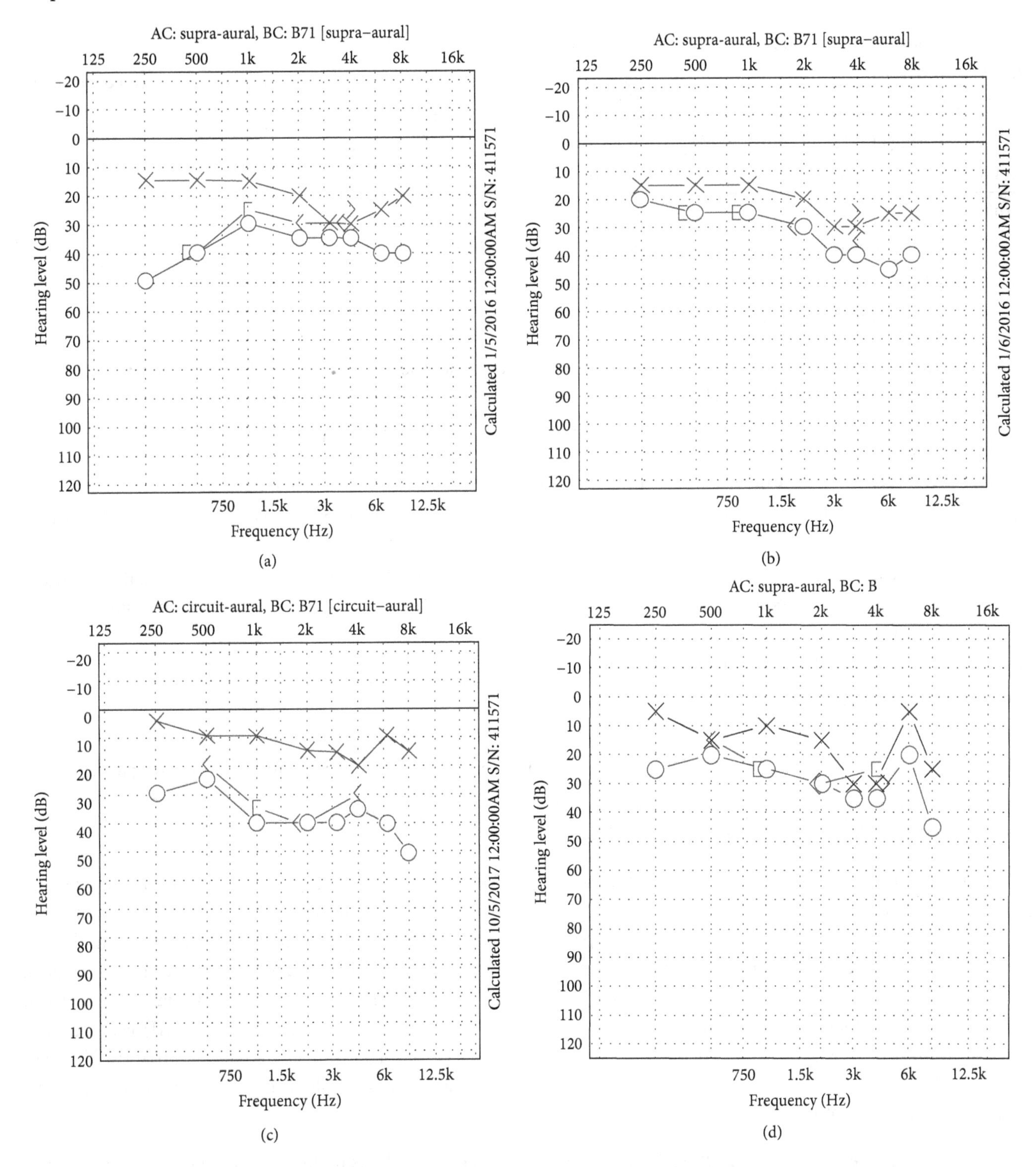

Figure 1: Fluctuating hearing levels affecting mainly the lowto midfrequencies in the right ear which corresponded to the fluctuating aural symptoms in the same ear. Audiogram done during the initial episode (a), after treatment with medications (b), during a subsequent episode (c), and after treatment with CPAP (d).

Table 1: AAO-HNS-amended (2015) diagnostic criteria for Meniere's disease.

Definite
(i)Two or more spontaneous episodes of vertigo, each lasting 20 min to 12 h
(ii) Audiometrically documented lowto midfrequency sensorineural hearing loss in 1 ear, defining the affected ear on at least 1 occasion before, during, or after 1 of the episodes of vertigo
(iii) Fluctuating aural symptoms (hearing, tinnitus, or fullness) in the affected ear
(iv) Not better accounted for by another vestibular diagnosis
Probable
(i) Two or more episodes of vertigo or dizziness, each lasting 20 min to 24 h
(ii) Fluctuating aural symptoms (hearing, tinnitus, or fullness) in the affected ear
(iii) Not better accounted for by another vestibular diagnosis

Table 2: Diagnostic criteria for vestibular migraine proposed by the Barany Society and the third International Classification of Headache Disorders (ICHD-3), 2012.

Vestibular migraine
(i) At least five episodes with vestibular symptoms of moderate[a] or severe[b] intensity, lasting 5 min to 72 h
(ii) Current or previous history of migraine with or without aura according to the International Classification of Headache Disorders (ICHD)
(iii) One or more migraine features with at least 50% of the vestibular episodes: (i) headache with at least two of the following characteristics: one-sided location, pulsating quality, moderate[a] or severe[b] pain intensity, and aggravation of routine physical activity; (ii) photophobia and phonophobia; (iii) visual aura
(iv) Not better accounted for by another vestibular or ICHD diagnosis
Probable vestibular migraine
(i) At least five episodes with vestibular symptoms of moderate or severe intensity, lasting 5 min to 72 h
(ii) Only one of criteria B and C for vestibular migraine is fulfilled (migraine history or migraine features during the episode)
(iii) Not better accounted for by another vestibular or ICHD diagnosis

[a]Usually interfere with daily activities. [b]Usually prohibit daily activities.

The patient in this case report, who is Chinese with a BMI of 23.1 kg/sq m, highlighted an important learning point. Concomitant OSAS in MD patients is not necessarily obvious to the clinician and can be easily missed. Nakayama and Kabaya also reported 2 patients who did not present with symptoms suggestive of sleep disturbances until when asked [6]. The 2 patients had moderate OSA but were not excessively overweight. Racial differences in craniofacial structures exist, and Asians may suffer from significant OSAS with lower weight gains as compared to Western patients [17–19]. In a larger series of 20 Asian patients with MD and OSAS, the body mass index (BMI) was found to range from 20.7 to 28.5 with an average of only 23.5 kg/sq m [7]. In a case report, Pisani et al. reiterated that the clinician must be mindful of the coexistence of "silent" OSAS among MD patients, especially those who were not responsive to standard medical treatment [8].

Th importance of identifying OSAS in MD patients is twofold. Firstly, as highlighted by Nakayama and Kabaya, failure to identify OSA can result in the use of medications than can adversely affect the outcomes [6]. MD patients are often prescribed sedatives such as benzodiazepines to relieve anxiety and insomnia. Th use of such sedatives which have muscle relaxant properties may inadvertently further aggravate OSA resulting in a vicious cycle of symptoms. Th could have been the case for our patient in this case report.

Secondly, it may not be possible to medically control the symptoms of MD unless the comorbidity of OSA is addressed. OSA is a source of body stress and can be a potent aggravating factor of the symptoms of MD. As illustrated by our patient, the symptoms of MD were eventually controlled by effective treatment of OSA using CPAP [6, 7, 10].

The pathophysiology linking OSA to MD remains controversial. Several reports have suggested that vascular occlusion played an important role in MD. In a transcranial Doppler sonographic study, compromise of the vertebrobasilar vascular circulation was found in 28% of MD patients [20]. Histologic studies of patients with MD revealed total or partial obstruction of small vessels around the endolymphatic sac [21]. This was substantiated by the observation that cochlear blood flow was impaired in experimentally induced endolymphatic hydrops in guinea pigs [22]. In fact, the cornerstone of the treatment protocol for MD patients at the University of Colorado was identification and control of disorders that impair cerebral and inner ear vascular perfusion [15].

Vascular occlusion is also closely associated with OSA. Night-time hypoxaemia from sleep apnoea can result in sympathetic overactivity during waking hours, endothelial damage, platelet aggregation, and chronic systemic and pulmonary hypertension [5]. Migraine, perhaps through the mechanism of ischaemia from vasospasm, frequently occurred in OSA particularly in the younger patients [15]. As hypertension and migraine are themselves risk factors for cerebrovascular and cardiovascular diseases, sleep apnoea is both a primary vascular risk factor and a secondary risk factor through these allied conditions [10].

Intermittent hypoxia itself could also contribute to the cardiometabolic consequences of OSA. Th molecular pathways and cellular interactions involved were recently studied by Arnaud et al. [23]. Th authors found that intermittent hypoxia resulted in sympathetic activation, low-grade inflammation, oxidative stress, and endoplasmic reticulum stress with the hypoxia-inducible factor-1 transcription factor and mitochondrial functional changes playing a role.

Oxidative stress could result in a breakdown of the blood-labyrinthine barrier, and the blood-labyrinthine barrier is critical in the maintenance of inner ear homeostasis [24]. Kim et al. believed that vascular occlusion and intermittent hypoxic events in OSA led to enhanced oxidative stress in the inner ear which could result in MD [9]. The symptoms of MD in such patients could then be possibly treated by CPAP which improves oxygenation to the inner ear leading to a reduction in hydropic distention of the endolymphatic system [7].

Besides MD, there have been some reports on other neurotological consequences of OSAS. Vestibular function had been demonstrated to be impaired in patients with OSAS [25, 26]. In 2010, Sowerby et al. first described a possible link between idiopathic dizziness, daytime somnolence, and sleep apnoea [27]. Kim et al. reiterated that sleep disturbance should be considered in patients with chronic subjective or nonspecific dizziness [28]. More recently, Foster and Machala reported that some OSA patients exhibited brief spells of nonpositional vertigo recurring throughout the day which responded to CPAP treatment [10]. OSAS has also been linked to sudden sensorineural hearing loss [29, 30]. However, in a large Korean study over 9 years, an association between OSAS and sudden sensorineural hearing loss could not be demonstrated [9].

Conclusion

The otologist/neurotologist must be mindful that some patients with MD may have concomitant OSA. Unless this comorbidity is treated, it may not be possible to control the symptoms of MD with standard medical therapies. Identification and successful treatment of OSA could potentially avoid the need for functionally destructive MD surgeries which are normally reserved for patients with uncontrolled disease. Symptoms suggestive of OSA must be proactively sought as these patients may not exhibit obvious phenotypic features of OSAS, especially in Asians.

Acknowledgments

The authors acknowledge the contributions of Mr. John Yanko Hevera for highlighting the link between Meniere's disease and obstructive sleep apnoea.

References

[1] T. Nakashima, I. Pyykko¨, M. A. Arroll et al., "Meniere's disease," *Nature Reviews Disease Primers*, vol. 2, pp. 1–8, 2016.

[2] A.-C. H. So¨derman, J. Mo¨ller, D. Bagger-Sjo¨ba¨ck, J. Bergenius, and J. Hallqvist, "Stress as a trigger of attacks in menie`re's disease. A case-crossover study," *The Laryngoscope*, vol. 114, no. 10, pp. 1843–1848, 2004.

[3] N. L. Yeo, M. P. White, N. Ronan, D. J. Whinney, A. Curnow, and J. Tyrrell, "Stress and unusual events exacerbate symptoms in menie`re's disease: a longitudinal study," *Otology & Neurotology*, vol. 39, no. 1, pp. 73–81, 2018.

[4] P. Le´vy, M. Kohler, W. T. McNicholas et al., "Obstructive sleep apnoea syndrome," *Nature Reviews Disease Primers*, vol. 1, pp. 1–21, 2015.

[5] B. K. Dredla and P. R. Castillo, "Cardiovascular consequences of obstructive sleep apnea," *Current Cardiology Reports*, vol. 21, p. 137, 2019.

[6] M. Nakayama and K. Kabaya, "Obstructive sleep apnea syndrome as a novel cause for Meniere's disease," *Current Opinion in Otolaryngology & Head and Neck Surgery*, vol. 21, no. 5, pp. 503–508, 2013.

[7] M. Nakayama, A. Masuda, K. B. Ando et al., "A pilot study on the efficacy of continuous positive Airway pressure on the manifestations of me´ni`ere's disease in patients with concomitant obstructive sleep apnea syndrome," *Journal of Clinical Sleep Medicine*, vol. 11, no. 10, pp. 1101–1107, 2015.

[8] L. R. Pisani, A. Naro, F. Caminiti, S. De Salvo, P. Bramanti, and S. Marino, "Obstructive sleep apnea syndrome with Me´nie`re's disease: a misdiagnosed case," *Sleep Medicine*, vol. 32, p. 284, 2017.

[9] J.-Y. Kim, I. Ko, B.-J. Cho, and D.-K. Kim, "Association of obstructive sleep apnea with the risk of me´ni`ere's disease and sudden sensorineural hearing loss: a study using data from the Korean national health insurance service," *Journal of Clinical Sleep Medicine*, vol. 15, no. 9, pp. 1293–1301, 2019.

[10] C. A. Foster and M. Machala, "The clinical spectrum of dizziness in sleep apnea," *Otology & Neurotology*, vol. 41, no. 10, pp. 1419–1422, 2020.

[11] M. Nakayama, M. Suzuki, A. Inagaki et al., "Impaired quality of sleep in me´nie`re's disease patients," *Journal of Clinical Sleep Medicine*, vol. 6, no. 5, pp. 445–449, 2010.

[12] J. A. Goebel, "2015 Equilibrium committee amendment to the 1995 AAO-HNS guidelines for the definition of me´nie`re's disease," *Otolaryngology-Head and Neck Surgery*, vol. 154, no. 3, pp. 403-404, 2016.

[13] T. Lempert, J. Olesen, J. Furman et al., "Vestibular migraine: diagnostic criteria," *Journal of Vestibular Research*, vol. 22, no. 4, pp. 167–172, 2012.

[14] K. C. Brennan and A. Charles, "Sleep and headache," *Seminars in Neurology*, vol. 29, no. 4, pp. 406–418, 2009.

[15] C. Foster, "Optimal management of Me´ni`ere's disease," *Therapeutics and Clinical Risk Management*, vol. 11, pp. 301–307, 2015.

[16] J. W. House, J. K. Doherty, L. M. Fisher, M. J. Derebery, and K. I. Berliner, "Meniere's disease: prevalence of contralateral ear involvement," *Otology & Neurotology*, vol. 27, no. 3, pp. 355–361, 2006.

[17] A. T. C. Villaneuva, P. R. Buchanan, B. J. Yee, and R. R. Grunstein, "Ethnicity and obstructive sleep apnoea," *Sleep Medicine Reviews*, vol. 9, no. 6, pp. 419–436, 2005.

[18] K. Ishiguro, T. Kobayashi, N. Kitamura, and C. Saito, "Relationship between severity of sleep-disordered breathing and craniofacial morphology in Japanese male patients," *Oral Surgery, Oral Medicine, Oral Pathology, Oral Radiology, and Endodontology*, vol. 107, no. 3, pp. 343–349, 2009.

[19] K. Sutherland, R. W. W. Lee, and P. A. Cistulli, "Obesity and craniofacial structure as risk factors for obstructive sleep apnoea: impact of ethnicity," *Respirology*, vol. 17, no. 2, pp. 213–222, 2012.

[20] D. Gortan, "Transcranial doppler sonography in patients with Menie´re's disease," *Acta Medica Croatica*, vol. 54, pp. 11–14, 2000.

[21] U. Friberg and H. Rask-Andersen, "Vascular occlusion in the endolymphatic sac in Meniere's disease," *Annals of Otology, Rhinology & Laryngology*, vol. 111, no. 3, pp. 237–245, 2002.

[22] Y. Yazawa, H. Kitano, M. Suzuki, H. Tanaka, and K. Kitajima, "Studies of cochlear blood flow in Guinea pigs with endolymphatic hydrops," *Okanagan Regional Library*, vol. 60, no. 1, pp. 4–11, 1998.

[23] C. Arnaud, T. Bochaton, J.-L. Pe´pin, and E. Belaidi, "Obstructive sleep apnoea and cardiovascular consequences: pathophysiological mechanisms," *Archives of Cardiovascular Diseases*, vol. 113, no. 5, pp. 350–358, 2020.

[24] G. Ishiyama, J. Wester, I. A. Lopez, L. Beltran-Parrazal, and A. Ishiyama, "Oxidative stress in the blood labyrinthine barrier in the macula utricle of meniere's disease patients," *Frontiers in Physiology*, vol. 9, p. 1068, 2018.

[25] S. Gallina, F. Dispenza, G. Kulamarva, F. Riggio, and R. Speciale, "Obstructive sleep apnoea syndrome (OSAS): effects on the vestibular system," *Acta otorhinolaryngologica Italica : organo ufficiale della Societa italiana di otorinolaringologia e chirurgia cervico-facciale*, vol. 30, no. 6, pp. 281– 284, 2010.

[26] S. Kayabasi, A. Iriz, M. Cayonu et al., "Vestibular functions were found to be impaired in patients with moderate-to-severe obstructive sleep apnea," *The Laryngoscope*, vol. 125, no. 5, pp. 1244–1248, 2015.

[27] L. J. Sowerby, B. Rotenberg, M. Brine, C. F. P. George, and L. S. Parnes, "Sleep apnea, daytime somnolence, and idiopathic dizziness-A novel association," *The Laryngoscope*, vol. 120, no. 6, pp. 1274–1278, 2010.

[28] S. K. Kim, J. H. Kim, S. S. Jeon, and S. M. Hong, "Relationship between sleep quality and dizziness," *PLoS One*, vol. 13, no. 3, Article ID e0192705, 2018.

[29] Y. Fischer, A. Yakinthou, and W. J. Mann, "Zur Prvalenz der obstruktiven Schlafapnoe (OSA) bei Patienten mit Hrsturz," *HNO*, vol. 51, no. 6, pp. 462–466, 2003.

[30] J.-J. Sheu, C. S. Wu, and H. C. Lin, "Association between obstructive sleep apnea and sudden sensorineural hearing Loss a population-based case-control study," *Archives of Otolaryngology-Head & Neck Surgery*, vol. 138, no. 1, pp. 55–59, 2012.

11

A Puzzle of Vestibular Physiology in a Meniere's Disease Acute Attack

Marta Martinez-Lopez, Raquel Manrique-Huarte, and Nicolas Perez-Fernandez

Department of Otorhinolaryngology, Clinica Universidad de Navarra, University of Navarra, Avenida P´ıo XII 36, 31008 Pamplona, Spain

Correspondence should be addressed to Nicolas Perez-Fernandez; nperezfer@unav.es

Academic Editor: Guangwei Zhou

ABSTRACT

The aim of this paper is to present for the first time the functional evaluation of each of the vestibular receptors in the six semicircular canals in a patient diagnosed with Meniere's disease during an acute attack. A 54-year-old lady was diagnosed with left Meniere's disease who during her regular clinic review suffers an acute attack of vertigo, with fullness and an increase of tinnitus in her left ear. Spontaneous nystagmus and the results in the video head-impulse test (vHIT) are shown before, during, and after the attack. Nystagmus was initially left beating and a few minutes later an upbeat component was added. No skew deviation was observed. A decrease in the gain of the vestibuloocular reflex (VOR) and the presence of overt saccades were observed when the stimuli were in the plane of the left superior semicircular canal. At the end of the crisis nystagmus decreased and vestibuloocular reflex returned to almost normal. A review of the different possibilities to explain these findings points to a hypothetical utricular damage.

INTRODUCTION

Meniere's disease (MD) crises are usually managed by patients at home or at a primary care facility. The characteristic features of the disease occur and usually hearing loss is best defined and sometimes audiometry is performed to confirm the deterioration in hearing loss.

Case reports of vestibular signs are infrequent because of the limited availability of equipment at emergency rooms. All of them provide interesting insight into the pathophysiology of the disorder by describing findings in terms of spontaneous and post-head-shake or vibration nystagmus, caloric test [1], and more recently head-impulse test (HIT) at bedside or assisted with video (vHIT) for the assessment of semicircular canal function [2] and vestibular evoked myogenic potentials (VEMP) for otolithic function [3].

We present a patient in whom an acute spell of vertigo has been seen while being at the hospital and in which the spontaneous nystagmus and the assessment of all 6 semicircular canals were possible.

Case Report

A 54-year-old woman was diagnosed with MD in her left ear. Vertigo spells begun 30 years ago, but after three years of activity the disease entered in a quiescent phase. In March 2013 vertigo recurred and since then has been unresponsive to medical treatment. When seen for the first time in July 2014, the number of typical vertigo spells in the 6 months previous was 12; also 4 additional ones were of the Tumarkin type, and her functional level score [4] was 4. PTA in the right ear was 5 dBHL and in her left ear 28 dBHL. CT scan and MRI were normal. After complete evaluation she was treated with intratympanic gentamicin ITG: August 5th and 11th and September 24th.

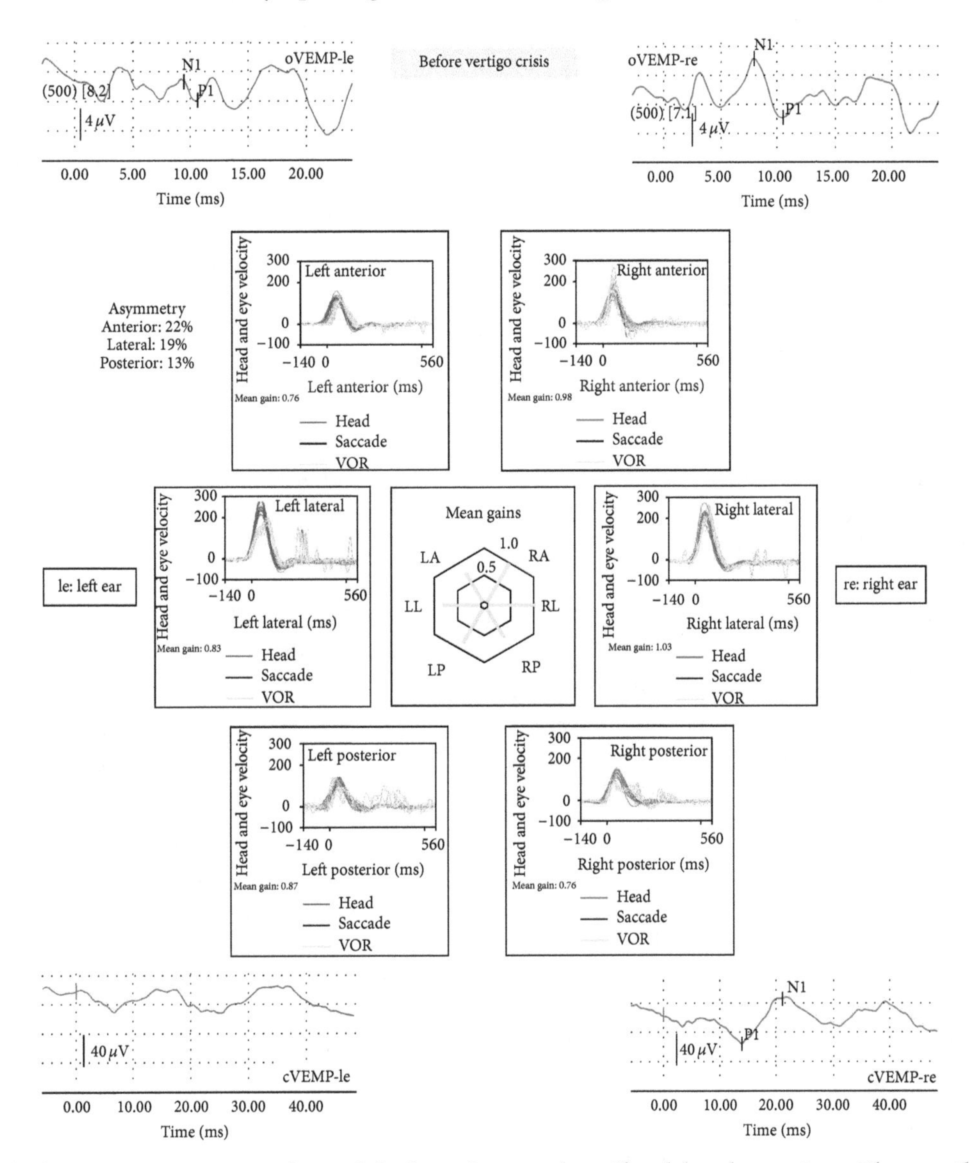

Figure 1: Vestibular examinations performed before the attack suff red by the patient. The vestibular myogenic evoked potentials for otolithic function, ocular (oVEMP) and cervical (cVEMP), are registered after bone vibration (500 Hz) with Bruel & Kjaer minishaker at the hairline (Fz); the response is abnormal on the left side/ear. The first component of the oVEMP (n10) is registered in the contralesional (right) eye that is very small or absent, whereas the n10 beneath the ipsilesional (left) eye is of normal amplitude. The sacculocollic cervical vestibular-evoked myogenic potential (cVEMP) is an uncrossed and predominantly sacculocollic response. The study of the vestibuloocular reflex with the video head-impulse test is normal except for the presence of reduced gain and overt saccades after left lateral semicircular canal stimulation.

It is interesting to mention that the external auditory canal is markedly anfractuous and the approach to the tympanic membrane is difficult; as such myringotomy was done in the anterior part of the inferior hemotympanum and a curved needle was used to deliver the gentamicin close to the round window niche. The treatment provided 1 month without any symptom and good equilibrium without increased hearing loss. Since then, vertigo spells have recurred scaling up in intensity and again one Tumarkin spell has occurred.

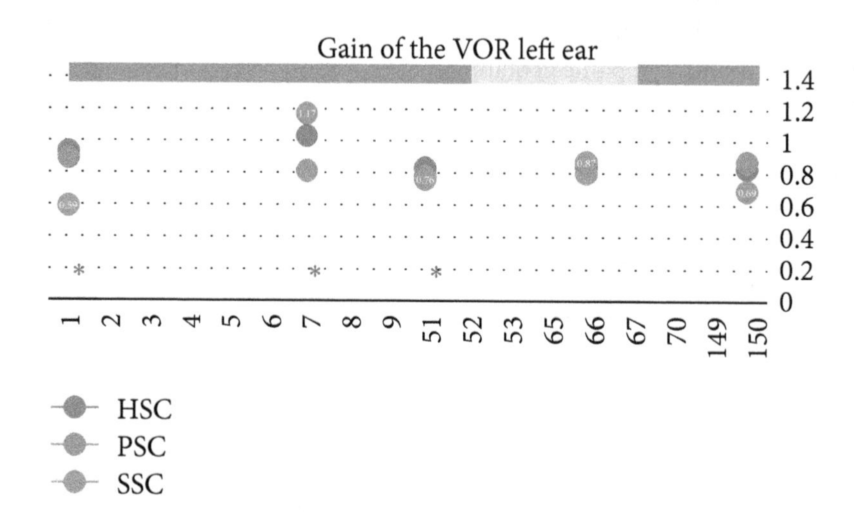

Figure 2: Gain of the vestibuloocular reflex in the left ear three semicircular canals at different follow-ups. Day 1 was the day of the first treatment with gentamicin intratympanically (that and the others are represented by ⁎). In light grey, the dates the patient felt steady and free of vertigo spells.

The date seen she was in good condition; last vertigo spell was 2 days before. Tympanic membrane had healed normally. There was no spontaneous nystagmus with or without visual fixation; neither gaze evoked nor post head-shake. The vHIT was normal in terms of gain of the vestibuloocular reflex (VOR), but overt saccades were clear for yaw-axis leftward head impulses as shown in Figure 1, suggesting a small reduction of VOR gain (changes in VOR at the different follows-up regarding the treatments are shown in Figure 2). Vestibular evoked myogenic potentials (VEMP) were performed with Fz 500 Hz vibration delivered with a Bruel & Kjaer minishaker. Results are shown to be normal for the right ear (both oVEMP and cVEMP) and abnormal for the left (both oVEMP and cVEMP) as shown in Figure 1. Hearing loss was mild to severe in her left ear (PTA was 48 dBHL).

After clinical and laboratory evaluation and when the patient was entering the office, she began to develop a vertigo spell and concurrently an intense tinnitus and pressure sensation in her left ar. At that timea left eating nystagmus with a mean slow phase velocity (mSPV) of 9.7°/s, and suppressed by visual fixation was seen under video-Frenzel glasses; 3 minutes latter a mild (mSPV = 4.3°/s) upbeat component was added (Figure 2). The nystagmus increased in leftward gaze and there was not skew deviation. In the vHIT there was an abnormal left superior VOR and this (leftanterior right-posterior) LARP plane of testing was repeated 3 times, in a period of 10 minutes, and was similar in all of them. The vertigo spell did not stop for 20 minutes and at that time was treated with sulpiride (100 mg I.M.). Three hours later the vertigo spell ended and the patient was able to return home; nystagmus was significantly reduced and vHIT returned to almost normal (precrisis) level (Figure 3).

Discussion

The situation that we present here is indicative of a complete, temporary dysfunction in the superior semicircular canal in the affected side and a unidirectional nystagmus beating ipsilaterally and upwards; in other words both horizontal and vertical components were present. These previously unreported findings while being in an acute vertigo spell in a patient with Meniere's disease deserve an explanation:

(1) While being in the vertigo crisis an acute deficit in the left superior canal was registered and confirmed not to be an artifact: the low gain was followed in each impulse by clear refixation saccades which had not been present during the earlier test in the quiescent phase.

(2) As the patient was seen in the very first minute of the crisis we can say that, in terms of nystagmus, this was unidirectional throughout the episode with a vertical component soon added and kept constant. In the case of unidirectional nystagmus most are paretic and very rarely irritative [3]. However the nystagmus in MD can change directions and the order of appearance heterogeneous. In general, an initial and brief period (<2 min) of irritative nystagmus is followed by a more prolonged period (20–30 min) during which nystagmus changes to paretic, being followed by a more prolonged period (days) of irritative nystagmus also called "recovery nystagmus." Different sequences can occur regarding the period of time the patient is seen. The origin for nystagmus has been claimed to be due to the irritative and paralytic action of potassium in the perilymph, respectively, for the first and second periods and to be due to a fast adapting response for the third one [5, 6]. Mechanical effects have been hypothesized to explain these findings too [7].

(3) Interestingly the spontaneous nystagmus has little effect on the assessment of both horizontal semicircular canals, either at the beginning or at the end of the crisis, probably because the SPV was so small relative to SPV of the VOR response.

(4) Regarding the treatment performed we can speculate that although some of the gentamicin could make its way to the inner ear the amount must be very small according to changes in the VOR in the different periods of time the patient was seen: the function from the horizontal and posterior semicircular canals in the left ear almost did not change, while that of the superior as mentioned above showed some fluctuations. This is also supported in the examination performed before the crisis: there were signs neither of the expected acute status nor of the compensated status after an appropriate damage to the left ear: spontaneous right beating nystagmus, biphasic post-head-shake nystagmus (first right and after left beating nystagmus).

The strong unidirectional nystagmus first raised the question of a deficit from the right side; however no difference to previous test was seen and during the crisis the patient mentioned neither symptoms pointing to a right side auditory deficit nor to pressure or tinnitus. Contrary to this an aggravation of pressure and tinnitus was attributed to her left ear. The finding of a reduction in right side posterior canal function (RP) is thought to occur due to the loss of concurrent inhibitory function from the left superior (LA) canal for head impulses in their plane. Alternatively an increase in the activity from the left horizontal canal could account for the right beating nystagmus; however as same as with the right side, no changes were seen form before to during the crisis for the function in this canal.

The need to focus on the superior canal is mainly due to the finding during the crisis but also is supported by a previous report that mentions marked fluctuations in activity for the canal function between the quiescent and acute attack states and in particular after gentamicin treatment [8]. In our patient in the different follow-ups in which vHIT was done, a fluctuation in the activity of the left superior canal function was registered. In the case of a deficient left superior semicircular canal the expected nystagmus should be a mixed vertical-torsional that from the examiner's point of view should be upward and counterclockwise with a small rightward component on VNG. However in our case only the vertical component fi s with this finding; the torsional component is very slow and the horizontal one is the contrary.

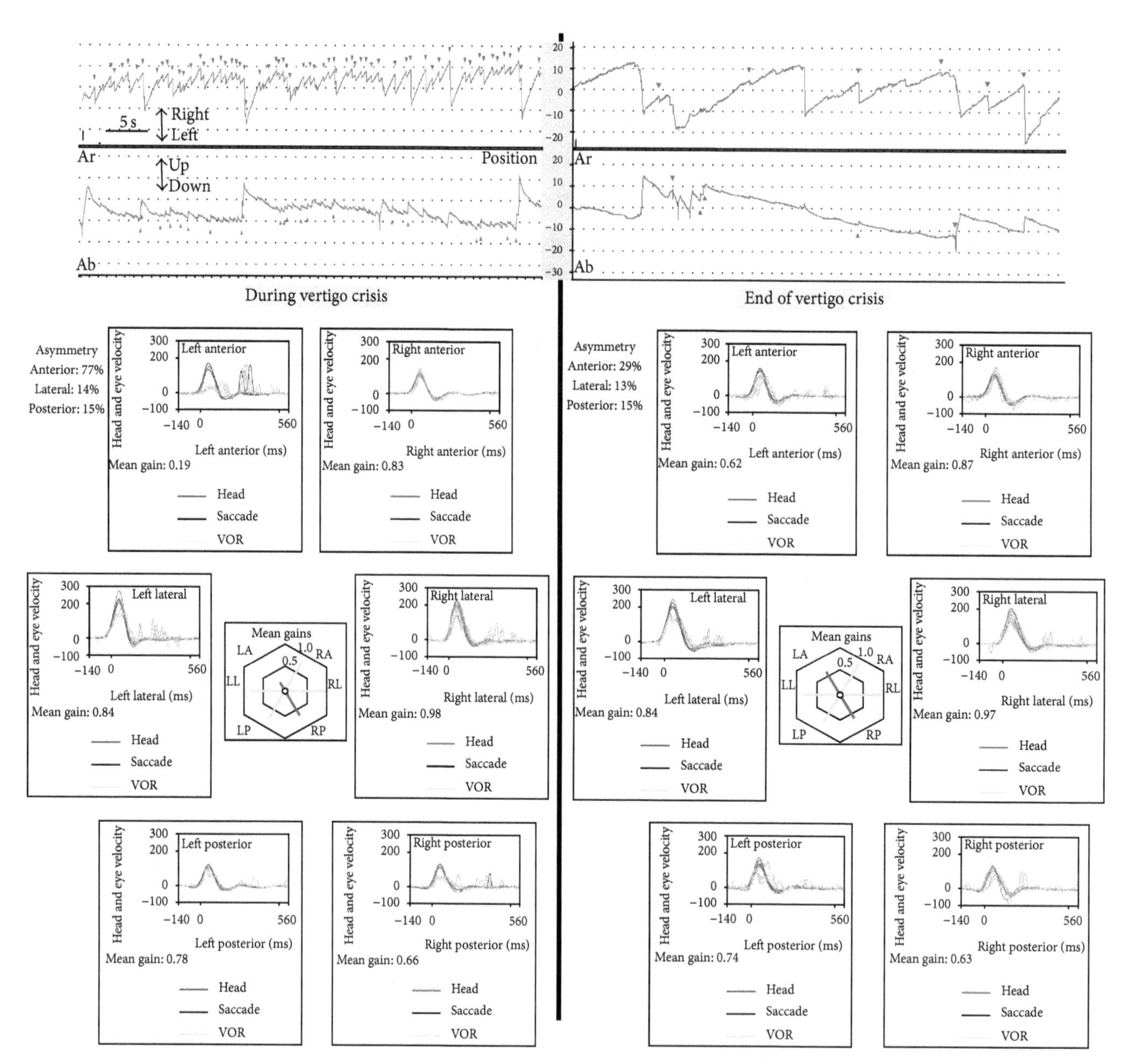

Figure 3: Spontaneous nystagmus and results of the video head-impulse test at the initiation of the crisis and at the end. Nystagmus is left beating with an upward component and there is a clear decrease in the gain of the vestibuloocular reflex in the plane of the left superior semicircular canal and right posterior canal (LARP) and the consequent presence of saccades. After the acute attack the same evaluation shows an increase of the gain and a significant decrease of the nystagmus.

A very similar pattern of nystagmus has been described in patients after surgery for superior semicircular canal dehiscence [9]. In all patients there is an abnormal HIT for impulses in the plane of the treated semicircular canal as expected for a surgery that prevents endolymph flow through that canal and abnormal pressure effects related to dilation of the canal and in 40% of the patients this combines also with a deficit in the posterior canal too; in these patients nystagmus, in the immediate postoperative period, was beating to the operated side. In the infrequent situation of a complete deficit for all the three semicircular canals nystagmus was typically paretic, beating to the nonoperated side [10]. For the situation in which an irritative nystagmus was found an exchange of potassium between endolymph and perilymph was proposed to occur through small leaks in the membranous canal.

This finding was also reported by others who also describe an acute event in a patient with Meniere-like symptoms but with superior semicircular canal dehiscence [11]. The pattern of the spontaneous nystagmus was similar as irritative both for the horizontal and torsional components. Concurrent with previous findings the authors presume an endolymphatic hydrops secondary to the action of prolapsing dura on membranous labyrinth through large canal dehiscences.

Another source of horizontal nystagmus has been shown to the utricle. Due to convergence of neural input from the otoliths onto horizontal canal neurons in the vestibular nuclei an ipsilesional nystagmus can occur in case of a deficit of the utricle [12]. In our case the previously done oVEMP both at the time of diagnosis (not shown) and at the day of last follow-up (Figure 1) is concurrent with a deficit from the ipsilateral utricle. However in the case of acute vertigo attacks in patients with Meniere's disease usually there is an enhancement of dynamic utricular function in the affected ear, contrary to what occurs in the case of Lermoyez crisis. We can speculate that this could have occurred in our patient and in particular because the modulation of nystagmus direction was very small when gaze was taken to right/left and up/down. Unfortunately her clinical situation was not good enough to proceed in more tests while being in the crisis.

As such, a combination of increased pressure in the left utricle (with concurrent amelioration of the n10 potential of the oVEMP, not found) generating a left beating nystagmus, transmitted to the superior semicircular canal with a concurrent utriculopetal displacement of the cupula (in the inhibitory direction) generating an upbeating nystagmus, could sum to generate the findings in our patient.

Acknowledgment

The authors wish to thank Professor Dr. I. Curthoys for his invaluable comments on the paper original form.

References

[1] H. Fushiki, M. Ishida, S. Sumi, A. Naruse, and Y. Watanabe, "Correlation between canal paresis and spontaneous nystagmus during early stage of acute peripheral vestibular disorders," *Acta Oto-Laryngologica*, vol. 130, no. 12, pp. 1352–1357, 2010.

[2] L. Manzari, H. G. MacDougall, A. M. Burgess, and I. S. Curthoys, "New, fast, clinical vestibular tests identify whether a vertigo attack is due to early Me´nie`re's disease or vestibular neuritis," *Laryngoscope*, vol. 123, no. 2, pp. 507–511, 2013.

[3] P. Du¨wel, L. E. Walther, J. Ilgner, and M. Westhofen, "Timedependent vestibular function loss of semicircular cannels and otolith organs in Menie`re's disease," *Laryngo-Rhino-Otologie*, vol. 84, no. 8, pp. 589–593, 2005.

[4] "Committee on Hearing and Equilibrium guidelines for the diagnosis and evaluation of therapy in Menie`re's disease," *Otolaryngology—Head and Neck Surgery*, vol. 113, no. 3, pp. 181– 185, 1995.

[5] T. K. Watanabe, "Nystagmus during an acute attack of Meniere's disese," *ENGReport*, pp. 1–3, 1996.

[6] J. A. McClure, J. C. Copp, and P. Lycett, "Recovery nystagmus in Meniere's disease," *Laryngoscope*, vol. 91, no. 10, pp. 1727–1737, 1981.

[7] J. Tonndorf, "Vestibular signs and symptoms in Meniere's disorder: mechanical considerations," *Acta Oto-Laryngologica*, vol. 95, no. 5-6, pp. 421–430, 1983.

[8] L. E. Walther, R. Huelse, K. Bla¨ttner, M. B. Bloching, and A. Blo¨dow, "Dynamic change of VOR and otolith function in intratympanic gentamicin treatment for Me´nie`re's disease: case report and review of the literature," *Case Reports in Otolaryngology*, vol. 2013, Article ID 168391, 5 pages, 2013.

[9] K. L. Janky, M. G. Zuniga, J. P. Carey, and M. Schubert, "Balance dysfunction and recovery after surgery for superior canal dehiscence syndrome," *Archives of Otolaryngology—Head and Neck Surgery*, vol. 138, no. 8, pp. 723–730, 2012.

[10] J. P. Carey, A. A. Migliaccio, and L. B. Minor, "Semicircular canal function before and after surgery for superior canal dehiscence," *Otology and Neurotology*, vol. 28, no. 3, pp. 356–364, 2007.

[11] C. Brandolini and G. C. Modugno, "Do signs of natural plugging of superior semicircular canal dehiscence exist?" *American Journal of Otolaryngology: Head and Neck Medicine and Surgery*, vol. 33, no. 2, pp. 268–271, 2012.

[12] L. Manzari, A. M. Burgess, and I. S. Curthoys, "Does unilateral utricular dysfunction cause horizontal spontaneous nystagmus?" *European Archives of Oto-Rhino-Laryngology*, vol. 269, no. 11, pp. 2441–2445, 2012.

12

Intratympanic Gentamicin Treatment for Ménière's Disease

Yongchuan Chai[1,2,3,4,5] and Hongzhe Li[1,2,6*]

[1]Research Service, VA Loma Linda Healthcare System, Loma Linda, CA, United States

[2]Loma Linda University School of Medicine, Loma Linda, CA, United States

[3]Department of Otorhinolaryngology—Head and Neck Surgery, Shanghai Ninth People's Hospital, Shanghai Jiao Tong University School of Medicine, Shanghai, China

[4]Ear Institute, Shanghai Jiao Tong University School of Medicine, Shanghai, China

[5]Shanghai Key Laboratory of Translational Medicine on Ear and Nose Diseases, Shanghai, China

[6]Department of Otolaryngology—Head and Neck Surgery, Loma Linda University School of Medicine, Loma Linda, CA, United States

*Address all correspondence to: hongzhe.li@va.gov; hongzhe@gmail.com

ABSTRACT

Ménière's disease (MD) is an inner-ear disease mostly characterized by frequent spontaneous vertigo and fluctuating sensorineural hearing loss. The main purpose of treatment for MD is to reduce or control the vertigo while maximizing the preservation of hearing. Among the various treatments, one that is effective for refractory MD, intratympanic gentamicin (ITG), relies on its ototoxic property to effectively control the vertigo symptoms of most patients. ITG treatment has relatively few side effects compared with surgically destructive treatments, but it also carries a nonnegligible risk of sensorineural hearing loss. So far, there is no consensus on the dosage and treatment duration of ITG. Most researchers recommend that intratympanic injection of gentamicin is more suitable for patients with unilateral onset and impaired hearing function, who are younger than 65 years old, as well as with frequent and severe vertigo attacks, and ineffective prior conservative treatment. Before an ITG treatment, patients should be adequately informed about the risk of hearing loss, and in order to reduce the risk of deafness, low drug dose and long intervals between injections are recommended. In short, to administer an ITG injection, multiple factors should be comprehensively considered including patient selection, pharmacological mechanism, drug dose, the interval of administration, complications, indications, and contraindications.

Keywords: intratympanic, gentamicin, Ménière's disease, management, aminoglycosides, vertigo, vestibulotoxicity, ototoxicity

INTRODUCTION

Ménière's disease (MD), also called idiopathic endolymphatic hydrops, is one of the most common causes of dizziness originating in the inner ear. The typical clinical manifestations are frequent spontaneous vertigo, fluctuating sensorineural hearing loss, tinnitus, and/or aural fullness. Vertigo is typically the most debilitating symptom, and control of vertiginous episodes is the primary goal of therapeutic interventions for most patients.

There are numerous available therapeutic options for MD including conservative treatments with dietary modifications, oral medication, procedural treatments with intratympanic therapies, and surgical treatments. A failure of conservative therapy often introduces the need for a more aggressive therapy on the treatment algorithm.

Surgical intervention or intratympanic aminoglycosides can be used in patients with intractable vertigo, which, ideally, should control the vertigo while preserving the hearing level and balance. The side effects of aminoglycosides are wellknow. The risks of vestibular and cochlear toxicity are mainly related to types of aminoglycosides, route of administration, duration of the therapy, total or cumulative dose, individual susceptibility, renal function, patient's age, etc.

In 1948, Fowler [1] first used systemic streptomycin to treat vertigo attacks in patients with intractable MD. The results showed that vertigo attacks could be well controlled, but treatment carried the risks of bilateral vestibulopathy, nephrotoxicity, and unpredictable results. In 1957, Schuknekt [2] may have been the first to use intratympanic streptomycin to alleviate vertigo attacks in patients with unilateral intractable MD, and it was firstly named "chemical labyrinthectomy". Intratympanic gentamicin (ITG) for the treatment of severe vertigo was reported by Lange [3]. The initial approach was complete vestibular ablation to control the vertigo. However, with this approach, the hearing was at a greater risk. Over the past decades, the pharmacological mechanisms of aminoglycosides have been progressively studied in depth and clinical trials have been extensively developed.

At present, intratympanic injection of gentamicin is probably the most effective non-surgical treatment to eradicate vertigo in MD and is gradually gaining popularity in the worldwide. Compared with the treatment regimen decades ago, several modifications for ITG treatment have emerged regarding the concentration of the gentamicin solution, the frequency of injections, and the method of delivery. In this chapter, the history, background, and progression of ITG treatment for MD are discussed, as well as the basic science, therapeutic method, treatment efficacy, indications, contraindications, and complications.

History of intratympanic gentamicin

Aminoglycosides are highly potent, broad-spectrum antibiotics and are widely used by various routes of injection to treat serious infections caused by Gram-negative bacteria (e.g., *Pseudomonas aeruginosa*, *Proteus* species, *Escherichia coli*, *KlebsiellaEnterobacter-Serratia* species, and *Citrobacter* species), and are sometimes used as an adjuvant treatment for infections caused by Gram-positive bacteria (e.g., *Staphylococcus* species). The basic chemical structure required for both potency and the spectrum of antimicrobial activity of aminoglycosides is that of one, or several, aminated sugars joined in glycosidic linkages to a dibasic cyclitol. Aminoglycosides act primarily by impairing bacterial protein synthesis through binding to prokaryotic ribosomes [4].

Streptomycin, which was discovered in 1944, is the first aminoglycoside antibiotic in human history and was thereafter marked by the successive introduction of a series of milestone compounds (kanamycin discovered in 1957, gentamicin in 1963, and neomycin in 1970s) which definitively established the usefulness of this class of antibiotics for the treatment of Gram-negative bacillary infections. From the 1960s to 1970s, aminoglycosides were widely used, but due to their serious ototoxicity and nephrotoxicity, their systemic application was limited, and they were gradually fading out of the ranks of first-line drugs. At the beginning, the most common side effect of streptomycin used by intravenous injection was temporary imbalance without vertigo or nystagmus. Higher systemic doses increased the chance of permanent imbalance and, occasionally, deafness. These early observations led to animal and cadaver studies which confirmed the vestibulotoxic and cochleotoxic effects of high-dose streptomycin.

Based on its vestibulotoxicity, streptomycin foremost unveiled its potential in the treatment of vestibular diseases. In 1948, about 4 years after streptomycin was discovered, Fowler [1] first used systemic streptomycin to treat vertigo attacks in patients with intractable MD which was refractory to traditional medical treatment. He and others used between 2 and 4 g of intramuscular streptomycin per day in patients with unilateral or bilateral MD, typically until onset of severe imbalance, and reported that vertigo attacks could be well controlled without loss of hearing. Often, and especially with higher dosing, vertigo control was accompanied with the troubling symptoms of permanent, severe imbalance, and oscillopsia.

In 1957, Schuknecht [2] may have been the first to use intratympanic streptomycin to alleviate vertigo attacks in patients with unilateral MD that was uncontrolled by traditional medical management. He conceived of this idea after noting that intratympanic formalin will readily pass into the inner ear and prevented postmortem degeneration of the inner ear membranous structures in patients. He correctly theorized that streptomycin could also pass into the inner ear and devised a cat animal model that demonstrated clinical and pathologic vestibulotoxicity with intratympanic streptomycin. Based on these results, he devised a clinical trial of intratympanic streptomycin administration to patients with uncontrolled unilateral MD. He administered variable amounts of streptomycin (between 0.125 and 0.5 g), either hourly or over 4 hours, over a variable amount of days. The first group of three patients who received 1 or 2 days of treatment achieved only brief control of their vertigo, but did not lose any hearing. Subsequently, an additional group of five patients received streptomycin for 3 days or longer. These patients had permanent resolution of their vertigo episodes, but at the cost of deafening the ear. Schuknekt coined the term "chemical labyrinthectomy" to describe this phenomenon. He concluded that intratympanic streptomycin at the therapeutic dosage failed to preserve hearing, and should only be considered for patients who are not good surgical candidates, but would otherwise be proper candidates for inner ear ablation [2].

With the administration of intratympanic aminoglycosides, chemical ablation of the inner ear via systemic administration of aminoglycosides fell into disfavor due to the side effects of bilateral vestibulopathy, nephrotoxicity, and unpredictable results. However, choosing which kind of aminoglycoside for intratympanic injection has gradually changed. In 1977, Lange [3] appears to be the first to have used IT administration of gentamicin. He reported about 55 patients suffering from severe unilateral MD, seen over a period of 3–10 years. Patients were treated with intratympanic administration of streptomycin or better, gentamicin. The medication was given using a plastic tube inserted behind the annulus within the transmeatal approach, and 0.1 ml gentamicin (earlier streptomycin) was instilled every 5 hours until the first signs of inner ear reaction (nystagmus or vertigo) appeared. In 90% of the cases, vertiginous attacks ceased after therapy, and hearing was preserved in 76%.

Entering the 1990s, intratympanic gentamicin had gained widespread popularity in the treatment of MD. Compared with streptomycin, ITG for treatment of MD provided equivalently excellent vertigo control while showing a lower incidence of hearing loss in early clinical data. Gentamicin gained popularity over streptomycin and gradually came to be the drug of choice for chemical ablation of inner ear.

In 1993, Nedzelski et al. [5] studied 50 patients with unilateral MD by treatment of microcatheter administration of streptomycin over a 5 h treatment, 4 treatments within 48 hours, and the rate of vertigo control was up to 96%; only 24% of his patients experienced various degrees of hearing loss. Although streptomycin was being used in the study, he advocated for using gentamicin instead for its theoretical reduction of cochleotoxicity.

Beck and Schmidt [6] reported on their 10 years of experience with intratympanally applied streptomycin and gentamicin in the therapy of MD. They theorized that the dosage might be a critical factor for hearing preservation with vertigo control. Aminoglycosides could be titrated to impede the secretory epithelium of the vestibular apparatus without destroying the sensory cells, thus achieving vertigo control while maintaining caloric response, that is, vestibulo-ocular reflex. More importantly, risk of deafness could potentially be eliminated. By reducing the dosage delivered and titrating, they were able to achieve excellent rates of vertigo control (92%) while also achieving respectable hearing preservation rates (15% hearing loss with no cases of deafness).

During the same era, around the early 1990s, two schools of thought emerged in an effort to standardize ITG treatment, dubbed the "shotgun" approach, and the "low-dose" approach. The shotgun approach, championed by Nedzelski and others [5], was characterized by daily IT injections to a fixed endpoint or to a clinical threshold that heralded damage to the inner ear. Proponents of this approach attempted to achieve adequate vestibular ablation for long-term vertigo control. The low-dose approach, championed by Magnusson and others [7], was characterized by weekly IT injections, also to a fixed endpoint or to clinical effect. Proponents of this approach tried to achieve vertigo control while minimizing damage to hearing and potentially preserving the caloric response as well.

Today, intratympanic injection of gentamicin is probably the most effective nonsurgical treatment to eradicate vertigo in MD. Yet, it is an ablative method that carries a non-negligible risk of hearing loss. Currently, gentamicin is usually instilled via IT injection or through a tympanostomy tube to the round window niche. These injections are repeated over a variable amount of time, typically between daily to weekly injections, until a clinical endpoint is achieved or until there is a decline in hearing. No consensus has been reached so far on the overall dosage, dosing methods, timing of delivery, treatment duration, clinical endpoint of therapy, or concentration of gentamicin. Both clinical evidence and basic science models should be further studied to scientifically elicit the most effective and safe regimen.

Mechanism of action

Aminoglycoside antibiotics have a well-documented history of cochleotoxic and vestibulotoxic effects. Administration of intratympanic aminoglycoside antibiotics to patients with MD is based on the notion that the patient's vestibular symptoms are due to the damaged and distorted vestibular signals emanating from their ear and that they are better off with no signal than with a damaged and distorted signal. The objective of ITG is to weaken vestibular signals in the Ménière's ear to the point at which they are no longer strong enough to generate a vertigo attack. Ideally, aminoglycosides would act to reduce vestibular function, and thus alleviate the patient's symptoms of vertigo, while preserving hearing. The degree to which a drug is cochleotoxic or vestibulotoxic differs among aminoglycosides. Gentamicin and streptomycin, for instance, are reported to be more vestibulotoxic. Other aminoglycosides, such as amikacin, are considered to be relatively more cochleotoxic and thus are not used transtympanically. The best evidence for this is the simple clinical observation that patients undergoing systemic gentamicin or streptomycin therapy experience vestibulopathy much more commonly than hearing loss. This feature has been used by otologists to control the vestibular symptoms of MD, initially provided through systemic delivery by Fowler [1] and subsequently through IT injections by Schuknecht [2, 8]. Use of streptomycin has been largely replaced by gentamicin which is thought to be more selectively vestibulotoxic and better able to preserve residual hearing in patients with unilateral MD refractory to medical management [9, 10].

Within the bony labyrinth, several studies have investigated the trafficking and distribution of aminoglycosides, finding different patterns of distribution dependent upon the dose, duration, and route of administration. IT-injected aminoglycosides appear to gain access to the inner ear via the oval window and the round window [11, 12], and uptake either by passive diffusion or by endocytosis [13, 14]. Salt et al. recently quantified diffusion of gentamicin through the oval (35%) versus the round window (57%) [12, 15]. Access to these membranous structures is however uncertain, partly due to their variable permeability in individuals, resulting in unpredictable drug exposure of the inner ear [16–18]. Similar mechanisms of cellular trafficking (active diffusion and endocytosis) have been proposed in the transport of aminoglycosides into cells of the inner ear [19].

Once the drug crosses the oval window and the round window, the situation becomes more complex and the precise mechanism by which aminoglycosides exert their toxic effects on hair cells is unknown, to date. Previous animal studies showed that in the cochlea, sensory hair cells, the spiral ligament including the stria vascularis, and spiral ganglion cells had a very early uptake of gentamicin. Similarly, hair cells, dark cells, and vestibular ganglion cells are the primary targets in the vestibular system. This may demonstrate that gentamicin most likely diffuses across the inner ear membranes, readily achieving concentrations within the scala vestibuli, cochlear duct, and vestibule and then exerts its cellular toxicity.

Multiple mechanisms, including disruption of calcium-dependent cytokine production resulting in the damage to hair cell membrane integrity, increased superoxide production, hair cell transduction blockage, glutamate decarboxylase inhibition, ornithine decarboxylase inhibition, and free radical damage, all have been developed to explain aminoglycosides' direct toxicity to hair cells [10, 20, 21]. While most cells of the inner ear demonstrate aminoglycoside penetration, several studies have identified preferential loss of the hair cells at the basal turn of the cochlea over the apical hair cells and vestibular type I hair cells over their type II counterparts [22–26]. Direct damage to the spiral ganglion has also been observed [27] and histologic studies in rhesus monkeys suggest relative sparing of the maculae [28].

In parallel to previous findings, several studies have demonstrated that direct application of gentamicin into the vestibular labyrinth also causes greater loss of type I versus type II vestibular hair cells [29, 30]. Recently, Lyford-Pike et al. [26] used the animal model, chinchilla, to provide the evidence that the selective loss of type I hair cells assuredly occurred because these cells preferentially accumulate gentamicin acutely after intratympanic administration. Type II hair cells and supporting cells concentrate substantially less gentamicin. These results might theoretically ameliorate the more profound symptom of vertigo (driven by type I hair cells) while preserving cochlear function.

Aminoglycosides may also act to inhibit production of endolymph, restoring the balance between endolymphatic and perilymphatic pressure. This would also act to alleviate all symptoms of endolymphatic hydrops. Additionally, aminoglycosides are theorized to cause selective damage to the cells of the cochlear stria vascularis and planum semilunatum in the cristae ampullae of the semicircular canals, which are involved in ionic regulation and endolymph production [31]. It is also known that gentamicin utilizes the cellular machinery of endolymph production to traffic into the inner ear after systemic administration [32]. The theory that vestibular dark cells and, thus, endolymphatic flow, are the targets by which aminoglycosides alleviate vertigo is of significant clinical interest because it suggests that it is not necessarily important to ablate the vestibule to achieve vertigo control in MD. This idea can explain why patients with intact caloric responses can still achieve significant vertigo control after intratympanic aminoglycoside administration.

In conclusion, direct toxicity to vestibular hair cells and direct toxicity to the endolymph producing apparatus might be the two major mechanisms of action by ITG. Most importantly, gentamicin has been proved to be more vestibulotoxic than cochleotoxic in humans. The inner ear toxicity of gentamicin might follow an order. Secretory dark cells of the vestibule might be the first to be damaged, followed by

the vestibular neuroepithelium and the afferent vestibular fibers, and finally, the hair cells of the organ of Corti are destroyed [33, 34].

Therapeutic method and treatment efficacy

Ménière's disease is manifested by episodic vertigo, tinnitus, aural fullness, and fluctuating hearing loss. The treatment of patients with MD is usually directed at the most disabling symptom, which is the debilitating vertigo. MD treatment protocols typically measure vertigo control according to AAO-HNS Committee on Hearing and Equilibrium guidelines for grading vertigo severity [35]. Often, clinical trials also attempt to assess other disease sequelae such as hearing loss, tinnitus, and aural fullness.

As a well-known relapsing-remitting disease, it is rather difficult to accurately evaluate the efficacy of ITG in treatment of MD. Firstly, the natural history of remission and exacerbation of symptoms make evaluation of the effectiveness of treatment remarkably difficult. Commonly, vertigo attacks can improve without treatment of any kind as periods of remission are not uncommon. Thus, a clinical trial without controls will not account for this finding. Another difficulty is that clinical researchers attempt to show hearing preservation with IT gentamicin protocol, but hearing tends to worsen over time in MD regardless of treatment. Finally, the variable nature of MD with fluctuation in levels of hearing and even frequency and severity of vertigo can make clinical trials difficult.

To date, there have only been a few interventional randomized controlled trials investigating the true efficacy of ITG in the treatment of MD. In 2004, the first prospective, double-blind, randomized clinical trial of intratympanic gentamicin versus intratympanic buffer solution (placebo) in patients with active MD was reported by Stokroos et al. [36]. They performed ITG injections with buffered gentamicin (30 mg/ml) every 6 weeks until the vertigo complaints disappeared (12 patients received gentamicin versus 10 for placebo), outcome measures included the number of vertiginous spells, degree of sensorineural hearing loss, labyrinthine function, and labyrinthine asymmetry. Compared to the placebo group, topical gentamicin provided a significant improvement in the number of vertiginous attacks per year at follow up which varied between 6 and 28 months. There was no statistically significant change in hearing or other outcomes in two groups. However, hearing had a tendency to deteriorate in the placebo-treated patients, due to the natural course of the disease, which suggests that early treatment with topical gentamicin may preserve residual sensorineural hearing in active MD.

In 2008, Postema et al. [37] reported another prospective, double-blind, randomized, placebo-controlled trial associated with ITG therapy for control of vertigo in unilateral MD. They used weekly injections of 0.4 ml of gentamicin (30 mg/ml). A total of 4 injections were given through a ventilation tube (16 patients received gentamicin and 12 received a placebo). The results showed that gentamicin treatment resulted in a significant reduction of the score for vertigo complaints (including vertigo severity) and the score for perceived aural fullness. They also noted that a small increase in hearing loss (average of losses at 0.5, 1, 2, and 4 kHz: 8 dB HL) was measured in the gentamicin group.

In 2016, Patel et al. [38] performed a randomized, double-blind, comparative effectiveness trial of intratympanic methylprednisolone (n = 30) versus gentamicin (n = 30) in patients with refractory unilateral MD. Patients were randomly assigned (1:1) to two intratympanic methylprednisolone (62.5 mg/ml) or gentamicin (40 mg/ml) injections given 2 weeks apart, and were followed up for 2 years. In the methylprednisolone group, complete vertigo control (Class A) was achieved in 21/30 patients (70%) compared to 25/30 (83.3%) in the gentamicin group. After methylprednisolone, 22 patients (78.5%) experienced an improved functional level score and 8 patients (28.7%) better pure-tone hearing and speech discrimination. There were also reductions for tinnitus, dizziness, and aural fullness. Fifteen patients (50%) required further courses of methylprednisolone. Two patients were deemed treatment failures and were assigned ITG treatment. The study showed no significant difference between the methylprednisolone and gentamicin for the control of vertigo, total number of injections, number of patients with relapsing vertigo, or the amount of pain from injection but better speech discrimination after methylprednisolone.

Based on the above prospective, double-blind, randomized controlled clinical trials, intratympanic gentamicin, as a medically ablative method, seems to be the most effective non-surgical treatment to eradicate vertigo in intractable MD, but with a potential risk of hearing loss. However, there is no consensus on the treatment protocol of ITG, especially for the concentration of gentamicin, dosage in each application, number of injection, and the time interval between two doses.

In the over 40 years of clinical trials in the treatment of MD by ITG, the majority are case series without controls, mainly because of the significant difficulties in conducting the randomized controlled clinical trials or case/control trials [33]. In earlier studies, the highest rate of vertigo control was reported with daily injections or multiple titrations. On the other hand, considerable hearing loss was experienced in several studies. Moller et al. [39] treated 15 patients with disabling MD with daily injections for periods ranging from 3 to 11 days. They achieved 93.4% of vertigo control, but also 33.4% of hearing loss. They reported that none of the patients were responsive to caloric stimulation. Laitakari [40] reported 90% of vertigo control and 45% of hearing loss in 20 patients who had daily ITG for a minimum of 3 consecutive days. Parnes and Riddell [41] reported 41.7% worsening of the hearing in their group of patients who received three daily injections within 4 days. Murofushi et al. [42], using several daily injections, reported hearing loss in 30% of cases. Corsten et al. [43] reported 81% vertigo control but 57% hearing loss in patients (n = 21) who had gentamicin instillation 3 times a day for 4 consecutive days. Kaplan et al. [44] reviewed the 10-year long-term results of 114 patients treated with gentamicin instillation 3 times a day for 4 consecutive days. They achieved 93.4% of vertigo control and 25.6% of hearing loss.

In the early 2000s, regarding patients with hearing deterioration and even those becoming deaf, there was a discussion about reducing the gentamicin dose or performing the application at longer intervals. Daily titration methods were abandoned. Transtympanic gentamicin therapy was modified to weekly or monthly intervals as "needed" or "on demand" to reduce the symptoms of MD, aiming to maintain cochlear as well as vestibular function. Harner et al. [45] reported a very high rate of vertigo control with preservation of hearing in 43 patients. There were no patients with changes in cochlear function and ablation of the labyrinth. All patients received one injection, and half of them received a repeat injection 1 month after therapy. Minor [46] used gentamicin on weekly intervals until the development of spontaneous nystagmus, head-shaking nystagmus, or head thrust sign. Vertigo was controlled in 91% of the patients, and profound hearing loss only occurred in 1 patient. Atlas and Parnes [47] reviewed the outcomes of 83 patients who received weekly injections. They reported hearing loss in 17% of the patients, with vertigo control in 84%. Martin and Perez [48] reported vertigo control in 83.1% of the patients and hearing loss in 15.5% of them after gentamicin at weekly intervals. De Beer et al. [49] reported 15.8% with hearing loss and 80.7% with vertigo control after, between 1 and 10, intratympanic injections at a minimum interval of 27 days. Casani et al. [50] reported 12% hearing loss after a maximum of 2 injections of gentamicin and 81% vertigo control.

Most recently, Vlastarakos et al. [51] published a systematic review looking at sustained-release delivery of IT gentamicin (dynamic-release versus sustainedrelease vehicles). Dynamic release (microcatheter at the round window) was found to provide satisfactory vertigo control in 89.3% (70.9% reporting complete control). Sustained-release preparations (gentamicin-soaked wick/pledget) provided 82.2% satisfactory control in the pool of patients (75% with complete control). In patients receiving sustained-release preparations, complete hearing loss was reported in 31.1% patients with another 23.3% of patients experiencing partial hearing loss. This adverse change in hearing was unacceptably high, reinforcing the suggestion of using a sustained-release vehicle only in patients who had failed IT gentamicin injections previously or those without serviceable hearing.

Commonly, intratympanic injection under otoscope or microscope is a simple and recommendable technique. The desired amount of gentamicin is injected over the round window through the posterosuperior quadrant of the tympanic membrane. There are two common doses of gentamicin for injection. The standard intravenous preparation of gentamicin is 40 mg/ml, which can be buffered with 8.4% sodium bicarbonate so that discomfort on injection is reduced. A total of 1.5 ml of gentamicin mixed with 0.5 ml of sodium bicarbonate at these concentrations will produce a final concentration of 26.6 mg/ml gentamicin. Approximately 0.3–0.5 ml of solution is usually adequate to bathe the round window in solution. Typically, patients will remain lying flat with the injected ear up for 10 min to 1 h. This procedure is generally well tolerated by patients, who should be told to expect brief pain on injection, followed by possible vertigo or disequilibrium. Warming the medication can help in this regard (preventing a cold caloric response).

Based on the combination of current clinical practice, basic science models, and results from clinical trials, low drug dose and long interval between injections, mainly in order to reduce the risk of deafness, are reasonably encouraged. The low dose method involves using 1–2 injections of gentamicin and waiting a month or 2 weeks between injections. The rate of vertigo control may be up to 80–90%, with no significant side effects. The second injection is given only if there has been a vertigo spell 2 weeks prior. In other words, instead of titrating to the onset of damage to the vestibular system, the criterion is a positive effect on the disease. Occasionally, a third dose is given.

In short, whatever technique is used, the goal is to apply gentamicin to the round window in sufficient concentration and over a sufficient amount of time that it achieves a therapeutic effect while avoiding both local and systemic side effects, especially hearing loss.

Indications and contraindications

Not all patients with MD can be treated with ITG. Based on the international consensus on treatment of MD obtained from the IFOS meeting 2017 [52], MD should be treated with a step-by-step therapy. The first line of treatment includes the medical conservative treatment, such as dietary modification and oral medicine. After this line of treatment, 80% of patients with MD are cured or in remission. When the vertigo of MD fails to be controlled by the first-line treatment for more than 6 months, it will be regarded as intractable MD. Then the second line is the IT injections, mainly IT steroids as a conservative treatment and ITG in the case of IT steroid failure, and preferentially in patients with hearing impairment. After the second line treatment, 90–95% of the total patients are cured or in remission. The third line is the surgical, either conservative or destructive, treatment. For unilateral intractable MD with serviceable hearing (i.e., speech reception threshold better than 50 dB HL and speech discrimination score of more than 50%) in the treated ear, treatment protocol with an injection repetition not shorter than 1 week between adjacent injections or one with injections on a monthly basis as "needed" is preferred. These methods provide the same level of vertigo control yet offer better preservation of hearing functions [33].

The best indication for ITG treatment appears to be the control of vertigo in profound hearing loss or non-serviceable ears, in which speech reception threshold is worse than 50 dB HL and speech discrimination score less than 50% [53, 54]. Under these scenarios, there is no need to consider the risk of deafness, and titration methods or multiple injections on a daily basis are preferred, since these methods have significantly elevated incidence of hearing loss [33]. Transmastoid labyrinthectomy has traditionally been offered for non-serviceable ears in patients with MD. This method has been the gold standard, and it is very effective in eradication of vertigo in more than 94% of patients. In comparison, ITG therapy provides a minimally invasive ambulatory substitute with low morbidity and fewer side-effects, which is also very cost effective to manage vertigo in these MD patients with non-serviceable ears [53].

Another important indicator is the control of vertigo in patients who have failed endolymphatic sac surgery. Marzo and Leonetti [55] have shown the effectiveness of ITG therapy for patients who have failed endolymphatic sac surgery, thus reducing the need for vestibular neurectomy in those with intractable disease.

To be allergic and hypersensitive to aminoglycosides are two absolute contraindications for ITG. It is worth noting that patients who carried the mitochondrial mutation of the gene MT-RNR1 (mitochondrially encoded 12S ribosomal RNA) are hypersensitive to aminoglycosides. A single injection of aminoglycosides results in complete and definitive deafness in subjects with this mutation [56]. A systematic genetic screening of MD patients is highly recommended to prevent the occurrence of bilateral deafness. The treatment is intended for the abolition of vestibular function; thus, administration of gentamicin must be done carefully in the elderly, who have difficulty attaining vestibular compensation, in patients with complications, or in those with bilateral MD. Taking also into consideration the fact that individual's drug sensitivity depends on their genetic background, investigation of appropriate drug levels according to evidence-based medicine remains a future task.

Complications

The complications of ITG treatment are primarily bi-fold: one is the risk caused by drug toxicity of gentamicin, the other is the risk caused by intratympanic injection. Undoubtedly, the main risk of ITG treatment for vertigo is the sensorineural hearing loss and associated prolonged disequilibrium and ataxia, which are common complaints after this treatment. Less common side effects include local hemorrhage, allergic response and tympanic membrane perforation (especially in an irradiated or otherwise damaged tympanic membrane), local discomfort, inflammation, otitis media or externa, and transient vertigo caused by a caloric reflex effect from the instilled fluid [38, 57]. It is also critical to educate all patients who are given intratympanic aminoglycosides that bilateral permanent hearing loss is possible, even from one single unilateral injection.

Conclusions

Intratympanic injection of gentamicin is probably the most effective nonsurgical treatment to eradicate vertigo in MD. But it is also an ablative method that carries a non-negligible risk of hearing loss. Gentamicin has been proved to be more vestibulotoxic than cochleotoxic; direct toxicity to vestibular hair cells and direct toxicity to the endolymph producing apparatus might be the two major mechanisms of action. To date, no consensus has been reached on the dosage, dosing methods, timing of delivery, treatment duration, clinical endpoint of therapy, and concentration of gentamicin. However, based on the combination of current clinical practice, basic science models, and results from clinical trials, low drug dose and long intervals between injections are reasonably recommended. The application of gentamicin-induced vestibular ablation has minimized the number of more invasive procedures such as unilateral labyrinthectomy and vestibular neurectomy. In comparison with surgery, the vertigo control is comparable, the overall cost is reduced, and complications are limited. ITG in treating intractable MD has gradually become a prevalent therapy during the past decades. However, to administer ITG treatment, multiple factors should be comprehensively considered including patient selection, pharmacological mechanism, drug dose, the interval of administration, complications, indications, and contraindications.

Acknowledgements

The authors thank Alisa Hetrick for her comments on an earlier version of the article.

References

[1] Fowler EP Jr. Streptomycin treatment of vertigo. Transactions of the American Academy of Ophthalmology and Otolaryngology. 1948;**52**:293-301

[2] Schuknecht HF. Ablation therapy in the management of Meniere's disease. Acta Oto-Laryngologica. Supplementum. 1957;**132**:1-42

[3] Lange G. The intratympanic treatment of Meniere's disease with ototoxic antibiotics. A follow-up study of 55 cases (author's transl). Laryngologie, Rhinologie, Otologie. 1977;**56**:409-414

[4] Mingeot-Leclercq MP, Glupczynski Y, Tulkens PM. Aminoglycosides: Activity and resistance. Antimicrobial Agents and Chemotherapy. 1999;**43**:727-737

[5] Nedzelski JM, Chiong CM, Fradet G, Schessel DA, Bryce GE, Pfleiderer AG. Intratympanic gentamicin instillation as treatment of unilateral Meniere's disease: Update of an ongoing study. The American Journal of Otology. 1993;**14**:278-282

[6] Beck C, Schmidt CL. 10 years of experience with intratympanally applied streptomycin (gentamycin) in the therapy of Morbus Meniere. Archives of Oto-Rhino-Laryngology. 1978;**221**:149-152

[7] Magnusson M, Padoan S. Delayed onset of ototoxic effects of gentamicin in treatment of Meniere's disease. Rationale for extremely low dose therapy. Acta Oto-Laryngologica. 1991;**111**:671-676

[8] Schuknecht HF. Ablation therapy for the relief of Meniere's disease. Laryngoscope. 1956;**66**:859-870

[9] Webster JC, McGee TM, Carroll R, Benitez JT, Williams ML. Ototoxicity of gentamicin. Histopathologic and functional results in the cat. Transactions of the American Academy of Ophthalmology and Otolaryngology. 1970;**74**:1155-1165

[10]Rudnick MD, Ginsberg IA, Huber PS. Aminoglycoside ototoxicity following middle ear injection. The Annals of Otology, Rhinology and Laryngology. Supplement. 1980;**89**:i-iii, 1-28

[11]Smith BM, Myers MG. The penetration of gentamicin and neomycin into perilymph across the round window membrane. Otolaryngology—Head and Neck Surgery. 1979;**87**:888-891

[12]Salt AN, Hartsock JJ, Gill RM, King E, Kraus FB, Plontke SK. Perilymph pharmacokinetics of locally-applied gentamicin in the guinea pig. Hearing Research. 2016;**342**:101-111

[13]Goycoolea MV. Clinical aspects of round window membrane permeability under normal and pathological conditions. Acta Oto-Laryngologica. 2001;**121**:437-447

[14]Becvarovski Z, Bojrab DI, Michaelides EM, Kartush JM, Zappia JJ, LaRouere MJ. Round window gentamicin absorption: An in vivo human model. The Laryngoscope. 2002;**112**:1610-1613

[15]Salt AN, Ma Y. Quantification of solute entry into cochlear perilymph through the round window membrane Hearing Research. 2001;**154**:88-97

[16]Silverstein H, Rowan PT, Olds MJ, Rosenberg SI. Inner ear perfusion and the role of round window patency. The American Journal of Otology. 1997;**18**:586-589

[17]Yoshioka M, Naganawa S, Sone M, Nakata S, Teranishi M, Nakashima T. Individual differences in the permeability of the round window: Evaluating the movement of intratympanic gadolinium into the inner ear. Otology and Neurotology. 2009;**30**:645-648

[18]Alzamil KS, Linthicum FH Jr. Extraneous round window membranes and plugs: Possible effect on intratympanic therapy. The Annals of Otology, Rhinology, and Laryngology. 2000;**109**:30-32

[19]Carey J. Intratympanic gentamicin for the treatment of Meniere's disease and other forms of peripheral vertigo. Otolaryngologic Clinics of North America. 2004;**37**:1075-1090

[20]Williams SE, Zenner HP, Schacht J. Three molecular steps of aminoglycoside ototoxicity demonstrated in outer hair cells. Hearing Research. 1987;**30**:11-18

[21]Schacht J. Biochemical basis of aminoglycoside ototoxicity. Otolaryngologic Clinics of North America. 1993;**26**:845-856

[22]Wersall J, Lundquist PG, Bjorkroth B. Ototoxicity of gentamicin. The Journal of Infectious Diseases. 1969;**119**:410-416

[23]Lindeman HH. Regional differences in sensitivity of the vestibular sensory epithelia to ototoxic antibiotics. Acta Oto-Laryngologica. 1969;**67**:177-189

[24]de Groot JC, Meeuwsen F, Ruizendaal WE, Veldman JE. Ultrastructural localization of gentamicin in the cochlea. Hearing Research. 1990;**50**:35-42

[25]Tsuji K, Velazquez-Villasenor L, Rauch SD, Glynn RJ, Wall C, Merchant SN. Temporal bone studies of the human peripheral vestibular system. Aminoglycoside ototoxicity. The Annals of Otology, Rhinology and Laryngology Supplement. 2000;**181**:20-25

[26]Lyford-Pike S, Vogelheim C, Chu E, Della Santina CC, Carey JP. Gentamicin is primarily localized in vestibular type I hair cells after intratympanic administration. Journal of the Association for Research in Otolaryngology: JARO. 2007;**8**:497-508

[27]Bae WY, Kim LS, Hur DY, Jeong SW, Kim JR. Secondary apoptosis of spiral ganglion cells induced by aminoglycoside: Fas–Fas ligand signaling pathway. The Laryngoscope. 2008;**118**:1659-1668

[28]Sun DQ , Lehar M, Dai C, Swarthout L, Lauer AM, Carey JP, et al. Histopathologic changes of the inner ear in Rhesus monkeys after intratympanic gentamicin injection and vestibular prosthesis electrode array implantation. Journal of the Association for Research in Otolaryngology: JARO. 2015;**16**:373-387

[29]Lopez I, Honrubia V, Lee SC, Schoeman G, Beykirch K. Quantification of the process of hair cell loss and recovery in the chinchilla crista ampullaris after gentamicin treatment. International Journal of Developmental Neuroscience. 1997;**15**:447-461

[30]Hirvonen TP, Minor LB, Hullar TE, Carey JP. Effects of intratympanic gentamicin on vestibular afferents and hair cells in the chinchilla. Journal of Neurophysiology. 2005;**93**:643-655

[31]Atlas J, Parnes LS. Intratympanic gentamicin for intractable Meniere's disease: 5-year follow-up. The Journal of Otolaryngology. 2003;**32**:288-293

[32]Li H, Steyger PS. Systemic aminoglycosides are trafficked via endolymph into cochlear hair cells. Scientific Reports. 2011;**1**:159

[33]Yetiser S. Intratympanic gentamicin for intractable Meniere's disease—A review and analysis of audiovestibular impact. International Archives of Otorhinolaryngology. 2018;**22**:190-194

[34]Sultemeier DR, Hoffman LF. Partial aminoglycoside lesions in vestibular epithelia reveal broad sensory dysfunction associated with modest hair cell loss and afferent calyx retraction. Frontiers in Cellular Neuroscience. 2017;**11**:331

[35]Monsell EM. New and revised reporting guidelines from the committee on hearing and equilibrium. Otolaryngology—Head and Neck Surgery. 1995;**113**:176-178

[36]Stokroos R, Kingma H. Selective vestibular ablation by intratympanic gentamicin in patients with unilateral active Meniere's disease: A prospective, double-blind, placebo-controlled, randomized clinical trial. Acta OtoLaryngologica. 2004;**124**:172-175

[37]Postema RJ, Kingma CM, Wit HP, Albers FW, Van Der Laan BF. Intratympanic gentamicin therapy for control of vertigo in unilateral Menire's disease: A prospective, double-blind, randomized, placebo-controlled trial. Acta Oto-Laryngologica. 2008;**128**:876-880

[38]Patel M, Agarwal K, Arshad Q, Hariri M, Rea P, Seemungal BM, et al. Intratympanic methylprednisolone versus gentamicin in patients with unilateral Meniere's disease: A randomized, doubleblind, comparative effectiveness trial. Lancet. 2016;**388**:2753-2762

[39]Moller C, Odkvist LM, Thell J, Larsby B, Hyden D. Vestibular and audiologic functions in gentamicintreated Meniere's disease. The American Journal of Otology. 1988;**9**:383-391

[40]Laitakari K. Intratympanic gentamycin in severe Meniere's disease. Clinical Otolaryngology and Allied Sciences. 1990;**15**:545-548

[41]Parnes LS, Riddell D. Irritative spontaneous nystagmus following intratympanic gentamicin for Meniere's disease. The Laryngoscope. 1993;**103**:745-749

[42]Murofushi T, Halmagyi GM, Yavor RA. Intratympanic gentamicin in Meniere's disease: Results of therapy. The American Journal of Otology. 1997;**18**:52-57

[43]Corsten M, Marsan J, Schramm D, Robichaud J. Treatment of intractable Meniere's disease with intratympanic gentamicin: Review of the University of Ottawa experience. The Journal of Otolaryngology. 1997;**26**:361-364

[44]Kaplan DM, Nedzelski JM, Al-Abidi A, Chen JM, Shipp DB. Hearing loss following intratympanic

instillation of gentamicin for the treatment of unilateral Meniere's disease. The Journal of Otolaryngology. 2002;**31**:106-111

[45]Harner SG, Kasperbauer JL, Facer GW, Beatty CW. Transtympanic gentamicin for Meniere's syndrome. The Laryngoscope. 1998;**108**:1446-1449

[46]Minor LB. Intratympanic gentamicin for control of vertigo in Meniere's disease: Vestibular signs that specify completion of therapy. The American Journal of Otology. 1999;**20**:209-219

[47]Atlas JT, Parnes LS. Intratympanic gentamicin titration therapy for intractable Meniere's disease. The American Journal of Otology. 1999;**20**:357-363

[48]Martin E, Perez N. Hearing loss after intratympanic gentamicin therapy for unilateral Meniere's disease. Otology and Neurotology. 2003;**24**:800-806

[49]De Beer L, Stokroos R, Kingma H. Intratympanic gentamicin therapy for intractable Meniere's disease. Acta OtoLaryngologica. 2007;**127**:605-612

[50]Casani AP, Piaggi P, Cerchiai N, Seccia V, Franceschini SS, Dallan I. Intratympanic treatment of intractable unilateral Meniere disease: Gentamicin or dexamethasone? A randomized controlled trial. Otolaryngolog—Head and Neck Surgery. 2012;**146**:430-437

[51]Vlastarakos PV, Iacovou E, Nikolopoulos TP. Is gentamycin delivery via sustained-release vehicles a safe and effective treatment for refractory Meniere's disease? A critical analysis of published interventional studies. European Archives of Oto-RhinoLaryngology. 2017;**274**:1309-1315

[52]Nevoux J, Barbara M, Dornhoffer J, Gibson W, Kitahara T, Darrouzet V. International consensus (ICON) on treatment of Meniere's disease. European Annals of Otorhinolaryngology, Head and Neck Diseases. 2018;**135**:S29-S32

[53]Bauer PW, MacDonald CB, Cox LC. Intratympanic gentamicin therapy for vertigo in nonserviceable ears. American Journal of Otolaryngology. 2001;**22**:111-115

[54]Sajjadi H, Paparella MM. Meniere's disease. Lancet. 2008;**372**:406-414

[55]Marzo SJ, Leonetti JP. Intratympanic gentamicin therapy for persistent vertigo after endolymphatic sac surgery. Otolaryngology—Head and Neck Surgery. 2002;**126**:31-33

[56]Prezant TR, Agapian JV, Bohlman MC, Bu X, Oztas S, Qiu WQ , et al. Mitochondrial ribosomal RNA mutation associated with both antibiotic-induced and non-syndromic deafness. Nature Genetics. 1993;**4**:289-294

[57]Liu YC, Chi FH, Yang TH, Liu TC. Assessment of complications due to intratympanic injections. World Journal of Otorhinolaryngology—Head and Neck Surgery. 2016;**2**:13-16

13

A Randomized Trial of Chinese Diaoshi Jifa on Treatment of Dizziness in Meniere's Disease

Yong-Xin Sun,[1] Yuan Wang,[1] Xunming Ji,[2] Xiaoguang Wu,[3] Yong Zhao,[4] Yuchuan Ding,[5] Mohammed Hussain,[5] Fei Yu,[1] Wenbo Zhao,[1] and Jianping Jia[1]

[1]Department of Neurology, Xuan Wu Hospital of Capital Medical University, Beijing 100053, China

[2]Department of Neurosurgery, Xuan Wu Hospital of Capital Medical University, Beijing 100053, China

[3]Evidence-Based Medicine Center, Xuan Wu Hospital of Capital Medical University, Beijing 100053, China

[4]Department of Neurology, Wangjing Hospital, China Academy of Chinese Medical Sciences, Beijing 100102, China

[5]Department of Neurological Surgery, Wayne State University School of Medicine, Detroit, MI 48201, USA

Correspondence should be addressed to Jianping Jia; jjp@ccmu.edu.cn

Academic Editor: Vernon A. Barnes

ABSTRACT

Background. Meniere's disease is characterized by refractory dizziness and hearing disturbance. We aimed to investigate the efficacy and tolerance of Diaoshi Jifa, a Chinese hand skill for treating dizziness in Meniere's disease. Methods. An open-labeled, randomized, controlled intervention trial was conducted. Twenty-seven patients diagnosed with Meniere's disease were randomly allocated to control group or experimental group. Both groups were assessed by DHI (dizziness handicap inventory (DHI)) questionnaire score before and within 24 hours of receiving treatment, respectively. Results. Twenty-six participants completed the study, and no adverse event was reported due to Diaoshi Jifa treatment. The difference in the DHI scores between baseline and posttreatment reached significant difference in both groups (63.88 ± 19.94 versus 10.25 ± 9.77 and 54.36 ± 17.97 versus 49.6 ± 20.50). Significant difference in DHI scores was observed between the two groups after treatment (10.25 ± 9.77 versus 49.6 ± 20.50). Further investigation of DHI subscales in the experimental group revealed significant improvement posttreatment in the physical domain, functional domain, and emotional domain. Although higher rate of improvement in the emotional domain compared to physical or functional domains was found, the difference was not statistically significant. Conclusions. Diaoshi Jifa might be a fast, effective, and well-tolerated method for alleviating dizziness in Meniere's disease.

INTRODUCTION

Meniere's disease is one of the major causes of dizziness syndrome of a peripheral vestibular origin. It is characterized by "recurrent, episodic vertigo associated with hearing fluctuation, hearing loss, aural fullness and tinnitus" [1]. Although Meniere's disease has been attributed to increased pressure within the endolymphatic system [2], the pathophysiology is still controversial [3]. As of now there is no effective medication that can completely treat Meniere's disease.

Diaoshi Jifa is a traditional Chinese approach to treat dizziness arising from various causes. Initiated by Dr. Diao, Diaoshi Jifa has been practiced in China for over 50 years with numerous patients reporting significant improvement in dizziness [4]. Diaoshi Jifa has an advantage of easy application, fast action, and good patient compliance. Although well accepted by the Chinese and widely practiced in traditional medicine, Diaoshi Jifa has not been objectively tested yet with well-designed clinical trials.

The aim of this randomized clinical trial was to examine the effectiveness and tolerance of Diaoshi Jifa in alleviating dizziness symptoms associated with Meniere's disease.

Methods

Study Design. This study was an open-labeled, randomized, and controlled intervention trial conducted at out-patient clinics of neurology and otorhinolaryngology in the Xuan Wu Hospital of Capital Medical University from January to November 2011. The study protocol was approved by the Ethical Review Board of Xuan Wu Hospital. All participants enrolled in the study signed the informed consent.

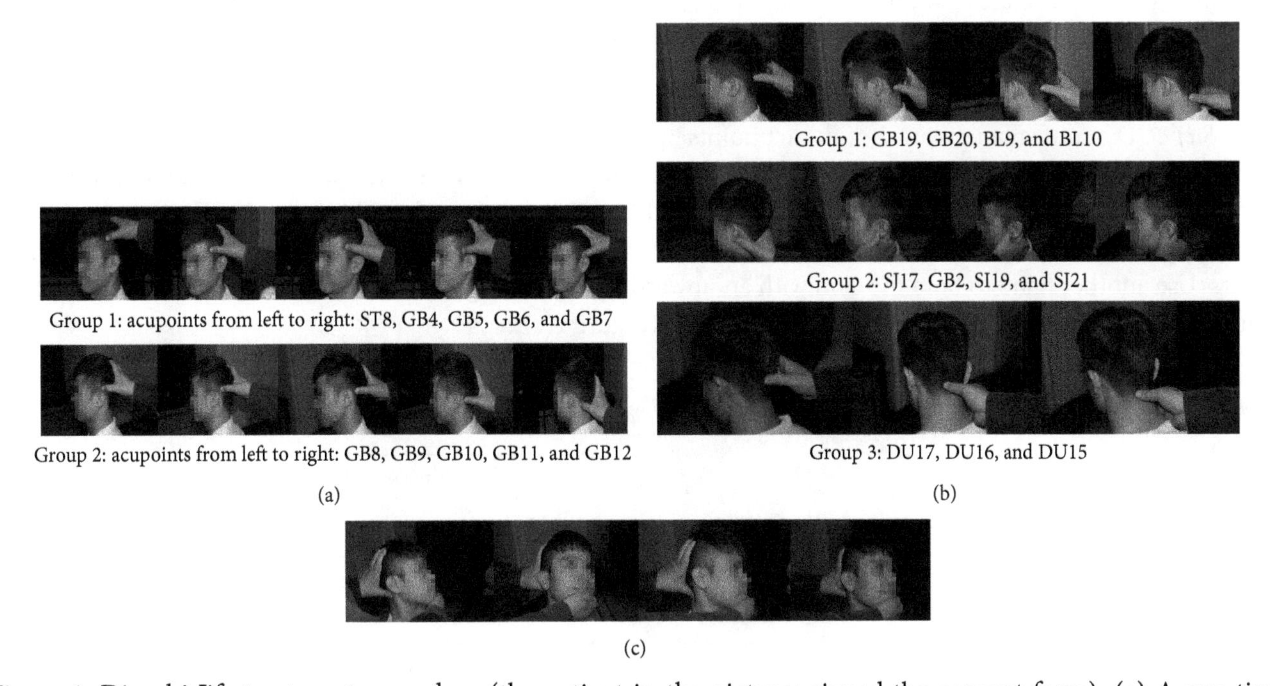

Figure 1: Diaoshi Jifa treatment procedure (the patient in the pictures signed the consent form). (a) A one-time finger press of the provided acupoints in sequence and repetition of the aforementioned motion 3 to 5 times. (b) Massaging of the acupoints clockwise for 3 cycles involving the provided sequence and repeating the sequence 3–5 times. (c) Dynamic manipulation of the acupuncture points in a two-step manner. Use thumb of one hand to press the acupoints "Wan Gu" GB12 (a) and "Tian Zhu" BL10 (b) and support the head with the other 4 fingers. Use the other hand to hold the chin 15° upward. Slightly rotate the head with both hands 2 to 3 times. One should feel the thumb move in the acupoint zones.

Study Participants. Subjects complaining of general dizziness, aged between 20 and 70 years, gave consent at the outpatient clinic and were then screened for inclusion criteria (meeting the American Academy of Otolaryngology-Head and Neck Surgery Committee on Hearing and Equilibrium criteria for probable Meniere's disease entailing a "washout period" of at least 5 days of any prior treatment before enrollment) [5] and exclusion criteria (illness of other systems that is not appropriate for manual treatment). A professional team consisting of 4 neurologists and 1 otolaryngologist performed physical examinations and prescribed pure tone audiometry and brain magnetic resonance imaging (MRI) for all subjects for the purpose of establishing a diagnosis or differential diagnosis. We collected the baseline characteristics of the participants, including sex, age, recurrent vertigo, family history, injury history, and smoking history.

Intervention. Participants in the control group received intravenous Ginkgo Injection (Ginkgo 20 mg, Beijing Double-Crane Pharmaceutical Business Co., Ltd., China) of 20 mL once a day and oral betahistine mesylate tablet (Merislon, Eisai Co., Ltd., China) of 6 mg 3 times a day. Participants in the experimental group received Diaoshi Jifa treatment, followed by the medicinal regimen identical to that used in the control group.

Diaoshi Jifa treatment consists of 3 major procedures: finger press of the acupuncture points, massage of the acupuncture points, and dynamic manipulation of the acupuncture points.

Step 1. A one-time finger press of the following acupoints in sequence and repetition of the aforementioned motion 3 to 5 times. (1) Press the first group of acupoints: from ST8 to GB4, GB5, GB6, and GB7. (2) Press the second group of acupoints: from GB8 to GB9, GB10, GB11, and GB12 (Figure 1(a)).

Step 2. Massage the acupoints clockwise for 3 cycles involving the following sequence and repeat the sequence 3–5 times. (1) Massage the first group of acupoints: from GB19 to GB20, BL9, and BL10. (2) Massage the second group of acupoints: from SJ17 to GB2, SI19, and SJ21. (3) Massage the third group of acupoints: from DU17 to DU16 and DU15 (Figure 1(b)).

Step 3. Dynamic manipulation of the acupoints ina two-step manner is as follows. (1) Use thumb of one hand to press the "Wan Gu" GB12 and support the head with the other 4 fingers. Use another hand to hold the chin with a tilt of 15° upward. Slightly rotate the head with both hands 2 to 3 times. One should feel the thumb move in the zone of the acupoint. (2) Use the thumb of one hand to press the "Tian Zhu" BL10 and support the head with the other 4 fingers. Use another hand to hold the chin with an upward tilt of 15°. Slightly rotate the head with both hands 2 to 3 times. One should feel the thumb move in the acupoint (Figure 1(c)).

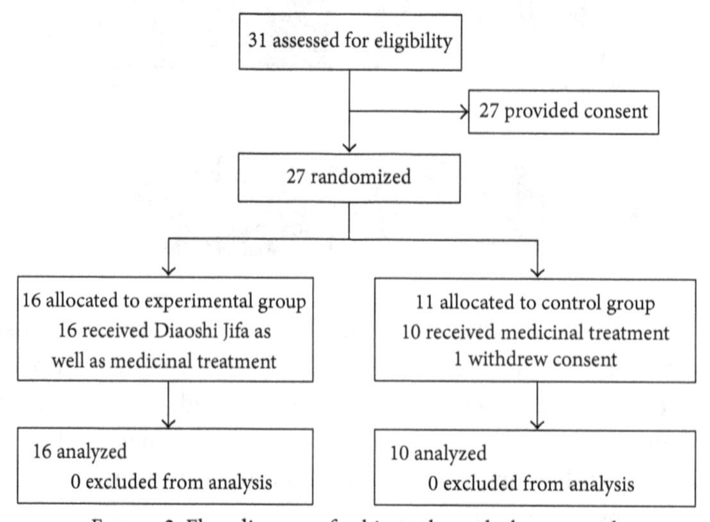

FIGURE 2: Flow diagram of subjects through the protocol.

Figure 2: Flow diagram of subjects through the protocol.

Outcome Measures and Quality Assurance Procedure. Participants were objectively assessed for dizziness by the dizziness handicap inventory (DHI) after randomization into either the experimental or control group [6]. DHI contains 25 items with a total score of 100 points (4 points for each item). Higher scores correlate with more severity of a handicap [7]. The scale is comprised of a mix of questions: 7 physical, 9 functional, and 9 emotional questions. DHI was assessed again within 24 hours of the first day's treatment.

Table 1: Demographic and clinical characteristics of the study participants at baseline.

Variables	Diaoshi Jifa group (n = 16)	Control group (n = 16)	P
Female sex: number (%)	11 (68.8)	5 (45.5)	0.264
Age	50.1 ± 15.6	54.2 ± 8.7	0.356
Recurrent vertigo: number (%)	11 (68.8)	7 (63.6)	1.000
Family history: number (%)	4 (26.7)	2 (18.2)	0.942
Injury history: number (%)	6 (37.5)	2 (18.2)	0.405
Smoking history: number (%) 4 (25.0)	5 (45.5)	0.411	

Plus–minus values are means ± SD. Differences in demographic and baseline variables were tested with a one-way analysis of variance and independentsample t-tests. There were no significant between-group differences in any baseline characteristics.

Various measures were implicated for quality assurance (external quality assessment (EQA)) involving the sampling scheme which was used to determine the sample size. The EQA was conducted by experts including statisticians from the Chinese Center for Disease Control and Prevention (CDC), Ethical Review Board Member from Xuan Wu Hospital, and clinicians from the Department of Neurology, Xuan Wu Hospital and Dongzhimen Traditional Chinese Hospital. Sampling for EQA was performed before, during, and at the end of the study, with each assessment meeting the quality standard. The information recorded by the interviewer was checked at the end of the study to ensure completeness. It was completed and met the quality standards.

Statistical Analysis. Statistical analysis was performed using SPSS 17.0 package. Between-group differences in demographic and baseline variables were tested using a one-way analysis of variance and independent-sample t-tests. Intervention effects after treatment were compared by means of independent-sample t-tests and paired t-tests (with 95% confidence intervals (CI)). Independent-sample t-tests were used to compare between experimental and control groups, and paired t-tests were used to examine within-group changes from baseline to posttreatment. The changes included the means of total DHI scores and three subscale scores. Subscale score changes were compared within the experimental group by means of change rate comparison: (posttreatment score − pretreatment score)/ pretreatment score × 100%. A two-sided P value of less than 0.05 was considered statistically significant.

Results

Twenty-seven subjects were enrolled and randomized in the study to receive either the medicinal treatment (control group) or Diaoshi Jifa in addition to medicinal treatment (experimental group). One participant in the control group voluntarily terminated his enrollment in the study before treatment started, leaving 26 participants. The flow of participants is illustrated in Figure 2.

Baseline Characteristics of the Participants. Table 1 shows the baseline data of the 27 participants. There were no significant differences seen in the baseline demographic variables between the experimental and control group.

Primary Outcomes. Table 2 shows the DHI evaluation data in the 26 participants before and after treatment application. The baseline DHI score was 63.88 ± 19.94 for the experimental group and 54.36 ± 17.97 for the control group, and there were no significant diff rences between the two groups ($P = 0.217$). In the experimental group, DHI score changed dramatically from 63.88±19.94 at baseline to 10.25±9.77 after application of both medicinal and Diaoshi Jifa treatments ($P < 0.001$); in the control group, the change in the DHI scores was less dramatic on comparing scores before and after medicinal treatment alone (54.36 ± 17.97 versus 49.6 ± 20.50, $P = 0.029$). On comparison of the DHI scores posttreatment, scores differed significantly between the two groups (49.6 ± 20.50 for the control group versus 10.25 ± 9.77 for the Diaoshi Jifa group). We further evaluated substratified scale scores in both groups, as shown in Table 3.

Table 2: Changes in dizziness handicap inventory (DHI) score in the participants.

DHI score	Diaoshi Jifa group ($N = 16$)	Control group ($N = 10$)	Between-group difference (95% CI)	P
Baseline	63.88 ± 19.94	54.36 ± 17.97	−9.51 (−24.98, 5.96)	0.217
After treatment	10.25 ± 9.77	49.6 ± 20.50	39.35 (24.20, 54.50)	<0.001*
Within-group difference (95% CI)	−53.63 (−42.87, −64.38)	−6.80 (−0.87, −12.73)		
P	<0.001**	0.029**		

Plus–minus values are means ± SD. The paired t-test was used for within-group comparison, while independent t-test was used for between-group difference. *Significantly different from the control group ($P < 0.01$). **Significantly different from the baseline ($P < 0.05$).

Table 3: Changes in dizziness handicap inventory (DHI) subscale scores in the participants.

DHI subscale scores	Diaoshi Jifa group ($N = 16$)	Control group ($N = 10$)	Between-group difference (95% CI)	P
Physical subscale (maximum 28 points)				
Baseline	19.13 ± 8.67	16.80 ± 8.60	−2.33 (−4.87, 9.52)	0.511
After treatment	2.25 ± 2.91	14.20 ± 8.30	11.95 (5.91, 17.99)	0.001*
Within-group difference (95% CI)	−16.88 (−12.35, −21.40)	−2.6 (−0.84, 6.04)		
P	<0.001**	0.122		
Functional subscale (maximum 36 points)				
Baseline	25.63 ± 8.17	23.00 ± 7.07	−2.63 (−3.84, 9.10)	0.411
After treatment	6.50 ± 5.90	21.20 ± 7.67	14.7 (9.19, 20.21)	<0.001*
Within-group difference (95% CI)	−19.13 (−14.41, −23.84)	−1.8 (−0.16, 3.76)		
P	<0.001**	0.068		
Emotional subscale (maximum 36 points)				
Baseline	19.13 ± 8.70	16.60 ± 8.75	−2.53 (−4.73, 9.78)	0.479
After treatment	1.50 ± 3.46	14.20 ± 9.97	12.7 (6.15, 19.25)	0.001*
Within-group difference (95% CI)	−17.63 (−13.36, −21.89)	−2.4 (−0.82, 5.62)		
P	<0.001**	0.126		

Plus–minus values are means ± SD. The paired t-test was used for within-group comparison, while independent t-test was used for between-group difference. Subscale score changes were compared within the experimental group by means of change rate comparison. *Significantly different from the control group ($P < 0.05$). **Significantly different from the baseline ($P < 0.05$).

Participants in the Diaoshi Jifa group showed significant improvement after treatment in physical domain (2.25 ± 2.91 versus 19.13 ± 8.67, $P < 0.001$), functional domain (6.50 ± 5.90 versus 25.63 ± 8.17, $P < 0.001$), and emotional domain (1.50 ± 3.46 versus 19.13 ± 8.70, $P < 0.001$). In contrast, participants in the control group showed no significant changes in DHI subscale scores in either physical domain ($P = 0.122$), functional domain ($P = 0.068$), or emotional domain ($P = 0.126$). Between-group analysis showed no significant difference between Diaoshi Jifa group and control group at baseline in any of the 3 subscales ($P = 0.511$ for physical domain, $P = 0.411$ for functional domain, and $P = 0.479$ for emotional domain, resp.). In contrast, posttreatment comparison of the subscale scores between the experimental and control group showed a significant difference in physical domain ($P = 0.001$), functional domain ($P < 0.001$), and emotional domain ($P = 0.001$), respectively.

An additional analysis was conducted to determine whether participants within the Diaoshi Jifa group had similar improvement in the 3 subscales of DHI after treatment. As shown in Figure 3, the absolute value of DHI score change rate was 88.3% for physical domain, 74.7% for functional domain, and 92.2% for emotional domain. Although the emotional domain was most affected by the treatment in the Diaoshi Jifa group when compared to the physical and functional domains, the difference was nevertheless statistically insignificant.

Discussion

This randomized, controlled trial shows that Diaoshi Jifa has a beneficial effect on alleviating dizziness in patients with Meniere's disease. It was seen that participants in control and experimental groups at baseline had similar DHI scores. After one day of treatment, patients in the experimental group showed significant improvement in DHI scoring, whilst a marginal improvement was seen in the control group. There was a significant difference in DHI scores between the experimental group and the control group within 24 hours after the first day's treatment. All the 16 participants in the experimental group completed the entire study and no adverse events were reported, validating the safety and good compliance of Diaoshi Jifa treatment for dizziness in patients with Meniere's disease.

Meniere's disease is a complex syndrome that originates from the inner ear; however, its etiology and pathophysiology remain controversial. Endolymphatic hydrops, endocrine dysfunction, congenital abnormalities, and psychosomatic factors have all been proposed to cause Meniere's disease, but an effective treatment to this condition still eludes [8]. From a long-term perspective Meniere's disease holds devastating consequences when it comes to hearing ability [9]. Each episode is rather self-limited and medicinal treatment such as betahistine and *Ginkgo biloba* has shown to have ambivalent results in alleviating dizziness [10]. Therefore we decided to evaluate the effectiveness of first-time application of Diaoshi Jifa over a short period (24 hours) of time.

Diaoshi Jifa stems from traditional Chinese approach to treat dizziness in patients with chronic disorders of multiple etiologies. Innovated by Dr. Diao, the method has been in practice in China for over 50 years. The principle theory explaining the effectiveness of Diaoshi Jifa stems from its ability to reconstitute a neurovascular response in the cervical and scapular areas based on muscle relaxation and acupuncture point manipulation [4]. Our data validated the effectiveness of Diaoshi Jifa by rapidly relieving dizziness in patients with Meniere's disease.

The self-perceived handicap in Meniere's disease patients was evaluated by 3 subscales of DHI: physical, functional, and emotional domains. In addition to the overall improvement in DHI scores, participants in the Diaoshi Jifa group showed significant improvement in each subscale after receiving treatment ($P \leq 0.001$ for all subscales). Though not statistically significant, emotional subscale had the greatest score change rate compared to the physical and functional subscales (−92.2% versus −88.3% and −74.7%, $P > 0.5$). In fact, after treatment with Diaoshi Jifa, most participants claimed to have felt a more relaxed feeling, especially in the cervical and scapular muscles, in addition to a clear mind and even better visual acuity. Jacobson and Newman [6], in their article of the development of 25-item DHI, reported that, although the overall internal reliability value (Cronbach's α coefficient) was rather high (0.89), the emotional subscale had the lowest Cronbach α coefficient (0.72 versus 0.78 for physical subscale and 0.85 for functional subscale). Emotional subscale was also affected significantly by the frequency of dizziness episodes [11]. Compared with the relatively objective questions listed in the physical subscale, subjects tended to respond variably to questions in the emotional subscale such as "Because of your problem, do you feel frustrated?" These results were in accordance with the widely reported psychosomatic property of Meniere's disease [12].

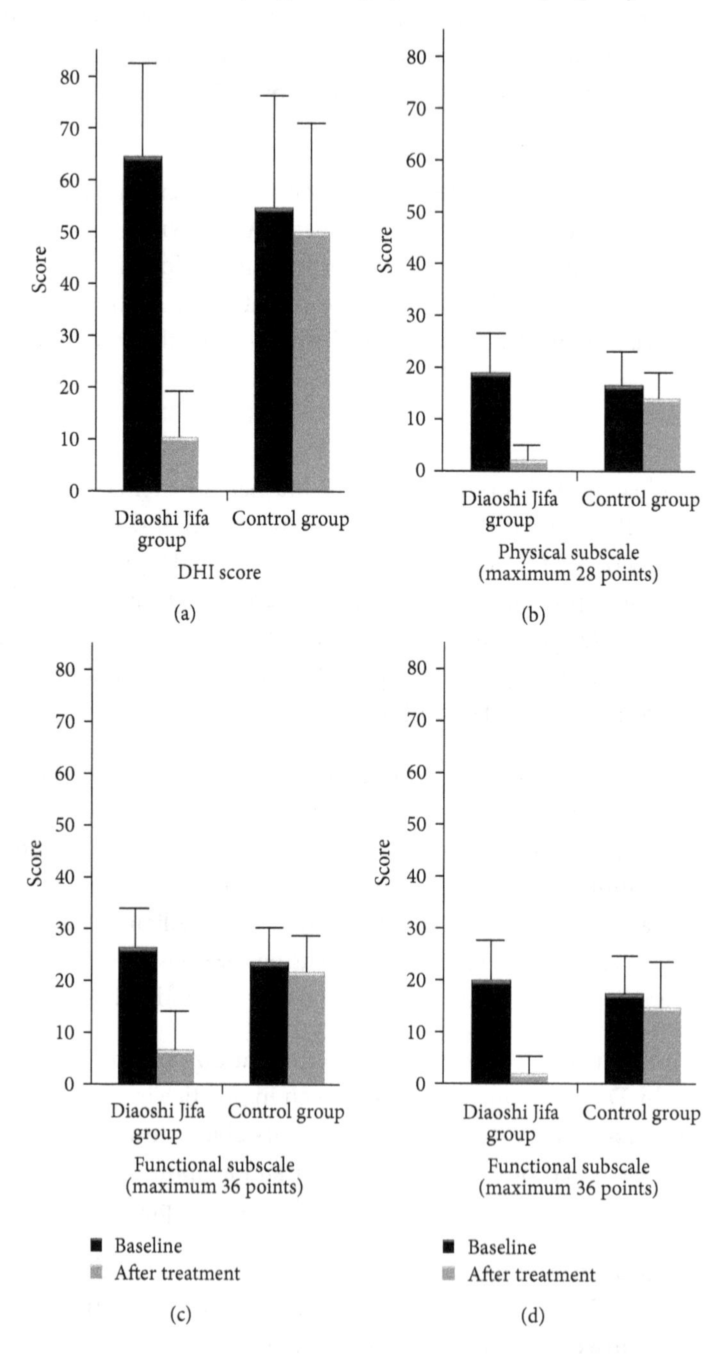

Figure 3: The DHI scores and the three subscale scores. In the Diaoshi Jifa group, the change rate was 88.3% for physical subscale, 74.7% for functional subscale, and 92.2% for emotional subscale.

The present study has some limitations. Firstly, the openlabeled property of the clinical trial made those patients who seek traditional Chinese medications more predisposed to enrolling, thus contributing towards a selection bias. Secondly, this study was designed to be conducted in a single clinical center instead of a multicenter clinical trial. The reason is attributed to Dr. Diao, being the innovator of Diaoshi Jifa, ensuring a homogenous manipulation to assess preliminary analysis of treatment effect and thus restricting the study to a single center to overlook a proper execution of the manipulation techniques. Thirdly, our study focused only on the short-term effectiveness of Diaoshi Jifa (within 24 hours after one-time treatment). Though positive results were seen rapidly by Diaoshi Jifa, it should be noted that patients usually get symptomatic alleviation after several days of initiating Meniere's disease medications.

In conclusion, our preliminary data showed that Diaoshi Jifa (a traditional Chinese approach) combined with medical regimen was effective in relieving dizziness symptoms in patients with Meniere's disease. In a short period of time (within 24 hours), patients showed symptomatic relief both functionally and emotionally from the treatment. The advantage of a relatively fast effect in addition to its safety makes Diaoshi Jifa a viable alternative to conventional medical treatment for Meniere's disease. Multicentered trial assessing its effectiveness on a larger scale is warranted.

Disclosure

Yuan Wang is the co-first author.

Acknowledgments

This work was partially supported by the Traditional Chinese Medicine Project (JJT2010-22) of Capital Medical Development Foundation, Beijing Outstanding Talents Cultivation Fund (2012D005018000007), and the High-Level Health Techonology Talent Construction Programme of Beijing Municiple Health Bureau (2013-3-092).

References

[1] E. M. Monsell, "New and revised reporting guidelines from the Committee on Hearing and equilibrium," *Otolaryngology— Head and Neck Surgery*, vol. 113, pp. 176–178, 1995.

[2] M. Kato, M. Sugiura, M. Shimono, T. Yoshida, H. Otake, K. Kato et al., "Endolymphatic hydrops revealed by magnetic resonance imaging in patients with atypical Meniere's disease," *Acta Otolaryngologica*, vol. 133, no. 2, pp. 123–129, 2013.

[3] I. Syed and C. Aldren, "Meniere's disease: an evidence based approach to assessment and management," *International Journal of Clinical Practice*, vol. 66, no. 2, pp. 166–170, 2012.

[4] Q. Dong, "Diaoshi Jifa and Dizziness," *China Healthcare & Nutrition*, vol. 8, pp. 120–121, 2009.

[5] E. M. Monsell, "Committee on Hearing and Equilibrium guidelines for the diagnosis and evaluation of therapy in Meniere's disease," *Otolaryngology—Head and Neck Surgery*, vol. 113, no. 3, pp. 181–185, 1995.

[6] G. P. Jacobson and C. W. Newman, "The development of the dizziness handicap inventory," *Archives of Otolaryngology—Head and Neck Surgery*, vol. 116, no. 4, pp. 424–427, 1990.

[7] J. Treleaven, "Dizziness handicap inventory (DHI)," *Australian Journal of Physiotherapy*, vol. 52, no. 1, article 67, 2006.

[8] W. P. R. Gibson, "Hypothetical mechanism for vertigo in meniere's disease," *Otolaryngologic Clinics of North America*, vol. 43, no. 5, pp. 1019–1027, 2010.

[9] S. S. Da Costa, L. C. A. De Sousa, and M. R. De Toledo Piza, "Meniere's disease: overview, epidemiology, and natural history," *Otolaryngologic Clinics of North America*, vol. 35, no. 3, pp. 455–495, 2002.

[10] M. M. Gananc¸a, H. H. Caovilla, M. S. L. Munhoz et al., "Optimizing the pharmacological component of integrated balance therapy," *Brazilian Journal of Otorhinolaryngology*, vol. 73, no. 1, pp. 12–18, 2007.

[11] P. Wu, H. Wang, and Z. Wu, "The assessment of anxiety and depression state in Meniere's disease patients," *Lin Chuang Er Bi Yan Hou Tou Jing Wai Ke Za Zhi*, vol. 26, pp. 516–518, 2012.

[12] S. E. Kirby and L. Yardley, "Understanding psychological distress in Me´nie`re's disease: a systematic review," *Psychology, Health and Medicine*, vol. 13, no. 3, pp. 257–273, 2008.

14

Meniere's Disease: Nonsurgical Treatment

Yetkin Zeki Yilmaz*, Begum Bahar Yilmaz and Aysegul Batioglu-Karaaltın

Istanbul University-Cerrahpasa Medical Faculty ENT, Istanbul, Turkey

*Address all correspondence to: dr_yzy@hotmail.com

ABSTRACT

Meniere's disease or syndrome is one of the most common inner ear diseases. Meniere's disease is characterized by episodic vertigo, sensorineural hearing loss that fluctuates during episodes, tinnitus, and ear fullness. Ideal treatment should stop vertigo attacks, restore hearing, get rid of tinnitus and ear fullness. Treatment options are decided upon the remaining hearing, severity, and intensity of vertigo attacks. Meniere's disease is progressive on hearing levels of the patient; some of them develop profound hearing loss that also could affect the other ear. In order to plan a treatment scheme for patient, these conditions should be assessed. It has a destructive and progressive nature, so the first step of treatment should contain more conservative treatment options. If symptom control could not be obtained, destructive treatment options should be considered.

Keywords: Meniere's disease, lifestyle changes, Meniett, vestibular rehabilitation, neuro-otology

INTRODUCTION

Meniere's disease was first described by Prosper Meniere in 1861 [1]. He described series of symptoms of a leukemic patient, and he suggested that vertiginous symptoms were caused by hemorrhage in the inner ear [2]. Knapp hypothesized inner ear hydrops, but its histologic confirmation was demonstrated in 1938 [3]. Still today, Meniere's disease etiology is not clear.

Meniere's disease is characterized by episodic vertigo, sensorineural hearing loss that fluctuates during episodes, tinnitus, and ear fullness. Some of the patients develop drop attacks called Tumarkin crisis, also known as otolithic crisis, and nausea [4, 5].

Meniere's disease or syndrome is one of the most common inner ear diseases. Its prevalence reported 3.5–513 per 100,000 in USA series [6]. It shows slightly female predominance 1.89:1 [7]. It is more common in white and older population; peak age is in the fourth and fifth decade but some early onset cases in children are reported [8, 9].

Meniere's usually starts in one ear, but bilateral disease is not uncommon. It may occur many years after the unilateral symptoms first started. Its prevalence is unclear and reported from 2 to 78% [9]. Familial Meniere's disease has been reported in 10–20% of cases [10]. Meniere's disease is strongly associated with Meniere's disease so as allergies.

Till this day, an effective treatment protocol is not established, because the pathogenesis of Meniere's disease is not clear.

Pathogenesis

Most common histopathologic finding is "endolymphatic hydrops" but the exact pathology is unknown. The Committee on Hearing and Equilibrium of American Academy of Otolaryngology Head and Neck Surgery's (AAO-HNS) definition of certain Meniere's disease contains histopathologial confirmation of endolymphatic hydrops [11].

Endolymph is produced by stria vascularis in the cochlea and by the dark cells in the vestibular labyrinth [12]. In autopsy studies, endolymphatic hydrops was observed in the temporal bones of patients who were diagnosed Meniere's disease, but not all individuals who had endolymphatic hydrops developed Meniere's disease symptoms [13, 14]. Perisaccular fibrosis and decreased endolymphatic duct size are observed in some of the patients. The CT images showed that individuals have hypoplastic endolymphatic sac and duct and inadequate periaqueductal pneumatization [15]. MRI studies showed that patients with Meniere's disease have significantly smaller and shorter drainage system [16]. After gadolinium enhancement, enhancement of endolymphatic sac and periventricular space was demonstrated in MRI [17, 18]. Nakashima et al. designed a study to demonstrate endolymphatic hydrops in Meniere's disease in 3 Tesla MRI. Gadolinium was injected transtympanically and MR images were taken a day after. They observed that the gadolinium moves first into the perilymphatic space and that can reveal the border between endolymph and perilymph. They successfully showed the endolymphatic hydrops in these patients [19]. Naganawa et al. study demonstrated same results with 1.5 Tesla MRI after intravenous administration of gadolinium. They reported their waiting time is much shorter (4 hours after contrast enhancement) and 95% success rate, while the intratympanic gadolinium method's rate of success is reported as 80–90% [20]. Imaging is also important as it helps in differential diagnosis of the other cases that could cause unilateral hearing loss, vertigo such as vestibular schwannoma.

It is hypothesized that the ruptures of membranous labyrinth and cicatrization in healing process could cause the drain blockage that leads to endolymphatic hydrops [21, 22]. Schuknect explained that, the ruptures of membranous labyrinth cause the leakage of potassium enriched endolymph to perilymph depolarize the nerve cells. Acute inactivation results with hearing loss and vertigo, after healing process of the chemical distribution of ions normalize; so the effects are reversible. Since the Meniere's disease takes its course through lifetime, the effects on the inner ear is irreversible at some point, so the hearing loss is permanent and vertigo attacks subdue [23]. However, this theory is not accepted by all; some authors suggested that ruptures are occurred rarely and not adequate to explain all the symptoms [24].

Etiology

Meniere's syndrome is the triad; fluctuating hearing loss, tinnitus, and episodes of vertigo; if the cause is unknown it is defined as Meniere's disease [25]. In experimental studies, the blockage of endolymphatic duct and its lead to endolymphatic hydrops is shown in animals. In order to create this, mechanical blockage, viral inoculation, and immune response-induced inflammation are used [26].

Some of the studies suggested that allergy and Meniere's disease could be linked. Derebery et al. studied patients who were diagnosed with Meniere's disease. The skin prick test results were positive of 41% of these patients, which were three times higher than general population [27]. Some mechanisms were proposed in order to explain the link between allergy and Meniere's disease.

1. The fenestrated blood vessels that are located in endolymphatic sac allow the antigen to enter that leads to mast cell degranulation. Inflammation around the perisaccular fibrous tissue and

release of histamine cause vasodilatation and increase the secretion that causes endolymphatic sac resorption capacity over rules.

2. Immune complexes that enter the endolymphatic sac circulation through this fenestrated vessels start inflammation and increase vascular permeability.

3. Waldeyer's ring stimulated by viral antigens triggers T-cell migration to endolymphatic sac and leads to inflammation and excession of fluid production [28].

In order to demonstrate this relationship, Derebery et al. investigated the effects of allergen immunotherapy and elimination of food allergens in Meniere's disease patients. Their results were surprisingly positive. They reported that the improvement of symptoms of Meniere's disease and allergic symptoms were significant [29].

Another mechanism that is suggested is viral infection; however, no specific virus is identified [30].

Ischemia is another factor that is suggested in Meniere's disease mechanism [31]. Migraine and Meniere's disease link by vascular mechanism [32].

Diagnosis

In order to plan a treatment algorithm for Meniere's disease, it is important to diagnose it accurately. Diagnostic investigation is not bound to only one test result. The Committee on Hearing and Equilibrium of the AAO-HNS has described the symptoms. As per AAO-HNS, the major symptoms of Meniere's disease are vertigo, hearing loss, and tinnitus [11].

Vertigo

Spontaneous, rotational vertigo that last at least 20 minutes accompanied usually with nausea and vomiting which are the definitive spells of Meniere's disease. During the spell, horizontal or horizontal rotatory nystagmus is observed.

Hearing loss

Fluctuating hearing loss, commonly in low frequencies, is the most common audiological finding. In some cases, hearing loss is progressive and is usually unilateral.

Hearing loss is described as:

- The arithmetic mean of hearing thresholds of 250, 500, and 1000 Hz which is 15 dB or higher than the average of 1000, 2000, and 3000 Hz; or,
- Average threshold of 500, 1000, 2000, and 3000 Hz which is 20 dB or higher in poorer ear in unilateral cases; or
- Average threshold of 500, 1000, 2000, and 3000 Hz which is higher than 25 dB in bilateral cases.

About 10 dB change or more or 15% or more change in speech discrimination rate is considered clinically significant.

One of the prognostic factors that affects hearing function is duration of the disease [33]. It is documented by most of the authors [34–36]. Age is also an independent prognostic factor to determine hearing function and its responsiveness to medical treatment [37].

Tinnitus and aural fullness

It could be confirmed with the patients' history. Tinnitus is commonly of a

low-frequency type [38]. Sometimes, patients describe it to be localized in affected ear or sense it in the whole head. Patients describe tinnitus differently from each other [39].

Clinical presentation

The initial symptom of Meniere's disease can be vertigo (37%), tinnitus (18%), fluctuating hearing loss (20%), or any combination of these. Only 25% of cases start with all of these symptoms [40].

Most of the patients describe recurrent vertigo attacks (96.2%) with tinnitus (91.1%) and ipsilateral hearing loss (87.7%) [41]. Most of the crippling symptom is vertigo. In an acute attack, it tends to stay 20 minutes to 24 hours [42].

The beginning of the Meniere's disease differs from patient to patient as well as the course of the disease. It is found that vertigo stops in 57% of the patients in 2 years and 71% of the cases in 8.3 years after the first onset [43].

Detailed clinical history should be taken as the first and most important step for diagnosis. Most of the distressing symptom is vertigo. It is usually present in horizontal axis, accompanied with nausea and vomiting. During this attack, horizontal or horizontal rotatory nystagmus could be observed.

Some of the patients could describe sudden drop attacks which were described by Tumarkin, and this symptom is named after him also called otolithic crisis of Tumarkin. This symptom is caused by utriculosaccular dysfunction [44]. Sudden changes in vertical gravity reference cause postural adjustments via vestibulospinal pathway and end up with sudden fall [45]. About 2–6% of patients with Meniere's disease were reported to experience drop attack [46].

Second common symptom is hearing loss usually accompanied with tinnitus and ear fullness sensation. Hearing loss is fluctuating, most in low frequencies and tends to be progressive; however, only 1–2% of patients end up with profound hearing loss [47]. Additionally, 43.6% of the patients have different perception of hearing between ears (diplacusis) and 56% recruitment [25].

Tinnitus description could be different between patients but it is usually nonpulsatile and could be continuous or appears only during the attack, or could get worse during the attacks.

The AAO-HNS Committee on Hearing and Equilibrium suggested staged diagnosis for Meniere's disease. They suggested to group patients in the order of their symptoms as possible, probable, definite, and certain Meniere's disease [11] (**Table 1**).

Possible Meniere's disease	• Episodic vertigo without documented hearing loss, or • *Sensor*ineural hearing loss (fluctuating or flat) with disequilibrium but *without definitive vertigo attacks*
Probable Meniere's disease	• One definite vertigo episode • Documented hearing loss at least once • Tinnitus or ear fullness
Definite Meniere's disease	• Two or more definite vertigo attacks lasted at least 20 minutes • Documented hearing loss at least one • Tinnitus or ear fullness
Certain Meniere's disease	• Definite Meniere's disease • Histopathological confirmation of endolymphatic hydrops

Table 1. *Diagnosis of Meniere's disease.*

Probable Meniere's disease	• Two or more spontaneous episodes of vertigo (each lasts 20 minutes to 24 hours) • Fluctuating aural symptoms on the affected ear (tinnitus, hearing loss, or aural fullness) • Other vestibular diseases were excluded
Definite Meniere's disease	• Two or more spontaneous episodes of vertigo (each lasts 20 minutes to 12 hours) • Lowto mid-frequency sensorineural hearing loss in affected ear (documented with audiometry) at least on one occasion (before, during, or after the vertigo episode) • Fluctuating aural symptoms on the affected ear (tinnitus, hearing loss, or aural fullness) • Other vestibular diseases were excluded

Table 2. *Amended 2015 criteria for diagnosis of Meniere's disease.*

The AAO-HNS Committee on Hearing and Equilibrium revised their diagnostic criteria in 2015. The new definition of "Definite" and "Probable" Meniere's disease is summed up in **Table 2** [48].

Diagnostic workup

To treat Meniere's disease successfully, diagnosis should be confirmed. There is not a single test exists to confirm Meniere's disease alone, so the patient should be evaluated with possible diagnostic tests.

Videonystagmography

Eye movements are observed after caloric or vestibular stimulation. Caloric response is found to decrease in 48–73.5% of the patients' affected ear, and complete absence is reported in 6–11% of patients [49, 50].

Electrocochleography

Summation potentials are larger and more negative in Meniere's disease. Most valuable ratio is summation potential/action potential. SP/AP ratio is found to be increased in Meniere's disease. However, this is not definitive, and only 62% of patients with Meniere's disease have elevated ratios [51].

Dehydrating agents

Dehydrating agent such as glycerol, urea used to reduce endolymph volume and improvement of symptoms were such as improved hearing, reduction of SP negativity in electrocochleography, trying to be observed. It is reported 60% sensitivity for Meniere's disease [52].

Vestibular evoked myopotentials

Loud clicks are used to stimulate stapedial movement in order to stimulate the saccule. Stimulation saccule triggers the pathway that relaxes sternocleidomastoid muscle. Normal ear response is recorded as 500 Hz, and affected ear's response is recorded in elevated thresholds with flattened tuning [53].

The AAO-HNS's guideline is suggested in 1995 and does not contain these diagnostic vestibular battery; it is only suggested to the use of full audiometric workup.

One of the recent guidelines for diagnosis and treatment of Meniere's disease is from French Otorhinolaryngology-Head and Neck Surgery Society (SFORL) in 2016. They describe that "definite" Meniere's disease could be diagnosed if another cause could not be described to explain the following four clinical findings;

- Two or more rotational vertigo attacks that last 2 minutes to 12 hours or, Tumarkin's crises;
- Low-frequency hearing loss on two consecutive frequencies, 30 dB or more if the other ear hearing is normal, or 35 dB or more if hearing is affected bilaterally; and
- Tinnitus or aural fullness; and
- Fluctuating otologic findings.

MRI of inner ear is suggested to rule out cerebellopontine angle or endolymphatic sac tumors, anatomic deformity, or a degenerative pathology such as multiple sclerosis that could mimic the symptoms of Meniere's disease. Also audiovestibular workup could lead the clinician to intralabyrintine pressure disorder. The workup should include at least pure-tone and speech audiometry with VNG or VEMP or VHIT [54].

Treatment

Ideal treatment should stop vertigo attacks, restore hearing, and get rid of tinnitus and ear fullness. Unfortunately, ideal treatment is absent nowadays. Our limited knowledge of pathophysiology of the disease makes it impossible to treat patients ideally. Also symptoms and course of the disease differ between patients, so treatment should be individualized.

The aim of the treatment is to reduce frequency and severity of vertigo attacks and improve hearing results [55]. All current treatment options are symptomatic.

Due to natural course of the disease, vertigo attacks of 60–80% of patients improve without any intervention [56, 57]. Patients who refused to take any medical or surgical assistance had spontaneous improvement of their symptoms at the rate of 71% [43]. Green et al. reported complete vertigo control in 50% of the patients, partial control in 28% of the patients, and only 17% of their patient needed medical treatment in their 14 years of follow-up [58].

Treatment options are decided upon the remaining hearing, severity, and intensity of vertigo attacks. Meniere's disease is progressive on hearing levels of the patient; some of them develop profound hearing loss which also could affect the other ear. In order to plan a treatment scheme for a patient, these conditions should be assessed. It has destructive and progressive nature, so the first step of treatment should contain more conservative treatment options. If symptom control could not be obtained, destructive treatment options should be considered.

AAO-HNS suggested a staging system based on a four-tone average of 500, 1000, 2000, and 3000 Hz on the worst pure-tone audiometry, and this system should be obtained to the patients who were diagnosed with "definite" or "certain" Meniere's disease (**Table 3**) [11].

International Consensus (ICON) on treatment of the Meniere's disease proposed a treatment algorithm in 2018 (**Figure 1**) [59].

ICON's proposal for treatment algorithm summarizes the logic of the treatment for Meniere's disease. When the course of the disease is considered, Meniere's disease could make the affected ear to deteriorate and also could affect the other ear at any time. Most logical approach for treatment is starting with less invasive option and assessing the patient periodically. If the suggested treatment fails, more invasive methods should be offered.

Stage	Four-tone average (dB)
I	25 or less
II	26–40
III	41–70
IV	>70

Table 3. *Staging of definite and certain Meniere's disease.*

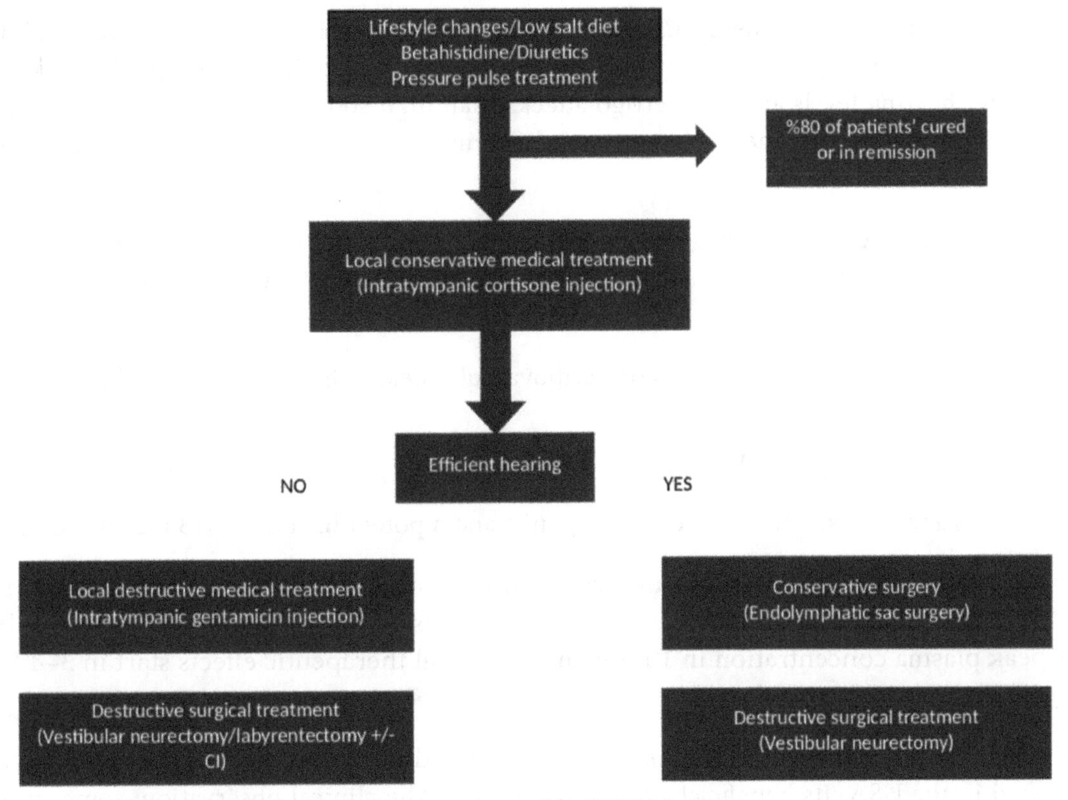

Figure 1. *Treatment algorithm of Meniere's disease proposed by ICON in 2018.*

Also in SFORL guideline of treatment, a step-by-step approach from conservative to destructive is suggested.

If a patient seeks for medical attention during vertigo attack, treatment is symptomatic. The rest of the chapter contains nonsurgical treatment options, acute attack treatment, and vestibular rehabilitation options.

Preventive treatment options

Lifestyle changes and low salt diet

The first line of treatment is to encourage the patient to change his lifestyle into a healthier one. Regulation of sleeping cycle, avoiding stress, caffeine, alcohol, and tobacco, and changing into a low salt diet should be advised [60–62]. Caffeine is accused to increase the endolymph volume due to its sympathomimetic actions, and it is suggested to be restricted to 100 mg/day by AAO-HNS [63]. More active lifestyle should be offered, like taking at least 20 minutes of walking.

Low salt diet has been suggested to Meniere's disease patients since the 1930s, where daily intake of sodium is recommended to be under 2 grams [64, 65]. Low salt intake increases serum aldosterone levels [66]. It has been found that endolymphatic sac contains receptors for mineral corticoids [67]. Aldosterone controls Na/K ATPase, thiazide-sensitive Na/Cl co-transporter, and epithelial Na channels which are also expressed on endolymphatic sac [68–73]. It has been shown that canrenoate, an aldosterone antagonist, reduced electrical potentials of endolymphatic sac after applied [74, 75]. Elevation of aldosterone levels may increase the endolymph absorption [70]. However, restriction of salt intake could not be proven to change the levels of sodium of plasma and endolymph [64, 65, 76].

In Miyashita et al.'s study, Meniere's disease patients were grouped in order to their sodium intake. After initiation of low sodium diet, patients were observed for 2 years. Low sodium group (daily intake of 3 grams or less) had better hearing levels and less vertigo attacks than high sodium group (daily intake more than 3 grams). However, serum aldosterone levels were not different although low sodium group had higher serum levels [77].

Also Tadros and colleagues investigated elder population and those who had higher serum aldosterone levels had better hearing levels, and they suggested that aldosterone might have a protective effect on hearing [78].

Low sodium intake has known benefits on cardiovascular health; hence, there is no harm to suggest it.

Betahistine

Betahistine is a weak histamine H1 receptor agonist and a potent histamine H3 receptor antagonist.

It is suggested to improve microvascular circulation in stria vascularis that reduces the endolymph pressure [79], and it inhibits vestibular nuclei activity that results longer and easier recovery [80, 81]. It reaches its peak plasma concentration in 1 hour, and maximal therapeutic effects start in 3–4 hours after intake [82].

Betahistine is a popular agent in Europe and Japan. FDA does not approve its use in vertigo as it is not commonly used in the USA. Its beneficial effects are based on the clinical observation; some studies report favorable results on vertigo control and hearing improvement and some studies do not. In betahistine's case, literature findings are controversial. In SFORL guideline, betahistine is suggested as the first line of treatment.

Tootoonchi et al. reported improvement of 6.35 dB in hearing levels after 6 months of betahistine administration [37]. However, patient's first hearing levels should be considered; if the patient has poor hearing levels at the first visit, he is less likely to benefit from the treatment [36]. Cochrane reviews support the positive effect of betahistine on vertigo attack frequency and hearing levels. They highlighted the fact that the investigated studies have serious study design flaws and tend to bias [83]. Therapeutic benefits of betahistine were reported in Nauta's meta-analysis [84].

BEMED study is a multi-central, placebo-controlled study that investigates the effects of betahistine. The results on vestibular symptoms were not any different compared to placebo [85]. In order to establish the benefits of betahistine, more well-designed, placebo-controlled studies are required.

Literature seems to be controversial but it is suggested as the first line of treatment in the European, French, and Japanese guidelines as its beneficial effects on patients are observed clinically.

Diuretics

Another treatment agent widely used for Meniere's disease treatment is diuretics. Thiazide group of diuretics is usually suggested. The cells that produce endolymph, such as dark cells and stria vascularis, contain carbonic anhydrase. Carbonic anhydrase inhibitors like acetazolamide are recommended in order to reduce the production endolymph [86].

Recent systematic review on diuretics was conducted by Crowson and colleagues. They reviewed four retrospective studies. One of the studies compared betahistine and diuretics and reported improved results on vertigo in both groups but lack of placebo group [87]. In another study, diuretics showed beneficial effects on vestibular symptoms compared to placebo [88]. Another placebo-controlled retrospective study reported beneficial effects of hydrochlorothiazide on hearing loss and vertigo control [89]. Most of the studies have low level of evidence.

Cochrane report in 2006 on diuretics reported beneficial but it highlighted the fact that most of the studies were lack of high quality of evidence [90]. However, studies indicate improvement in vertigo and lesser effect on hearing. Still they are suggested as the first line of treatment options in many guidelines.

Pulse pressure treatment

Around three decades ago, it has been reported that positive pressure to middle ear could have helped release of Meniere's disease's symptoms [91]. The underlying mechanism is still unclear. Meniett device was introduced by Medtronic company in 2000 and approved by FDA for Meniere's disease treatment. After insertion of a ventilation tube, the device is placed to external ear canal and sends low-pressure pulses.

There are many studies about Meniett's effect on Meniere's disease and symptom control. Gates et al.'s randomized controlled studies showed benefits of Meniett device in short term. They demonstrated a significant decrease of vertigo attacks in first 3 months but this could not be observed in long term [92]. Other studies reached different conclusions about Meniett.

Ahsan et al. suggested that Meniett could be useful for Meniere's disease treatment, but Syed and van Sonsbeek were unable to show this effect in their randomized controlled studies where they compared the device effect to placebo [93–95]. Recent meta-analysis reported that Meniett device provided complete remission of 52% of patients and 34% of patients had not complete but significant release of symptoms [96]. This meta-analysis also investigated the suggested treatment protocols. Initiation of Meniett after 2 weeks of ventilation tube insertion seemed to have better control over the symptoms. Effects on vertigo seem to begin in first 6 months, reach its peak in 6–18 months, and stabilize after 18 months. Also it was observed that the shorter initiation of the therapy after placement of ventilation tube had a better effect on hearing preservation and vertigo control [96].

However, some authors have different opinions when it comes to ventilation tubes. They suggest that ventilation tube insertion alone could control Meniere's disease symptoms [97–100]. In hypoxia theory, it is hypothesized that vertigo attacks are triggered by anoxia in inner ear, which can decrease endolymphatic potentials and microcirculation of cochlea [101, 102]. Ventilation tube enriches middle ear oxygenation and helps anoxic environment of inner ear [103]. Also ventilation tube decreases the middle ear pressure, and it is hypothesized that this could help to balance the increased inner ear pressure that could lead to Meniere's attack [104]. It remains inconclusive that the decrease of symptoms after Meniett device is only from the ventilation tube or ventilation tube insertion alone. However, Zhang et al.'s meta-analysis reviewed studies that compare Meniett to placebo device and reached a conclusion. They report that if the interval between ventilation tube insertion and Meniett device is longer than 2 weeks, beneficial effects may be due to Meniett device alone [96].

Recent Cochrane database reviewed Meniett device-based studies that were published until 2014. Randomized controlled trials that compare Meniett and placebo devices were included in their study. Due to heterogeneity of data, calculation of outcome was reported not possible. Most of the studies found no significant difference between Meniett and placebo on vertigo control. Only one study showed a significant vertigo control after 8 weeks of usage of Meniett. Secondary outcomes like improvement on hearing, Meniett group significantly had better outcomes with 7.38 dB increase, effects on tinnitus and aural fullness could not be determined due to heterogeneity of data. Their conclusion is that data due to these studies are not adequate to determine the beneficial effects of Meniett [95].

Long-term results of Meniett device was published by Dornhoffer et al. Treated patients' improvement rates reported 75%, similar of untreated patients [105]. University of Colorado stated that the device is expensive and lacks costbeneficiality [106].

None of the studies that investigated Meniett device reported any complications. Therefore it is harmless to propose this treatment. It is advised as the first-line treatment of ICON's guideline as well as Italian and Australian treatment algorithms [59, 95]. It is reported as the most common second-line treatment option in the USA [107]. With its potential benefits and low risk of complication rates, Meniett device could be advised to patients.

Ventilation tubes

Though it is a surgical procedure, it is minimally invasive so its effects on Meniere's disease will be discussed in this chapter. After myringotomy of the anteroinferior quadrant of tympanic membrane, ventilation tube could be inserted as an office procedure. Sugawara et al. and Montandon et al. reported that ventilation tube insertion has control over Meniere's disease symptoms without further treatment [97, 98].

Kimura and Hutta's experimental study on guinea pigs is that the middle ear ventilation reduced endolymphatic hydrops. It is hypothesized that ventilation of middle ear decreases the pressure in middle and inner ear [103].

Tumarkin was the first physician who introduced ventilation tubes as a treatment option in 1966. Tumarkin also reported that eustachian tube dysfunction is correlated with endolymphatic hydrops and his data was supported by Lall [108, 109]. However, Cinnamond, Hall, and Brackmann reported that eustachian tube dysfunction was not always observed with Meniere's disease patients and insertion of ventilation tube could worsen the symptoms of patients [110, 111].

Montadon et al. reported that complete remission or improvement rates of their patients were 82%. They also reported that the patient whose ventilation tube blocked had recurrence of symptoms and immediate relief after reinsertion of ventilation tubes [98]. Thomsen published results of patients who received transmastoid endolymphatic decompression surgery compared with patients who were inserted ventilation tube. Each group had significant control over their symptoms but found no difference between these groups [112].

Among the most recent studies in literature in 2015, Ogawa et al. studied ventilation tube insertion and its effects on intractable Meniere's disease patients. All of their patients were treated medically at least 6 months before ventilation tube insertion was advised. After a year, 20% of their patients had complete remission, 47% had partial remission. Two years later, complete vertigo control rates increased to 47%. Secondary benefits of procedure on hearing levels had no significant difference. They reported that ventilation tube insertion could be beneficial and postponed more invasive procedures [100]. Therefore, it could be advised as a first-line surgical procedure to patients who have symptoms after medical treatment.

The SFORL guideline does not recommend this procedure due to lack of evidence [54]. Not considered in ICON's guideline or the European Position Statement on diagnosis and Treatment of Meniere's disease [59, 113].

However, it is worthwhile to try because literature findings of some authors showed beneficial effects and it is minimally invasive and has low-complication rates.

Intratympanic steroid injections

Intratympanic steroid treatment will be discussed in later chapters.

Treatment of acute attacks

It is important to control the effects and related vegetative symptoms of vertigo during acute attack. Meniere's attacks are sudden onset and could last 20 minutes to 24 hours. In order to suppress the symptoms, benzodiazepines, meclizine, or other antihistamines could be used [106]. Drugs that are used to suppress the symptoms of Meniere's disease have no effect on progression of the disease.

Antihistamines, such as dimenhidrate, meclizine, benzodiazepines, and scopolamine, and anti-dopamines, which had antiemetic effects, such as metoclopramide and fenotiazines, are used to suppress the vestibular symptoms. These agents also have sedative effects that could help to reduce the patients' anxiety. Diazepam is effective on GABA receptors in vestibular nucleus and inhibits their response. It should only be used during acute attack because the long-term usage decreases vestibular compensation mechanisms. Dimenhidrate could also provide relief during acute attack but it could affect concentration and cause dizziness in long term [114].

Diazepam inhibits vestibular response with its effect on GABA-ergic receptors located in cerebellar system [115]. However, clinical and experimental studies show that the long-term usage of diazepam prolongs the vestibular compensation [116, 117].

Meclizine is useful to reduce vegetative symptoms like nausea, benzodiazepines are also well tolerated anxiolytic, in order of intractable vomiting promethazine suppositories could be used [106].

Transdermal scopolamine patches reaches therapeutic blood level 4 hours after placement and release drug to system 72 hours; however, this could not be useful because of the attacks' sudden onset nature [118].

Intravenous lidocaine has found to be effective during acute attack of Meniere's disease [119].

Vestibular rehabilitation and psychological support

Meniere's disease is a chronic attack characterized by their sudden onset. It is observed by most of the physicians that it also burdens patients psychologically. Also it is observed that stress and anxiety could trigger the attacks. Increase of vertigo severity is associated with worse quality of life scores of Meniere's disease [120]. Most of the guidelines suggest psychological support and behavioral therapy for the patients so they could have a better understanding of their condition and help themselves to cooperate with this condition.

Van Cruijsen et al. suggested that the symptoms could be worsened in negative emotional state [121]. Many studies reported the relation between symptoms and behavioral characteristics; the worse perception of the disease could create a vicious circle [122–124]. Patients suffering from Meniere's disease were found to be having more stress-causative behavioral characteristics than normal controls. This information leads to hypothesis that higher stress-related hormone levels could cause endolymphatic hydrops [124]. Another study by Van Cruijsen that assesses the psychological state of Meniere's disease patients compared to patients who had chronic vestibular diseases documented that 63% of Meniere's disease patients had psychologic pathology, such as depression or anxiety, but found no significant difference between non-Meniere's disease patients. It is also reported that Meniere's disease patients quality of life questionnaire results were worse than normal results [125].

Yokota et al. studied the treatment outcomes of both surgical and nonsurgical treatment due to patients' psychological status. Patients who had no mental distress had benefitted from both of the treatments more than the patients who had mental problems. Also surgical treatment options tend to have been found more beneficial over nonsurgical treatment among the patients who had psychological disorders. In order to improve treatment results of both surgical and nonsurgical options, it is advised that psychological support is necessary [126].

Better understanding of the disease and psychological state and their relation with better results seem to be beneficial for patients. Healthier psychology, encouragement to participate in active life, and providing psychological support in any chronic illness are important to help patients to remain as functional individuals in the society.

Traditionally, vestibular rehabilitation is ineffective in episodic vertigo patients. Stable conditions are better candidates for successful rehabilitation. Due to its chronic and progressive nature, rehabilitation of these patients is tricky. In order to obtain rehabilitation, physical therapy must be customized. It is not advised to initiate a rehabilitation program in acute onset.

The success of rehabilitation depends on the patient. First step of a successful rehabilitation program is education of the patient. Each patient is unique, and their characteristics, mental status, and understanding capacity differ between each other. Patients have to be informed about their disease, its nature and treatment options. Detailed explanation should be given about the effectiveness of physical therapy, coping mechanisms, and possible sequels for each person's understanding level. It is also important to correct the patient if they were misinformed [127].

Before customizing a rehabilitation program, the patient should be examined systemically. Mecagni et al.'s study demonstrated that limited ankle motion range affects the patient's performance on balance tests [127]. Lower extremities should be examined on their functional levels and sense of proprioception. Impaired vision could affect oculomotor functions negatively. In order to determine relationships between the input mechanisms of balance system, posturography could be used if it is available [128]. It is reported that static platform posturography is more sensitive and specific in Meniere's disease than caloric and rotational tests, both in diagnosing and detecting other deficits that accompany these patients' vestibular system [129, 130].

Although there is not a test battery that could predict the effects of attacks on patients daily life, most of the patients describe the attacks debilitating [131]. Most of the time attacks occur suddenly and being prepared for those attacks is important. It should be discussed with the patient about special sensations or feelings before the attack. At least half of the patients could identify a trigger [132]. In order to identify these conditions, a symptom diary could be advised.

Some protective advices should be given to the patient to be performed during the attack. Also most of the patients tend to close their eyes during the attack, and it should be taught that keeping their eyes open and targeting them onto something would help them to suppress nystagmus [127]. Instead of panicking over symptoms, they should be advised to stay calm and sit or lie down in order to prevent themselves from further injuries.

When the attack subdued, refractory effects could continue to debilitate the patient. The patient should be advised to avoid any sudden movements. In order to minimize the effects on their personal lifestyles, some modifications should be advised like performing daily activities, sitting instead of standing while cooking, dressing up, etc.

In order to prevent patients' social isolation, patients should be encouraged about informing their social circle about their condition. Also series of exercises should be programmed for each patient's current status, and patients should be encouraged to participate in social life. In our clinic, we advise our patients to go to a mall for window shopping. It helps patients to overcome their fear to be in public, helps them to use visual object to train their vestibulo-ocular system, and also improves their walking and sense of proprioception. In addition to these advises, if a specific problem was found on their posturography, it is consulted with related departments.

Rehabilitation and its importance are well documented in Meniere's disease patients who received a destructive protocol [133–135]. However, studies about the effects of vestibular rehabilitation on patients who suffer from post-vertigo disequilibrium are limited. Clendaniel and Tucci reported the importance of vestibular rehabilitation of patients after vertigo attack [136].

Gottshall et al.'s study demonstrated the beneficial effects of vestibular exercises on post-vertigo symptoms with unilateral Meniere's disease. Patients reported that their balance function was significantly improved, only experiencing subtle discomfort [137]. In bilateral disease, it is reported by Cohen et al. that vestibular rehabilitation was not effective and advised to evaluate other adaptive strategies with these patients [138].

Vestibular rehabilitation between attacks could help patients to cooperate with disease and help them to keep their functionality levels up. Vestibular rehabilitation's effect on patients' mental status is not reported in the current literature but logically it could improve mental health. Recent guidelines recommend behavioral therapies and vestibular rehabilitation programs.

Hearing loss and tinnitus in Meniere's disease

Meniere's disease symptoms are episodic vertigo attacks, fluctuating hearing loss, tinnitus, and ear fullness. Most disturbing symptom of this condition is vertigo according to most of the studies that evaluated the quality of life scores of the patients. So the preservation of hearing function and reducing the tinnitus intensity are always evaluated as secondary outcomes in studies. During follow-up of the patients, it is important to document hearing levels because remained hearing function is the key factor in decision-making process of the treatment.

One of the diagnostic criteria of Meniere's disease according to AAO-HNS's guideline is hearing loss.

It is recommended to stage the disease and underline as an important factor to monitor the treatment results [11].

In ICON's guideline, destructive treatment options are recommended if there is no functional hearing left [59]. Hearing loss is usually located in lower frequencies, and in early stages of the disease, it has a fluctuating pattern [139, 140]. In later phases, it could decrease, and after 5–10 years, hearing thresholds usually settle to 50–60 dB as well as speech discrimination scores decrease to 50–60% [141]. Tinnitus is mostly a low-frequency type due to hearing loss, which could be localized to affected ear and could be described globally [38]. Low-frequency tinnitus is difficult to be masked with environmental sounds [142].

Havia et al. reported the relationship between vertigo, hearing loss, and tinnitus. Patients with more profound hearing loss had worse outcomes on their posturography tests and caloric test responses found decreased on the affected ear [35]. Recent studies demonstrated that hearing loss in these patients is associated with sensory element degeneration [143].

The intensity of tinnitus reported to increase with duration symptoms. Intense tinnitus is found to be related with hearing loss specifically at 500 Hz. However, vertigo attack frequency or duration of the attacks was not related with tinnitus intensity [35]. Gentamicin injections proven to be effective to reduce the tinnitus but surgical interventions found to be ineffective on tinnitus control [144, 145]. In order to compensate with tinnitus, behavioral therapy should be advised. Betahistine and nasal oxytocin were studied in Meniere's disease and they reported to decrease tinnitus perception but data are limited [146, 147]. Cochlear implants have reported that they decrease tinnitus significantly; although the data are limited and still relatively new, it is reported to decrease tinnitus of patients after 6 months [148].

Treatment of bilateral Meniere's disease

Bilateral Meniere's disease prevalence is reported in 2–47% of the cases, and it could occur after several years of the first onset of the disease [9]. Temporal bone studies suggest that bilateral Meniere's disease incidence is higher and bilateral endolymphatic hydrops observed 25–30% of the inspected temporal bones [149– 151]. Bilateral Meniere's disease should be treated conservatively; bilateralization could occur at any time, and there is no test that could prevent this. This condition is the main reason of the emphasis on being conservative while choosing the treatment option.

Meniere's disease rarely start bilaterally, it usually starts with unilaterally [152–154]. Most of the cases, contralateral involvement occurs after 2–5 years after the first initiation of symptoms [155]. Clinical presentation of these cases is different from each other. Most important step in diagnosis is suspicion and knowledge of the possible nature of the disease could affect the contralateral side at some point of patients' follow-up. Severity of the disease should be established independently for each ear, in pure-tone audiometry average of 500, 1000, 2000, and 3000 Hz >25 dB [11]. Tinnitus is reported to be more intense in bilateral Meniere's patients. Also they reported that patients who had bilateral Meniere's disease had significantly longer history of disease and worse pure-tone average [35].

In EcoG, Iseli and Gibson reported that summation potential/action potential ratio has a limited value to determine endolymphatic hydrops and should be combined with summation potential amplitude ans summating potential bias ratio [156]. Lin et al. proposed to combine VEMP tuning and VEMP thresholds to detect the hydrops in the contralateral ear before the symptoms' onset [157]. In imaging, studies suggest that affected side has endolymphatic dilatation and due to this perilymph volume seem decreased [158]. Combination of these diagnostic strategies could help physicians to detect bilateral involvement and avoid from destructive procedures in suspected patients.

In ICON's guideline, they reported that the bilateral tendency of the disease attributed as an important factor of most clinic treatment protocol shift from intratympanic gentamicin to intratympanic steroid. Also as a surgical treatment option, endolymphatic sac procedures are recommended for bilateral Meniere's disease [59]. In SFORL guideline, gentamicin injections are contraindicated in single intact ear or bilateral Meniere's disease. They recommend endolymphatic sac surgery if medical treatments failed in bilateral Meniere's disease. Destructive surgeries such as vestibular neurectomy and labyrinthectomy are not recommended in bilateral Meniere's disease [54].

Treatment options of bilateral disease are restricted. Conservative treatment options should be advised and symptomatic treatment should be prescribed during attack. Peterson et al. conduct a survey study among American otorhinolaryngologists about their choice of treatment with patient who had only hearing ear and most common option is Meniett device when other conservative treatment options failed. After Meniett, intratympanic steroid injection comes second in their choice of treatment. Endolymphatic sac procedures come in third; first decompression is advised than shunt procedures. Selective vestibular nerve section comes later [107].

Intratympanic steroid injection could be advised to patients with bilateral Meniere's disease. Recent randomized controlled study conducted in 2005 reported that intratympanic steroid injections are the effective way of treatment [159]. However, another study found no difference between intratympanic steroid injection and saline injection [160, 161]. The literature findings are controversial.

Intravenous streptomycin sulfate in debilitating bilateral Meniere's disease reported to reduce the symptoms [162–164]. If complete or near complete bilateral hypo-function has occurred, streptomycin sulfate is found to be effective [163]. Immune-mediated bilateral Meniere's disease is a subgroup of Meniere's disease, and methotrexate treatment is found to be effective on symptom control [165]. Another treatment option for immune-mediated group is systemic steroids, its efficacy is reported in a few studies [153, 166–170]. Prospective study on treatment of bilateral Meniere's disease with systemic steroids reported significant improvement on decrease in vertigo attacks but had no effect on hearing loss or tinnitus or aural fullness [170].

Surgical option of these patients is endolymphatic sac surgery; it has lowest complication rates on sensorineural hearing loss, <2% [171]. Kitahara et al.'s study reported the results of patients who had endolymphatic sac drainage with and without insertion of steroid induced silastic and nonsurgical group. The vertigo control rates were similar in surgery groups with or without steroid, but hearing levels of steroid group had better long-term results than nonsteroid surgery group and nonsurgical group [172]. Their findings were also supported with review of Wetmore. In order of retractable disease ablative surgeries combined with cochlear implant insertion should be considered.

References

[1] Pearce JMS. Marie-Jean-Pierre Flourens (1794-1867) and cortical localization. European Neurology. 2009; **61**(5):311-314. DOI: 10.1159/000206858

[2] Baloh RW. Prosper Ménière and his disease. Archives of Neurology. 2001. DOI: 10.1001/archneur.58.7.1151

[3] Knapp HJ. A Clinical Analysis of the Inflammatory Affections of the Inner Ear.; 1871

[4] Perez-Fernandez N, Montes-Jovellar L, Cervera-Paz J, Domenech-Vadillo E. Auditory and vestibular assessment of patients with Ménière's disease who suffer Tumarkin attacks. Audiology and Neurotology. 2010. DOI: 10.1159/ 000310899

[5] Hägnebo C, Andersson G, Melin L. Correlates of vertigo attacks in Meniere's disease. Psychotherapy and Psychosomatics. 1998. DOI: 10.1159/ 000012296

[6] Alexander TH, Harris JP. Current epidemiology of Meniere's syndrome. Otolaryngologic Clinics of North America. 2010. DOI: 10.1016/j. otc.2010.05.001

[7] Shojaku H, Watanabe Y, Fujisaka M, et al. Epidemiologic characteristics of definite Ménière's disease in Japan: A long-term survey of Toyama and Niigata prefectures. ORL; Journal for Oto-rhino-laryngology and its Related Specialties. 2005. DOI: 10.1159/ 000089413

[8] Choung YH, Park K, Kim CH, Kim HJ, Kim K. Rare cases of Ménière's disease in children. The Journal of Laryngology and Otology. 2006. DOI: 10.1017/S0022215106000569

[9] House JW, Doherty JK, Fisher LM, Derebery MJ, Berliner KI. Meniere's disease: Prevalence of contralateral ear involvement. Otology & Neurotology. 2006. DOI: 10.1097/00129492-200604000-00011

[10] Morrison AW, Mowbray JF, Williamson R, Sheeka S, Sodha N, Koskinen N. On genetic and environmental factors in Menière's disease. The American Journal of Otology. 1994

[11] Committee on Hearing and Equilibrium. Committee on hearing and equilibrium guidelines for the diagnosis and evaluation of therapy in Meniere's disease. Otolaryngology–Head and Neck Surgery. 1995;**113**(3):181-185. DOI: 10.1016/S0194-5998(95)70102-8

[12] Jansson B, Rask-Andersen H. Erythrocyte removal and blood clearance in the endolymphatic sac. An experimental and TEM study. Acta Oto-Laryngologica. 1996

[13] Rauch SD, Merchant SN, Thedinger BA. Meniere's syndrome and endolymphatic hydrops: Double-blind temporal bone study. The Annals of Otology, Rhinology, and Laryngology. 1989. DOI: 10.1177/000348948909801108

[14] Wackym PA. Histopathologic findings in Meniere's disease. Otolaryngology and Head and Neck Surgery. 1995. DOI: 10.1016/S0194-5998 (95)70307-1

[15] Valvassori GE, Dobben GD. Multidirectional and computerized tomography of the vestibular aqueduct in Meniere's disease. The Annals of Otology, Rhinology, and Laryngology. 1984. DOI: 10.1177/000348948409300604

[16] Albers FWJ, Van Weissenbruch R, Casselman JW. 3DFT-magnetic resonance imaging of the inner ear in Meniere's disease. Acta Oto-Laryngologica. 1994. DOI: 10.3109/ 00016489409126111

[17] Fitzgerald DC, Mark AS. Endolymphatic duct/sac enhancement on gadolinium magnetic resonance imaging of the inner ear: Preliminary observations and case reports. The American Journal of Otology. 1996

[18] Carfrae MJ, Holtzman A, Eames F, Parnes SM, Lupinetti A. 3 Tesla delayed contrast magnetic resonance imaging evaluation of Meniere's disease. The Laryngoscope. 2008. DOI: 10.1097/ MLG.0b013e31815c1a61

[19] Nakashima T, Naganawa S, Sugiura M, et al. Visualization of endolymphatic hydrops in patients with Meniere's disease. The Laryngoscope. 2007;**117**(3):415-420. DOI: 10.1097/ MLG.0b013e31802c300c

[20] Naganawa S, Nakashima T. Visualization of endolymphatic hydrops with MR imaging in patients with Ménière's disease and related pathologies: Current status of its methods and clinical significance. Japanese Journal of Radiology. 2014; **32**(4):191-204. DOI: 10.1007/ s11604-014-0290-4

[21] Schuknecht HFIM. Pathophysiology of Meniere's disease. In: Pfaltz CR, editor. Controversial Aspects of Meniere's Disease. New York: Georg Thieme; 1986

[22] Flock Å, Flock B. Micro-lesions in Reissner's membrane evoked by acute hydrops. Audiology & Neuro-Otology. 2003. DOI: 10.1159/000069002

[23] Schuknecht HF. The pathophysiology of Meniere's disease. The American Journal of Otology;**5**(6): 526-527

[24] Brown DH, McClure JA, DownarZapolski Z. The membrane rupture theory of Menière's disease–is it valid? The Laryngoscope. 1988. DOI: 10.1288/ 00005537-198806000-00003

[25] Paparella MM. Pathogenesis of Meniere's disease and Meniere's syndrome. Acta Oto-Laryngologica. 1983. DOI: 10.3109/00016488309122996

[26] Kimura RS. Animal models of inner ear vascular disturbances. American Journal of Otolaryngology Head and Neck Medicine and Surgery. 1986. DOI: 10.1016/S0196-0709(86)80042-4

[27] Derebery MJ, Berliner KI. Prevalence of allergy in Meniere's disease. Otolaryngology-Head and Neck Surgery. 2000. DOI: 10.1016/S0194-5998(99)80287-3

[28] Derebery MJ, Berliner KI. Allergy and its relation to Meniere's disease. Otolaryngologic Clinics of North America. 2010. DOI: 10.1016/j. otc.2010.05.004

[29] Derebery MJ. Allergic management of Meniere's disease: An outcome study. Otolaryngology-Head and Neck Surgery. 2000. DOI: 10.1016/S0194-5998(00)70235-X

[30] Bergström T, Edström S, Tjellström A, Vahlne A. Ménière's disease and antibody reactivity to herpes simplex virus type 1 polypeptides. American Journal of Otolaryngology and Head and Neck Surgery. 1992. DOI: 10.1016/0196-0709 (92)90051-T

[31] Lee KS, Kimura RS. Ischemia of the endolymphatic sac. Acta OtoLaryngologica. 1992. DOI: 10.3109/ 00016489209137456

[32] Radtke A, Lempert T, Gresty MA, Brookes GB, Bronstein AM, Neuhauser H. Migraine and Ménière's disease: Is there a link? Neurology. 2002. DOI: 10.1212/01.WNL.0000036903. 22461.39

[33] Paparella MM, Mcdermott JC, Sousa LCA. Meniere's disease and the peak audiogram. Archives of Otolaryngology. 1982. DOI: 10.1001/ archotol.1982.00790570021005

[34] Katsarkas A. Hearing loss and vestibular dysfunction in Meniere's disease. Acta Oto-Laryngologica. 1996. DOI: 10.3109/00016489609137819

[35] Havia M, Kentala E, Pyykkö I. Hearing loss and tinnitus in Meniere's disease. Auris, Nasus, Larynx. 2002; **29**(2):115-119. DOI: 10.1016/S0385-8146(01)00142-0

[36] Sato G, Sekine K, Matsuda K, et al. Long-term prognosis of hearing loss in patients with unilateral Ménière's disease. Acta Oto-Laryngologica. 2014. DOI: 10.3109/00016489.2014.923114

[37] Seyed Tootoonchi SJ, Ghiasi S, Shadara P, Samani SM, Fouladi DF. Hearing function after betahistine therapy in patients with Ménière's disease. Brazilian Journal of Otorhinolaryngology. 2015. DOI: 10.1016/j.bjorl.2015.08.021

[38] Vernon J, Johnson R, Schleuning A. The characteristics and natural history of tinnitus in Meniere's disease. Otolaryngologic Clinics of North America. 1980. DOI: 10.1002/nur.20223

[39] Stouffer JL, Tyler RS. Characterization of tinnitus by tinnitus patients. The Journal of Speech and Hearing Disorders. 1990. DOI: 10.1044/ jshd.5503.439

[40] Pfaltz C, Matefi L. Meniere's disease-or syndrome? A critical review of diagnose criteria. In: Vosteen K-H, Schuknecht H, Pfaltz C, et al., editors. Meniere's Disease, Pathogenesis, Diagnosis and Treatment. Stuttgart: Georg Thieme Verlag; 1981. pp. 1-10

[41] Paparella MM, Mancini F. Vestibular Meniere's disease. Otolaryngology-Head and Neck Surgery. 1985. DOI: 10.1177/ 019459988509300203

[42] Oosterveld W. Meniere's disease, signs and symptoms. The Journal of Laryngology and Otology. 1980;**94**(8): 885-892. DOI: 10.1017/ S0022215100089647

[43] Silverstein H, Smouha E, Jones R. Natural history vs. surgery for Meniere's disease. Otolaryngology–Head and Neck Surgery. 1989. DOI: 10.1177/ 019459988910000102

[44] Tumarkin A. The otolithic catastrophe. British Medical Journal. 1936. DOI: 10.1136/bmj.2.3942.175

[45] Ödkvist LM, Bergenius J. Drop attacks in Meniere's disease. Acta Oto-Laryngologica, Suppl. 1988

[46] Oku R, Shigeno K, Kumagami H, Takahashi H. Otolith dysfunction during vertiginous attacks in Meniere's disease. Acta Oto-Laryngologica. 2003. DOI: 10.1080/00016480310000377

[47] Friberg U, Stahle J, Svedberg A. The natural course of Meniere's disease. Acta Oto-Laryngologica. 1983. DOI: 10.3109/ 00016488309123007

[48] Goebel JA. 2015 equilibrium committee amendment to the 1995 AAO-HNS guidelines for the definition of Ménière's disease. Otolaryngology– Head and Neck Surgery. 2016. DOI: 10.1177/0194599816628524

[49] Black FO, Kitch R. A review of vestibular test results in Meniere's disease. Otolaryngologic Clinics of North America. 1980. DOI: Pm: 18686702

[50] Maire R, Van Melle G. Vestibuloocular reflex characteristics in patients with unilateral Ménière's disease. Otology & Neurotology. 2008. DOI: 10.1097/MAO.0b013e3181776703

[51] Goin DW, Staller SJ, Asher DL, et al. Summating potential in Meniere's disease. The Laryngoscope. 1982. DOI: 10.3757/ jser.55.419

[52] Klockhoff I. Diagnosis of Menière's disease. Archives of Oto-RhinoLaryngology. 1976. DOI: 10.1007/ BF00453679

[53] Rauch SD, Zhou G, Kujawa SG, Guinan JJ, Herrmann BS. Vestibular evoked myogenic potentials show altered

tuning in patients with Ménière's disease. Otology & Neurotology. 2004. DOI: 10.1097/00129492-200405000-00022

[54] Nevoux J, Franco-Vidal V, Bouccara D, et al. Diagnostic and therapeutic strategy in Menière's disease. Guidelines of the French Otorhinolaryngology-Head and Neck Surgery Society (SFORL). European Annals of Otorhinolaryngology, Head and Neck Diseases. 2017;**134**(6):441-444. DOI: 10.1016/j.anorl.2016.12.003

[55] Van Esch BF, Van Der Zaag-Loonen HJ, Bruintjes TD, Van Benthem PPG. Interventions for Menière's disease: Protocol for an umbrella systematic review and a network meta-analysis. BMJ Open. 2016. DOI: 10.1136/bmjopen-2015-010269

[56] Hamill TA. Evaluating treatments for Meniere's disease: Controversies surrounding placebo control. Journal of the American Academy of Audiology. 2006. DOI: 10.3766/jaaa.17.1.4

[57] Torok N. Old and new in Ménière disease. The Laryngoscope. 1977. DOI: 10.1002/lary.1977.87.11.1870

[58] Green JD, Blum DJ, Harner SG. Longitudinal follow up of patients with Meniere's disease. Otolaryngology–Head and Neck Surgery. 1991. DOI: 10.1177/ 019459989110400603

[59] Nevoux J, Barbara M, Dornhoffer J, Gibson W, Kitahara T, Darrouzet V. International consensus (ICON) on treatment of Ménière's disease. European Annals of Otorhinolaryngology, Head and Neck Diseases. 2017. DOI: 10.1016/j. anorl.2017.12.006

[60] Holgers K-M, Finizia C. Health profiles for patients with Meniere's disease. Noise & Health. 2001

[61] Nakayama M, Masuda A, Ando KB, et al. A pilot study on the effi cacy of continuous positive airway pressure on the manifestations of Ménière's disease in patients with concomitant obstructive sleep apnea syndrome. Journal of Clinical Sleep Medicine. 2015. DOI: 10.5664/jcsm.5080

[62] Luxford E, Berliner KI, Lee J, Luxford WM. Dietary modification as adjunct treatment in Ménière's disease: Patient willingness and ability to comply. Otology & Neurotology. 2013. DOI: 10.1097/MAO.0b013e3182942261

[63] Sánchez-Sellero I, San-Román-Rodríguez E, Santos-Pérez S, Rossi-Izquierdo M, Soto-Varela A. Caffeine intake and Menière's disease: Is there relationship? Nutritional Neuroscience. 2017

[64] Coelho DH, Lalwani AK. Medical management of Ménière's disease. The Laryngoscope. 2008. DOI: 10.1097/MLG.0b013e31816927f0

[65] Sharon JD, Trevino C, Schubert MC, Carey JP. Treatment of Menière's disease. Current Treatment Options in Neurology. 2015;**17**(4). DOI: 10.1007/ s11940-0150341-x

[66] He FJ, Li J, Macgregor GA. Effect of longer-term modest salt reduction on blood pressure. Cochrane Database of Systematic Reviews. 2013. DOI: 10.1002/14651858.CD004937.pub2

[67] Furuta H, Sato C, Kawaguchi Y, Miyashita T, Mori N. Expression of mRNAs encoding hormone receptors in the endolymphatic sac of the rat. Acta Oto-Laryngologica. 1999. DOI: 10.1080/ 00016489950181936

[68] Kim G, Masilamani S, Turner R, et al. The thiazide-sensitive Na-Cl cotransporter is an aldosterone-induced protein. Proceedings of the National Academy of Sciences of the United States of America. 1998. DOI: 10.1093/icb/23.2.347

[69] Rossier BC, Baker ME, Studer RA. Epithelial sodium transport and its control by aldosterone: The story of our internal environment revisited. Physiological Reviews. 2015. DOI: 10.1152/physrev.00011.2014

[70] Miyashita T, Tatsumi H, Hayakawa K, Mori N, Sokabe M. Large Na+ influx and high Na+, K+-ATPase activity

in mitochondria-rich epithelial cells of the inner ear endolymphatic sac. Pflügers Archiv European Journal of Physiology. 2007. DOI: 10.1007/s00424-006-0166-2

[71] Akiyama K, Miyashita T, Mori T, Inamoto R, Mori N. Expression of thiazide-sensitive Na+-Clcotransporter in the rat endolymphatic sac. Biochemical and Biophysical Research Communications. 2008. DOI: 10.1016/j.bbrc.2008.04.081

[72] Kim SH, Park HY, Choi HS, Chung HP, Choi JY. Functional and molecular expression of epithelial sodium channels in cultured human endolymphatic sac epithelial cells. Otology & Neurotology. 2009. DOI: 10.1097/MAO.0b013e31819a8e0e

[73] Matsubara A, Miyashita T, Inamoto R, Hoshikawa H, Mori N. Cystic fibrosis transmembrane conductance regulator in the endolymphatic sac of the rat. Auris, Nasus, Larynx. 2014. DOI: 10.1016/j. anl.2014.02.005

[74] Mori N, Uozumi N, Yura K, Sakai SI. Effect of aldosterone antagonist on the DC potential in the endolymphatic SAC. The Annals of Otology, Rhinology, and Laryngology. 1991. DOI: 10.1177/ 000348949110000112

[75] Mori N, Uozumi N, Yura K, Sakai S. The difference in endocochlear and endolymphatic sac d.c. potentials in response to furosemide and canrenoate as diuretics. European Archives of Oto-Rhino-Laryngology. 1990. DOI: 10.1007/BF00179010

[76] Thai-Van H, Bounaix MJ, Fraysse B. Menière's disease: Pathophysiology and treatment. Drugs. 2001. DOI: 10.2165/ 00003495-200161080-00005

[77] Miyashita T, Inamoto R, Fukuda S, et al. Hormonal changes following a low-salt diet in patients with Ménière's disease. Auris, Nasus, Larynx. 2017; **44**(1):52-57. DOI: 10.1016/j. anl.2016.03.001

[78] Tadros SF, Frisina ST, Mapes F, Frisina DR, Frisina RD. Higher serum aldosterone correlates with lower hearing thresholds: A possible protective hormone against presbycusis. Hearing Research. 2005. DOI: 10.1016/j.heares.2005.05.009

[79] Martinez DM. The effect of serc (betahistine hydrochloride) on the circulation of the inner ear in experimental animals. Acta OtoLaryngologica. 1972. DOI: 10.3109/ 00016487209122697

[80] Lacour M, van de Heyning PH, Novotny M, Tighilet B. Betahistine in the treatment of Ménière's disease. Neuropsychiatric Disease and Treatment. 2007

[81] Timmerman H. Pharmacotherapy of vertigo: Any news to be expected? Acta Oto-Laryngologica. 1994. DOI: 10.3109/ 00016489409127323

[82] Betahistine dihydrochloride. Electronic Medicines Compendium. 2015. Available from: https://www.med icines.org.uk/emc/medicine/266172015

[83] Murdin L, Hussain K, Schilder AGM. Betahistine for symptoms of vertigo. Cochrane Database of Systematic Reviews. 2013. DOI: 10.1002/14651858.CD010696

[84] Nauta JJP. Meta-analysis of clinical studies with betahistine in Ménière's disease and vestibular vertigo. European Archives of Oto-RhinoLaryngology. 2014. DOI: 10.1007/ s00405-013-2596-8

[85] Adrion C, Fischer CS, Wagner J, Gürkov R, Mansmann U, Strupp M. Efficacy and safety of betahistine treatment in patients with Meniere's disease: Primary results of a long term, multicentre, double blind, randomised, placebo controlled, dose defining trial (BEMED trial). BMJ. 2016;**352**. DOI: 10.1136/bmj.h6816

[86] Shinkawa H, Kimura RS. Effect of diuretics on endolymphatic hydrops. Acta Oto-Laryngologica. 1986. DOI: 10.3109/00016488609108606

[87] Petermann W, Mulch G. Long-term therapy of Meniere's disease. Comparison of the effects of betahistine dihydrochloride and hydrochlorothiazide. Fortschritte der Medizin. 1982

[88] Van Deelen GW, Huizing EH. Use of a diuretic (Dyazide®) in the treatment of ménière's disease: A double-blind cross-over placebocontrolled study. ORL; Journal for Otorhino-laryngology and its Related Specialties. 1986. DOI: 10.1159/ 000275884

[89] Klockhoff I, Lindblom U. Meniére's disease and hydrochlorothiazide dichlotride® —A critical analysis of symptoms and therapeutic effects. Acta Oto-Laryngologica. 1967. DOI: 10.3109/ 00016486709128769

[90] Thirlwall AS, Kundu S. Diuretics for Meniere's disease or syndrome. Cochrane Database of Systematic Reviews. 2006. DOI: 10.1002/14651858. CD003599.pub2

[91] Ingelstedt S, Ivarsson A, Tjernström Ö. Immediate relief of symptoms during acute attacks of Meniere's disease, using a pressure chamber. Acta OtoLaryngologica. 1976. DOI: 10.3109/ 00016487609120921

[92] Gates GA, Green JD, Tucci DL, Telian SA. The effects of transtympanic micropressure treatment in people with unilateral Ménière's disease. Archives of Otolaryngology – Head & Neck Surgery. 2004. DOI: 10.1001/ archotol.130.6.718

[93] Ahsan SF, Standring R, Wang Y. Systematic review and meta–Analysis of Meniett therapy for Meniere's disease. The Laryngoscope. 2015;**125**(1): 203-208. DOI: 10.1002/lary.24773

[94] Syed MI, Rutka JA, Hendry J, Browning GG. Positive pressure therapy for Meniere's syndrome/disease with a Meniett device: A systematic review of randomised controlled trials. Clinical Otolaryngology. 2015. DOI: 10.1111/ coa.12344

[95] van Sonsbeek S, Pullens B, van Benthem PP. Positive pressure therapy for Ménière's disease or syndrome. Cochrane Database of Systematic Reviews. 2015. DOI: 10.1002/14651858. CD008419.pub2

[96] Zhang S-L, Leng Y, Liu B, Shi H, Lu M, Kong W-J. Meniett therapy for Meniere's disease: An updated Metaanalysis. Otology & Neurotology. 2016; **37**(3):290-298. DOI: 10.1097/ MAO.0000000000000957

[97] Sugawara K, Kitamura K, Ishida T, Sejima T. Insertion of tympanic ventilation tubes as a treating modality for patients with Meniere's disease: A shortand long-term follow-up study in seven cases. Auris, Nasus, Larynx. 2003. DOI: 10.1016/S0385-8146(02)00105-0

[98] Montandon PB, Guillemin P, Häusler R. Prevention of vertigo in Mèniér's syndrome by means of transtympanic ventilation tubes. ORL: Journal for Oto-rhino-laryngology and its Related Specialties. 1988. DOI: 10.1159/000276016

[99] Ballester M, Liard P, Vibert D, Häusler R. Menière's disease in the elderly. Otology & Neurotology. 2002

[100] Ogawa Y, Otsuka K, Hagiwara A, et al. Clinical study of tympanostomy tube placement for patients with intractable Ménière's disease. The Journal of Laryngology and Otology. 2015;**129**(2):120-125. DOI: 10.1017/ S0022215115000079

[101] Masutani H, Nakai Y, Kato A. Microvascular disorder of the stria vascularis in endolymphatic hydrops. Acta Oto-Laryngologica. 1995. DOI: 10.3109/00016489509121874

[102] Yazawa Y, Kitano H, Suzuki M, Tanaka H, Kitajima K. Studies of cochlear blood flow in Guinea pigs with endolymphatic hydrops. ORL; Journal for Oto-rhino-laryngology and its Related Specialties. 1998. DOI: 10.1159/ 000027554

[103]Kimura RS, Hutta J. Inhibition of experimentally induced endolymphatic hydrops by middle ear ventilation. European Archives of Oto-RhinoLaryngology. 1997. DOI: 10.1007/ BF00874091

[104]Chi FL, Liang Q, Wang ZM. Effects of hyperbaric therapy on function and morphology of Guinea pig cochlea with endolymphatic hydrops. Otology & Neurotology. 2004. DOI: 10.1097/00129492-200407000-00024

[105]Dornhoffer JL, King D. The effect of the Meniett device in patients with Ménière's disease: Long-term results. Otology & Neurotology. 2008. DOI: 10.1097/MAO.0b013e318182025a

[106]Foster CA. Optimal management of Ménière's disease. Therapeutics and Clinical Risk Management. 2015. DOI: 10.2147/TCRM.S59023

[107]Peterson WM, Isaacson JE. Current management of Ménière's disease in an only hearing ear. Otology & Neurotology. 2007;**28**(5):696-699. DOI: 10.1097/mao.0b013e3180577963

[108]Tumarkin A. Thoughts on the treatment of labyrinthopathy. The Journal of Laryngology and Otology;**80** (10):1041-1053. DOI: 10.1017/ S0022215100066366

[109]Lall M. Meniere's disease and the grommet (survey of its therapeutic effects). The Journal of Laryngology and Otology. 1977;**83**(8):787-791. DOI: 10.1017/S002221510007095X

[110]Cinnamond MJ. Eustachian tube function in Meniére's disease. The Journal of Laryngology and Otology. 1975. DOI: 10.1017/S0022215100080075

[111]Hall CM, Brackmann DE. Eustachian tube blockage and Meniere's disease. Archives of Otolaryngology – Head & Neck Surgery. 1977;**103**(6): 355-357. DOI: 10.1001/ archotol.1977.00780230077012

[112]Thomsen J, Bonding P, Birgit B. The non-specific effect of endolymphatic sac surgery in treatment of Meniere's disease: A prospective, randomized controlled study comparing "classic" endolymphatic sac surgery with the insertion of a ventilating tube in the tympanic membrane. Acta OtoLaryngologica. 1998;**118**(6):769-773. DOI: 10.1080/00016489850182413

[113]Magnan J, Ozgirgin ON, Trabalzini F, et al. European position statement on diagnosis, and treatment of Meniere's disease*. The Journal of International Advanced Otology. 2018;**14**(2):317-321. DOI: 10.5152/iao.2018.140818

[114]Guneri EA. Endolenfatik hidrops ve Meniere hastaligi. In: Onerci M, editor. Kulak Burun Boğaz Baş Boyun Cerrahisi Cilt 2 Nörootoloji. Ankara: Matsa Basimevi; 2016. pp. 523-536

[115]Bienhold H, Flohr H. Role of cholinergic synapses in vestibular compensation. Brain Research. 1980. DOI: 10.1016/0006-8993(80)90083-9

[116]Ishikawa K, Igarashi M. Effect of diazepam on vestibular compensation in squirrel monkeys. Archives of OtoRhino-Laryngology. 1984. DOI: 10.1007/BF00464344

[117]Schaefer K, Meyer D. Aspects of vestibular compensation in Guinea pig. In: Flohr H, Precht E, editors. LesionInduced Neuronal Plasticity in Sensorimotor System. New York: Springer; 1981. pp. 197-297

[118]Antor MA, Uribe AA, ErminyFalcon N, et al. The effect of transdermal scopolamine for the prevention of postoperative nausea and vomiting. Frontiers in Pharmacology. 2014. DOI: 10.3389/fphar.2014.00055

[119]Gejrot T. Intravenous xylocaine in the treatment of attacks of Meniere's disease. Acta Oto-Laryngologica. 1976. DOI: 10.3109/00016487609120911

[120]Orji F. The influence of psychological factors in Meniere's disease. Annals of Medical and Health Sciences Research. 2014;**4**(1):3. DOI: 10.4103/2141-9248.126601

[121]Van Cruijsen N, Wit H, Albers F. Psychological aspects of Ménière's disease. Acta Oto-Laryngologica. 2003. DOI: 10.1080/0036554021000028125

[122]House JW, Crary WG, Wexler M. The inter-relationship of vertigo and stress. Otolaryngologic Clinics of North America. 1980

[123]Eagger S, Luxon LM, Davies RA, Coelho A, Ron MA. Psychiatric morbidity in patients with peripheral vestibular disorder: A clinical and neuro-otological study. Journal of Neurology, Neurosurgery, and Psychiatry. 1992. DOI: 10.1136/ jnnp.55.5.383

[124]Takahashi M, Ishida K, Iida M, Yamashita H, Sugawara K. Analysis of lifestyle and behavioral characteristics in Ménière's disease patients and a control population. Acta Oto-Laryngologica. 2001. DOI: 10.1080/000164801300043721

[125]Van Cruijsen N, Jaspers JPC, Van De Wiel HBM, Wit HP, Albers FWJ. Psychological assessment of patients with Menière's disease. International Journal of Audiology. 2006. DOI: 10.1080/14992020600753239

[126]Yokota Y, Kitahara T, Sakagami M, et al. Surgical results and psychological status in patients with intractable Ménière's disease. Auris, Nasus, Larynx. 2016;**43**(3):287-291. DOI: 10.1016/j. anl.2015.10.007

[127]Dowdal-Osborn M. Early vestibular rehabilitation in patients with Meniere's disease. Otolaryngologic Clinics of North America. 2002;**35**(3):683-690. DOI: 10.1016/S0030-6665(02)00026-9

[128]Di Fabio RP. Sensitivity and specificity of platform posturography for identifying patients with vestibular dysfunction. Physical Therapy. 1995. DOI: 10.1093/ptj/75.4.290

[129]Black FO, Wall C. Comparison of vestibulo-ocular and vestibulospinal screening tests. Otolaryngology-Head and Neck Surgery. 1981. DOI: 10.1177/ 019459988108900523

[130]Di Fabio RP. Meta-analysis of the sensitivity and specificity of platform posturography. Archives of Otolaryngology – Head & Neck Surgery. 1996. DOI: 10.1001/archotol. 1996.01890140036008

[131]Cohen H, Ewell LR, Jenkins HA. Disability in Meniere's disease. Archives of Otolaryngology-Head and Neck Surgery. 1995. DOI: 10.1001/ archotol.1995.01890010017004

[139]Antoli Candela F Jr. The histopathology of Meniere's disease. Acta Oto-Laryngologica. 1976

[140]Lee CS, Paparella MM, Margolis RH, Le C. Audiological profiles and Meniere's disease. Ear, Nose, & Throat Journal. 1995

[141]Stahle J, Friberg U, Svedberg A. 's

[132]Haybach P. Meniere's disease— What you need to know. In: Vestibular Disorders Association. Portland, Oregon; 1998

[133]Odkvist L. Gentamicin cures Vertigo, but what happens to hearing? The International Tinnitus Journal. 1997

[134]Gottshall K, Hoffer ME, Kopke R. Vestibular physical therapy rehabilitation after low dose microcatheter administered gentamicin treatment for Meniere's disease. In: 4th International Symposium on Meniere's Disease. Hauge (Netherlands): Kuglar Publications; 2000. pp. 663-668

[135]Suryanarayanan R, Cook JA. Long-term results of gentamicin inner ear perfusion in Ménière's disease. The Journal of Laryngology and Otology. 2004. DOI: 10.1258/ 0022215041615083

[136]Clendaniel RA, Tucci DL. Vestibular rehabilitation strategies in Meniere's disease. Otolaryngologic Clinics of North America. 1997

[137]Gottshall KR, Topp SG, Hoffer ME. Early vestibular physical therapy rehabilitation for Meniere's disease. Otolaryngologic Clinics of North America. 2010;**43**(5):1113-1119. DOI: 10.1016/j.otc.2010.05.006

[138]Cohen H. Vestibular rehabilitation improves daily life function. American Journal of Occupational Therapy. 1994. DOI: 10.1097/ IGC.0b013e31828b4f19 Long-term progression of Meniere disease. Acta Oto-Laryngologica. 1991. DOI: 10.3109/00016489109128047

[142]Kolbe U, Brehmer D, Schaaf H, Hesse G, Laubert A. Tinnitus and morbus Meniere. In: Sterkers O, Ferrary E, Dauman R, Sauvage JP, Tran Ba Huy P, editors. Meniere's Disease 1999-Update. Kugler Publications; 2000. pp. 459-462

[143]Vasama JP, Linthicum FH. Meniere's disease and endolymphatic hydrops without Meniere's symptoms: Temporal bone histopathology. Acta Oto-Laryngologica. 1999. DOI: 10.1080/ 00016489950181279

[144]Sala T. Transtympanic gentamicin in the treatment of Meniére's disease. Auris, Nasus, Larynx. 1997

[145]Kaasinen S, Pyykkö I, Ishizaki H, Aalto H. Effect of intratympanically administered gentamicin on hearing and tinnitus in Meniere's disease. Acta OtoLaryngologica. 1995. DOI: 10.3109/ 00016489509125223

[146]Ganança MM, Caovilla HH, Gazzola JM, Ganança CF, Ganança FF. Betahistine in the treatment of tinnitus in patients with vestibular disorders. Brazilian Journal of Otorhinolaryngology. 2011. DOI: 10.1590/S1808-86942011000400014

[147]Azevedo AA, Figueiredo RR, Elgoyhen AB, Langguth B, Penido NDO, Schlee W. Tinnitus treatment with oxytocin: A pilot study. Frontiers in Neurology. 2017. DOI: 10.3389/ fneur.2017.00494

[148]Langguth B, Kreuzer PM, Kleinjung T, De Ridder D. Tinnitus: Causes and clinical management. Lancet Neurology. 2013. DOI: 10.1016/S1474-4422(13)70160-1

[149]Perez R, Chen JM, Nedzelski JM. The status of the contralateral ear in established unilateral Menière's disease. The Laryngoscope. 2004. DOI: 10.1097/ 00005537-200408000-00010

[150]Yazawa Y, Kitahara M. Bilateral endolymphatic hydrops in Meniere's disease: Review of temporal bone autopsies. The Annals of Otology, Rhinology, and Laryngology. 1990. DOI: 10.1177/000348949009900705

[151]Tsuji K, Velazquez-Villasenor L, Rauch S, Glynn R, Wall CI, Merchant S. Temporal bone studies of the human peripheral vestibular system. Meniere's disease. The Annals of Otology, Rhinology, and Laryngology. 2000. DOI: 10.1177/00034894001090S502

[152]Kitahara M. Bilateral aspects of Meniere's disease: Meniere's disease with bilateral fluctuant hearing loss. Acta Oto-Laryngologica. 1991. DOI: 10.3109/00016489109128046

[153]Agrawal S, Parnes L. Systemic treatment of bilateral Meniere's disease. In: Roland P, Rutka J, editors. Ototoxicity. Hamilton, Canada: BC Decker; 2004

[154]Mizuta K, Furuta M, Ito Y, et al. A case of Meniere's disease with vertical nystagmus after administration of glycerol. Auris, Nasus, Larynx. 2000. DOI: 10.1016/S0385-8146(00) 00050-X

[155]Paparella MM, Griebie MS. Bilaterality of Meniere's disease. Acta Oto-Laryngologica. 1984. DOI: 10.3109/ 00016488409130984

[156]Iseli C, Gibson W. A comparison of three methods of using transtympanic electrocochleography for the diagnosis of Meniere's disease: Click summating potential measurements, tone burst summating potential amplitude measurements, and biasing of the summating potential using a low frequency tone. Acta OtoLaryngologica. 2010. DOI: 10.3109/ 00016480902858899

[157]Lin MY, Timmer FCA, Oriel BS, et al. Vestibular evoked myogenic potentials (VEMP) can detect asymptomatic saccular hydrops. The Laryngoscope. 2006. DOI: 10.1097/01. mlg.0000216815.75512.03

[158]Fukuoka H, Tsukada K, Miyagawa M, et al. Semi-quantitative evaluation of endolymphatic hydrops by bilateral intratympanic gadoliniumbased contrast agent (GBCA) administration with MRI for Meniere's disease. Acta Oto-Laryngologica. 2010. DOI: 10.3109/00016480902858881

[159]Garduño-Anaya MA, De Toledo HC, Hinojosa-González R, PanePianese C, Ríos-Castañeda LC. Dexamethasone inner ear perfusion by intratympanic injection in unilateral Ménière's disease: A two-year prospective, placebo-controlled, doubleblind, randomized trial. Otolaryngology-Head and Neck Surgery. 2005. DOI: 10.1016/j. otohns.2005.05.010

[160]Silverstein H, Isaacson JE, Olds MJ, Rowan PT, Rosenberg S. Dexamethasone inner ear perfusion for the treatment of Meniere's disease: A prospective, randomized, double-blind, crossover trial. American Journal of Otolaryngology. 1998. DOI: 10.1111/ j.1467-6494.1954.tb02338.x

[161]Alles MJRC, Der Gaag MA, Stokroos RJ. Intratympanic steroid therapy for inner ear diseases, a review of the literature. European Archives of Oto-Rhino-Laryngology. 2006. DOI: 10.1007/s00405-006-0065-3

[162]Balyan FR, Taibah A, De Donato G, et al. Titration streptomycin therapy in Meniere's disease: Long-term results. Otolaryngology-Head and Neck Surgery. 1998. DOI: 10.1016/S0194-5998 (98)80028-4

[163]Graham MD. Bilateral Meniere's disease. Treatment with intramuscular titration streptomycin sulfate. Otolaryngologic Clinics of North America. 1997

[164]Kilpatrick JK, Sismanis A, Spencer RF, Wise CM. Low-dose oral methotrexate management of patients with bilateral Meniere's disease. Ear, Nose, & Throat Journal. 2000

[165]Schessel D, Minor L, Nedzelski J. Meniere's disease and other peripheral vestibular disorders. In: Cummings C, Flint P, Haughey B, editors. Cummings Otolaryngology: Head and Neck Surgery. 4th ed. Philadelphia: Elsevier Inc; 2005

[166]Shea JJJ, Ge X. Dexamethasone perfusion of the labyrinth plus intravenous dexamethasone for Meniere's disease. Otolaryngologic Clinics of North America. 1996

[167]Shea JJ. The role of dexamethasone or streptomycin perfusion in the treatment of Meniere's disease. Otolaryngologic Clinics of North America. 1997

[168]Hirvonen TP, Peltomaa M, Ylikoski J. Intratympanic and systemic dexamethasone for Meniere's disease. ORL; Journal for Oto-rhino-laryngology and its Related Specialties. 2000. DOI: 10.1159/000027730

[169]Morales-Luckie E, Cornejo-Suarez A, Zaragoza-Contreras MA, GonzalezPerez O. Oral administration of prednisone to control refractory vertigo in Ménière's disease: A pilot study. Otology & Neurotology. 2005. DOI: 10.1097/01.mao.0000185057.81962.51

[170]Paparella M. Revision of endolymphatic sac surgery for recurrent Meniere's disease. Otolaryngologic Clinics of North America. 2002;**35**(3): 607-619. DOI: 10.1016/S0030-6665(02) 00032-4

[171]Kitahara T, Kubo T, Okumura SI, Kitahara M. Effects of endolymphatic sac drainage with steroids for intractable Ménière's disease: A long-term followup and randomized controlled study. The Laryngoscope. 2008. DOI: 10.1097/ MLG.0b013e3181651c4a

[172]Wetmore SJ. Endolymphatic sac surgery for Ménière's disease: Longterm results after primary and revision surgery. Archives of Otolaryngology – Head & Neck Surgery. 2008. DOI: 10.1001/archotol.134.11.1144

15

Menière's Disease: Etiopathogenesis

Carlos A. Oliveira

Brasília University Medical School, Brasília, DF, Brazil

*Address all correspondence to: cacpoliveira@brturbo.com.br

ABSTRACT

This chapter will discuss idiopathic Menière's syndrome. That is to say—Menière's disease. We will start with a brief recall on the History of Menière's disease begin- ning with the description of the syndrome by Prosper Menière in 1861, the descrip- tion of endolymphatic hydrops in temporal bone studies by Hallpike and Cairns in 1938 and by Yamakaua in the same year. Endolymphatic hydrops became a patho- logic correlate for Menière's syndrome. Theories that considered endolymphatic hydrops as the cause of the syndrome will be discussed. More recent studies ques- tioning the old theories and thinking of endolymphatic hydrops as an epiphenom-enon in the course of the syndrome rather than the cause of the symptoms will be discussed. Temporal bone studies were the basis of these new theories too. Familial Menière's disease will be discussed and several families will be described in detail. Because the phenotype of siblings on each family studied was variable and migraine was present in many affected members of these families a spectrum was postulated going from migraine alone to full blown Menière's disease. Some siblings had what has been described recently as vertiginous migraine and a detailed description of this syndrome will be provided and the differences between this syndrome and Menière's disease will be made clear. About 20% of Menière's disease patients have a familial history. Sporadic Meniere's disease might have a genetic predisposition and other environmental and behavioral factors contribute for the surfacing of the disease (multifactorial etiology). Because migraine is a central phenomenon and the vertiginous episodes and auditory symptoms are peripheral a hypothesis is presented for the pathophysiology of Menière's disease. Recent research comparing vestibular migraine and Manière's disease reinforcing the concept of these syndromes repre- senting a continuum process with similar etiology are discussed at the end.

Keywords: Menière's disease (MD), endolymphatic hydrops (EH), migraine, familial Menière's syndrome, continuum, vertiginous migraine (VM)

INTRODUCTION

This chapter will present the etiopathogenesis and pathophysiology of Menière's disease (MD). It is necessary therefore to make clear the definition of Menière's disease that will be considered here.

We consider Menière's disease the Menière's syndrome without a clear etiology. Because vertigo, tinnitus and hearing loss are present in most of the insults to the inner ear there are many known causes for these symptoms. However, there is the Menière's syndrome present in some patients without any definable etiology. This is Menière's disease and will be our subject in this chapter.

1.1 History of Menière's disease

Let us start with following the History of MD. In 1861 Prosper Menière sug- gested that vertigo, tinnitus and hearing loss were symptoms of vestibular organs injury rather than of brain apoplexy. This paper marked the starting point of a discussion that is now almost 180 years old [1].

In 1938 Hallpike and Cairns described in temporal bone histopathology study hydrops of the endolymphatic compartment in patients who had the Menière's symptoms during life. This was a material proof of the inner ear origin of the Menière's syndrome as stated by Menière in 1861 [2]. In the same year Yamakawa in Japan described the same histopathological findings in temporal bones of patients with the Menière's syndrome [3].

From then on, several temporal bone histopathologists [4–6] found endolym- phatic hydrops (EH) in temporal bones of patients with the Menière's syndrome. So, EH was established as the pathological correlate of MD.

Schuknecht [7] in 1978 observed rupture of endolymphatic membranes in patients with EH (**Figures 1** and **2**) in temporal bones of patients who had the Menière's syndrome during their life time. Lawrence in 1864 [8] had shown that rupture of Reisner's membrane in one segment of the chinchilla's cochlear duct and consequent mixing of endolymph with perilymph would cause permanent damage to the organ of Corti in the involved segment.

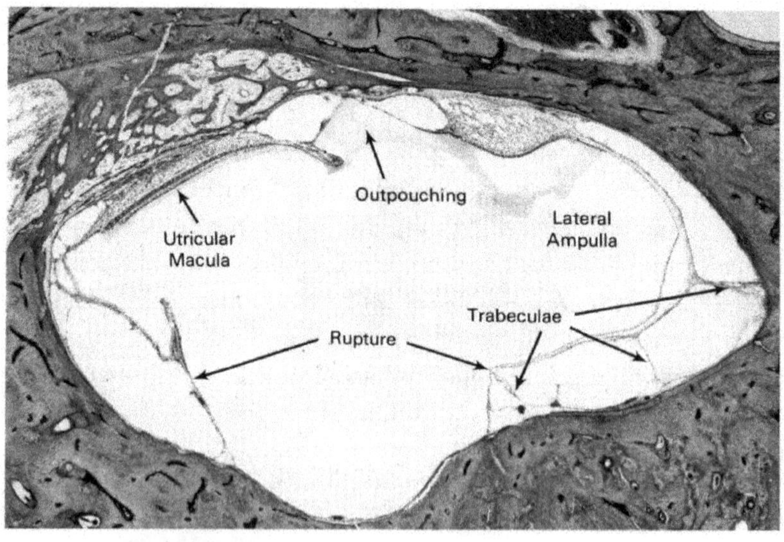

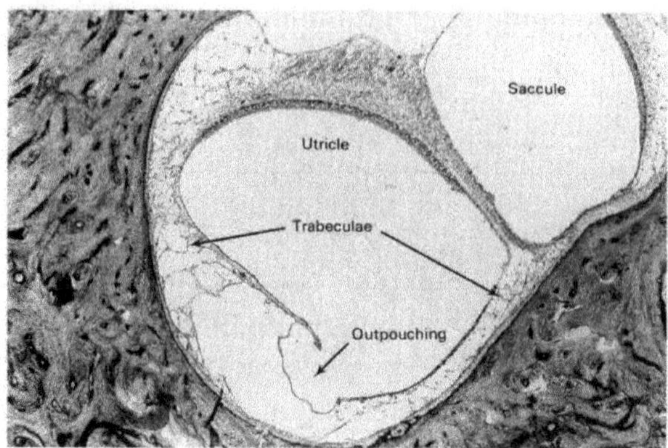

Figure 1. *Membrane rupture in the vestibular labyrinth. Reprinted with permission from Ref. [7].*

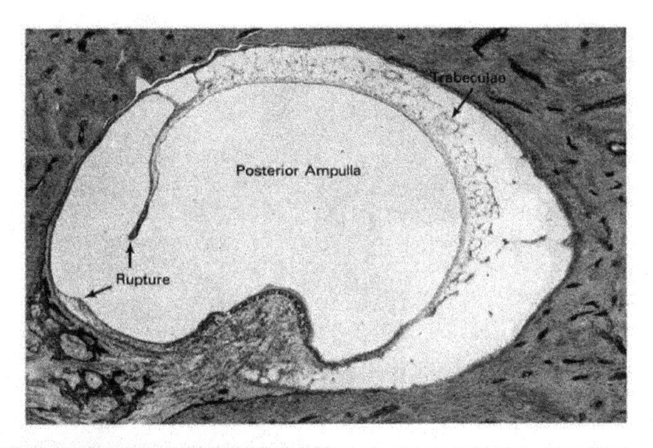

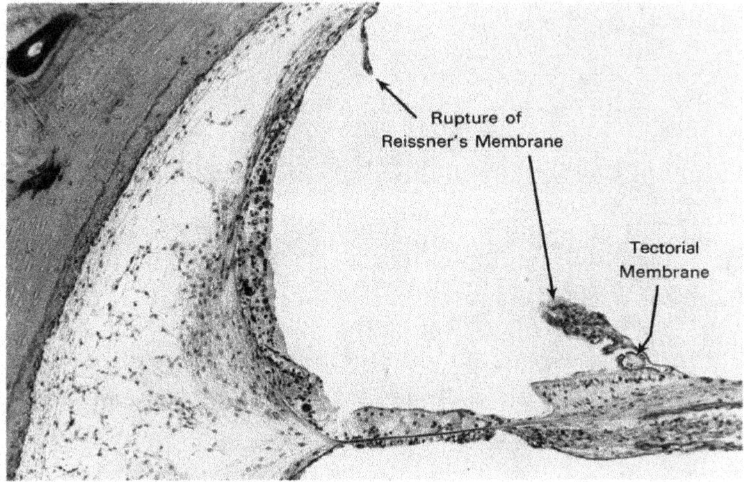

Figure 2. *Membrane ruptures in the semicircular canal and cochlea duct. Reprinted with permission from Ref. [7].*

Based on the ruptures of cochlear and vestibular membranes in the hydropic ears Schuknecht proposed that these ruptures and the consequent mixing of endolymph and perilymph would cause the acute Menière's attack.

After the Schuknecht paper EH became more than a pathologic correlate. It was the cause of the Menière's symptoms. For one decade this theory was accepted as true and things appeared to be settled down regarding the etiopathology of Menière's disease.

However, during the year of 1989 Oliveira selected 83 temporal bones of patients who had significant tinnitus during life and tried to find a pathologic correlate for this symptom. Thirty-seven temporal bones had normal histology (44.5%), 23 had EH (27.7%). Among the normal histology bones there were 13 patients who also had episodic vertigo during life. It was notable that 72.2% of the bones had normal histology and EH. He thought of a common cause for MD and EH. In that case EH would not be the cause for MD but both would have a common cause [8].

Rauch et al. in 1989 [9] studied 26 temporal bones from patients who had MD during their life's time but only 13 of them had EH. **Figures 3** and **4** are from Rauch's paper and express the change in position of EH: from the cause of the symptoms to an epiphenomenon also caused by an unknown primary event.

Fraysse in 1990 [10] pointed out that EH may be present in several diseases of the inner ear and that MD patients may not have EH present. Merchant et al. in 1995 found 28 temporal bones from patients with MD who had EH but 19 other patients with EH never had MD symptoms during life [11].

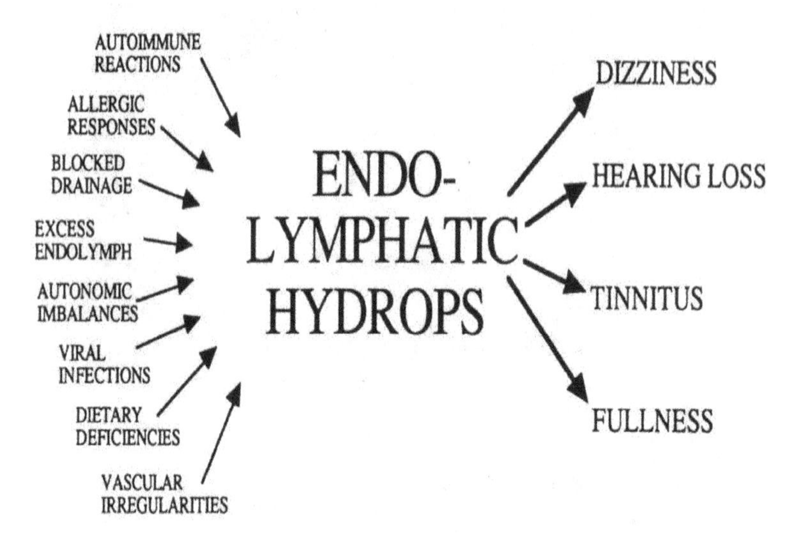

Figure 3. *Reprinted with permission from Ref. [9]. See text for explanation.*

In this way the rupture theory put forward by Schuknecht is now discarded.

Summarizing what has been said above:

1. EH is present in most cases of MD but it is not the cause of the Menière's symptoms. At most it can be taken as a pathologic correlate for MD. A primary unknown cause produces first the symptoms and later EH as an epiphenomenon.
2. Menière's syndrome is indeed a reaction of the inner ear to many insults (infec- tion, trauma, tertiary syphilis, otosclerosis, autoimmune diseases).
3. EH may be found in the temporal bones from patients with all the above-mentioned insults: it is therefore a common pathologic correlate to many inner ear injuries.
4. We consider as MD the Menière's syndrome without a known cause.

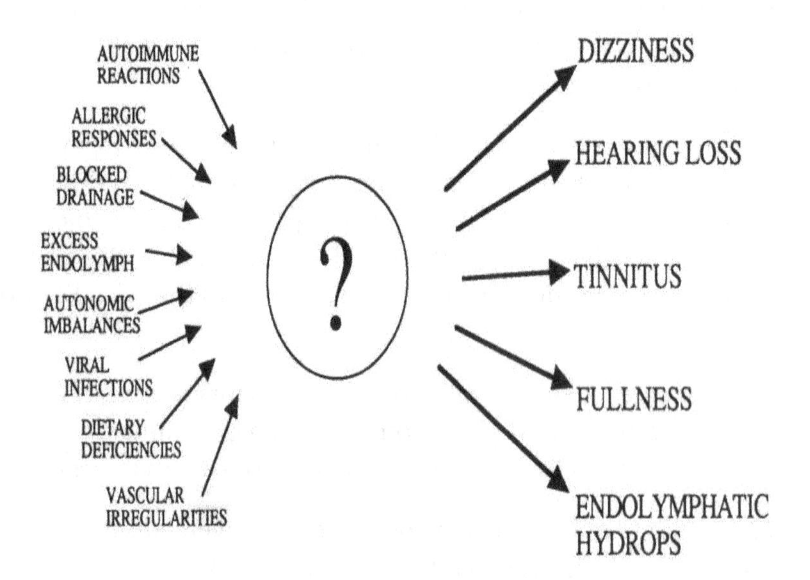

Figure 4. *Reprinted with permission from Ref. [9]. See text for explanation.*

Familial Menière's disease

Familial MD is not a rare finding. The presence of MD in several siblings of a family points to a genetic etiology for the disease. Studying these families is a way to learn about MD etiology. In this section we will discuss our experience with MD occurring in families.

This research line started up in 1992 [12]. By that time, we saw a patient who was 69 years old and had a full blown Menière's syndrome: severe episodic rota- tory vertigo with drop (falling) attacks, tinnitus and fluctuating hearing loss in his right year. These symptoms started up 5 years before we saw him. His drop attacks were severe and several times he hearts himself during falls. Right sided headaches usually preceded the crisis. Audiogram showed low tone sensorineural hearing loss bilateral and flat severe sensorineural hearing loss on the right ear. Left ear had hearing preserved in the frequencies above 500 Hz (**Figure 5A**). VDRL test was negative and glycerol test was positive bilaterally. An endolymphatic sac procedure was performed in his right ear and the drop attacks disappeared. Mild dizziness attacks and headache continued but were controlled on medication. Ten years later in June 1090 his hearing in the right ear had worsened (**Figure 5B**) considerably but the drop attacks had not come back and his dizziness was under control. His headache was unchanged.

The heredogram of this family (**Figure 6**) shows that six of seven sons and daughters of this man had the same complaints as their father and the audiograms on four available siblings showed low tone sensorineural hearing loss (**Figure 5C–F**). One offspring from a second marriage of the index patients also had the same com- plaints. We did not give attention to the headache these patients complained about so we did not classify this symptom properly.

We found several reports of headache associated with both familial and sporadic Menière's syndrome [13–15] but the headache was not well characterized in any.

Two questions were in our minds after we studied the family described above: (1) how often a family history could be elicited from patients with classic Menière's syndrome; (2) what kind of headache was associated with Menière's syndrome? We started to apply to all the patients with Menière's syndrome seen in our clinic a questionnaire with questions about the presence of similar symptoms in their fam- ily members as well as about the presence of migraine symptoms.

Through this questionnaire we identified a large family who had typical Menière's syndrome present in some siblings, migraine and Menière's syndrome in others, and only migraine symptoms in others. Considering all siblings affected with these symptoms we arrived to the heredogram displayed in **Figure 7**. The mode of genetic transmission was clearly autosomal dominant [17]. Of course, we knew that in every day clinic work we find more patients with incomplete than with full blown Menière's syndrome. To consider patients with migraine only as affected siblings was an assumption that was supported by continuing the line of thought.

The summary of all symptoms present on 19 affected members of the family is in **Table 1**. It can be seen there the spectrum of symptoms with some of them present and others absent in different patients. The index patient had full blown Menière's syndrome and fluctuating low tone sensorineural hearing loss (**Figure 8**). Three of his sons had intractable migraine who needed hospitalization for treatment some-times but they lacked Menière's syndrome symptoms at that point. We concluded that: there was a strong association between migraine and Menière's syndrome in this family and both seemed to be transmitted by a single gene in an autosomal dominant mode. From a physiopathology stand point we do not know how the migraine (central) relates to the Menière's symptoms (peripheral).

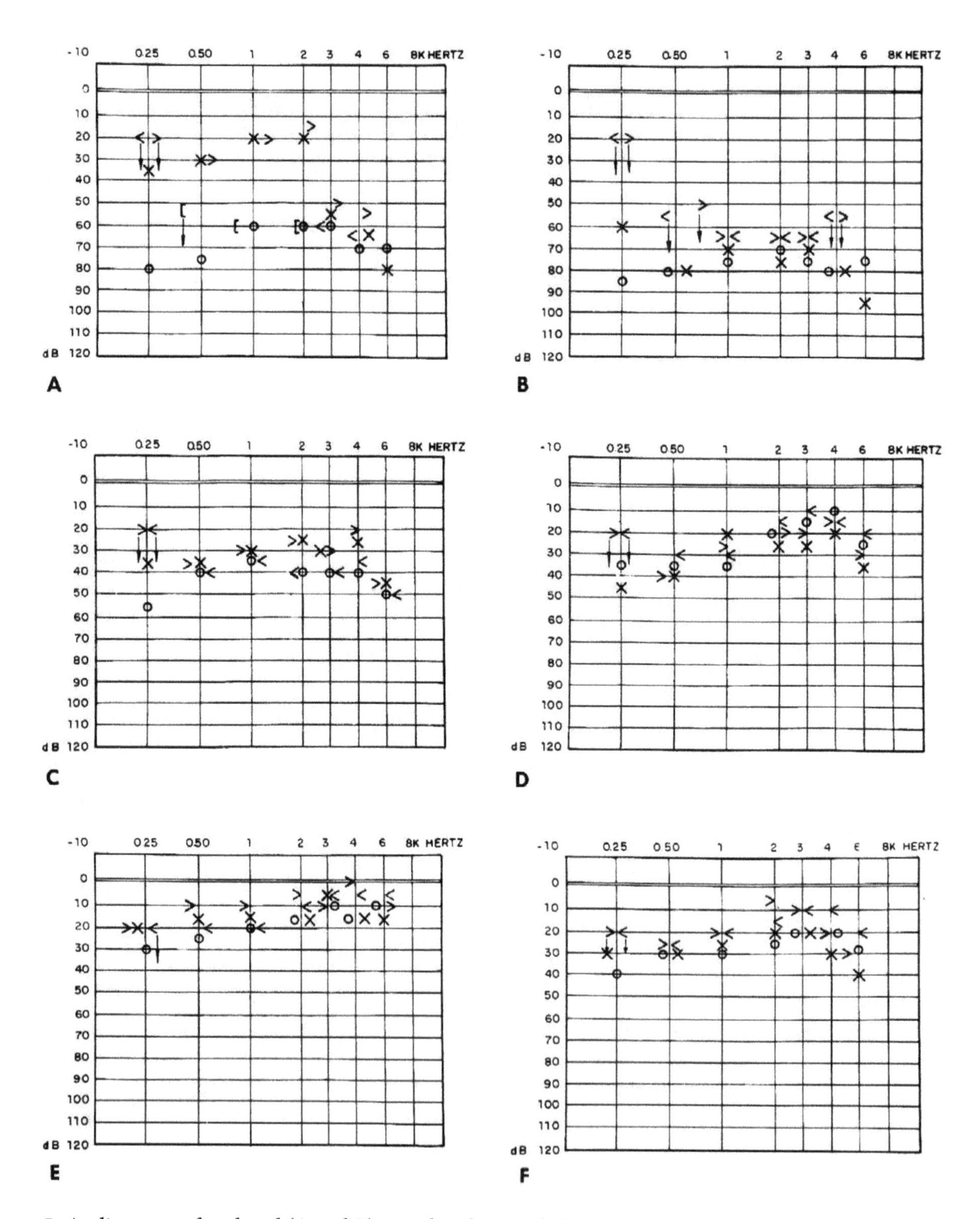

Figure 5. *Audiograms of proband (A and B), one daughter and three sons of his (C–F). Reprinted with permission from Ref. [13].*

Now we had a hypothesis: migraine and Menière's syndrome are related and transmitted in an autosomal dominant mode. To further this hypothesis, we set up to answer two questions: (1) How often is the occurrence of familial Migraine–Menière's syndrome in our population? (2) How is the evolution of these symptoms as time goes by? In other words: what is the Natural History of this symptom's complex?

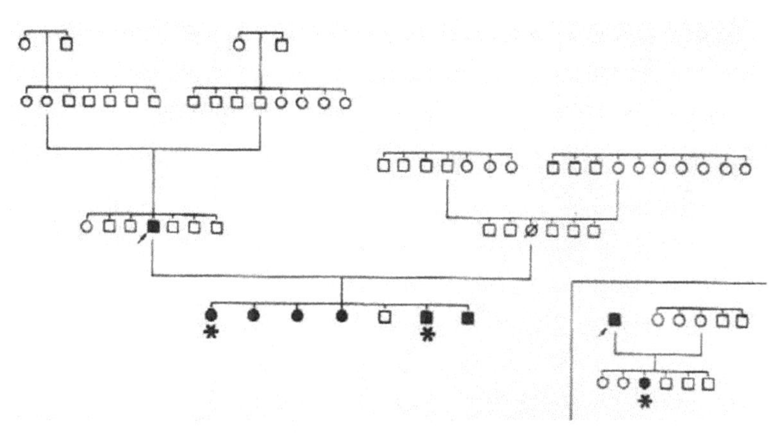

Figure 6. *Heredogram of the 1992 family. Reprinted with permission from Ref. [13]. Black symbols are affected siblings. Circles are male and square are females.*

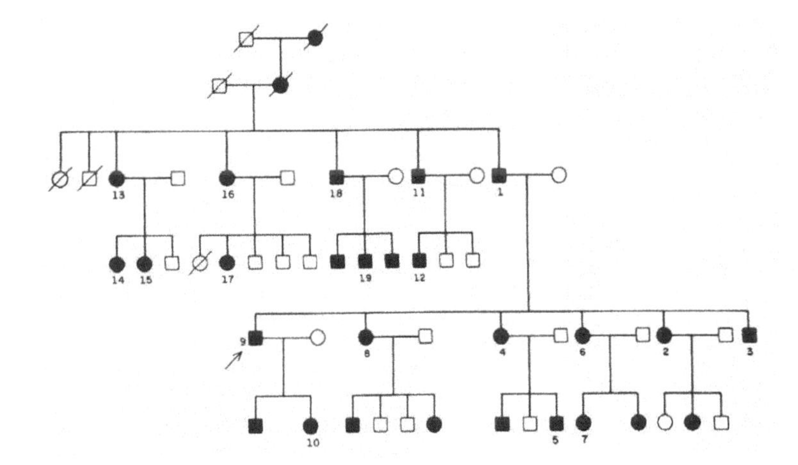

Figure 7. *Heredogram of 1997 family. Reprinted with permission from Ref. [16]. Black symbols are affected siblings. Circles are males and square are females.*

We then started to apply a questionnaire inquiring about the family history of every patient with typical Menière's syndrome seen in our Otology Clinic prospec- tively beginning in January 1997 and finishing in December 1998.

All index patients were required to have typical Menière's syndrome according to the American Academy of Otolaryngology—Head and Neck Surgery criteria. The work up included audiometry, tympanometry, vectoeletronystagmography and a glycerol test in order to seal the diagnosis of idiopathic typical Menière's syndrome (Menière's disease). At this point the included patients were questioned about migraine symptoms. Next the questionnaire about their family history regarding Menière's and migraine's symptoms present in other family members was applied. It is worth to mention that any symptom of one of these syndromes were noted and used to construct the heredogram of each family. Every available affected member of these families went through the same work up of the index patients.

Eight patients with typical, complete Menière's syndrome were collected in 2 years from our otology clinic in Brasília. Six of the eight had positive family his- tory for Menière's and/or migraine. **Table 2** shows that only one index patient had low tone sensorineural hearing loss. All others displayed high tone sensorineural hearing loss in between crisis. **Table 3** shows the presence/absence of Menière's and migraine symptoms in the affected members as well as demographic data.

Age of the index patients varied from 26 to 63 years old. Symptoms appeared between 15 and 40 years. Six patients had unilateral symptoms and two had both ears affected. Most of the time migraine occurred before the vestibular symptoms, sometimes it came after the vestibular crisis and a minority had migraine unrelated to the vertiginous attack. In six of the eight indices patient's headache fit the classification of the International Headache Society of 1988 as migraine. There were six female and two male probands [16].

Figures 9–11 show heredograms of the six affected families. It is clear from them that the pattern of genetic transmission is autosomal dominant and there is great variability with some siblings having typical Menière's disease and migraine, others having migraine alone and others having symptoms of Menière's syndrome incom- plete with or without migraine. If we assume a monogenetic transmission then variable penetrance of the gene is probably the cause of this variability.

Patient	*Age*	*Sex*	*Tinnitus*	*Hearing Loss*	*Vertigo*	*Headache*	*Vomiting*	*Nausea*	*Scotomas*
1	22	M	+	+	+	–	+	+	–
2	41	F	+	+	+	+*	+	+	+
3	50	M	+	+	+	+*	+	+	+
4	46	F	+	+	+	+*	+	+	+
5	17	M	–	–	–	+*	+	+	+
6	41	F	+	+	+	+	+	+	+
7	19	F	–	–	–	+*	+	+	+
8	56	F	+	–	+	+	–	+	+
9	58	M	+	+	+	+*	+	+	+
10	15	F	+	–	+	+*	+	+	+
11	77	M	+	+	+	–	+	+	–
12	51	M	+	+	+	+*	–	–	+
13	71	F	+	+	+	+	+	+	–
14	49	F	–	–	–	+*	–	–	–
15	47	F	+	+	+	+	–	–	–
16	80	F	+	–	+	+	–	–	–
17	59	F	+	+	+	+*	–	+	+
18	75	M	+	+	+	+	+	+	+
19	45	M	–	–	–	+*	–	–	–

ENG — electronystagmography, N — normal, SNHL — sensorineural hearing loss, ND — not done, MS — Meniere's syndrome, HL — hyperactive labyrinth.

*Headache was described by patient as typical migraine.

Patient	Anopsia	Pares-thesia	Age (y) at Which Symptoms Appeared	Time Sequence of Headache and Vertigo	Blood Tests	Audiometry	Tympa-nometry	ENG
1	+	–	30		N	SNHL, bilateral, down-sloping	N	ND
2	+	–	10	Headache precedes vertigo	ND	ND	ND	ND
3	–	–	10	Variable	ND	ND	ND	ND
4	–	+	13 migraine, 30 MS	Migraine only for 17 years, MS only afterward	N	Mild SNHL, bi-lateral, 500 and 1,000 Hz	N	N
5	+	–	15		ND	Mild SNHL, bi-lateral, 500 and 1,000 Hz	ND	N
6	–	+	14	Headache precedes vertigo	N	Bilateral moderate SNHL, down-sloping	N	HL left side
7	–	–	10		ND	ND	N	N
8	+	+	9	Headache and scotomas precede vertigo	N	Mild SNHL, 500 and 1,000 Hz, right	N	HL left side
9	–	–	39	Headache precedes vertigo	N	Bilateral moderate SNHL, down-sloping	N	HL left side
10	–	–	7	Headache precedes vertigo	ND	ND	ND	ND
11	–	–	18		ND	Bilateral moderate SNHL, down-sloping	N	HL left side
12	+	–	17 migraine, 25 MS	Migraine only for 8 years, then MS only	ND	Bilateral moderate SNHL, down-sloping	N	HL bilateral
13	–	–	30	Variable	N	Bilateral mixed hearing loss, worse on left	ND	HL bilateral
14	–	–	20		ND	ND	ND	ND
15	–	–	35	Variable	N	Mild SNHL, left	N	HL bilateral
16	–	–	21	Variable	ND	ND	ND	ND
17	+	+	43	Variable	ND	ND	ND	ND
18	–	–	15	Headache precedes vertigo	ND	ND	ND	ND
19	–	–	20		ND	ND	ND	ND

ENG — electronystagmography, N — normal, SNHL — sensorineural hearing loss, ND — not done, MS — Meniere's syndrome, HL — hyperactive labyrinth.

*Headache was described by patient as typical migraine.

* *Reprinted with permission from Ref. [16].*

Table 1. *Summary of clinical, laboratory, audiometric, and electronystagmographic findings in 19 affected members of family studied in 1997.**

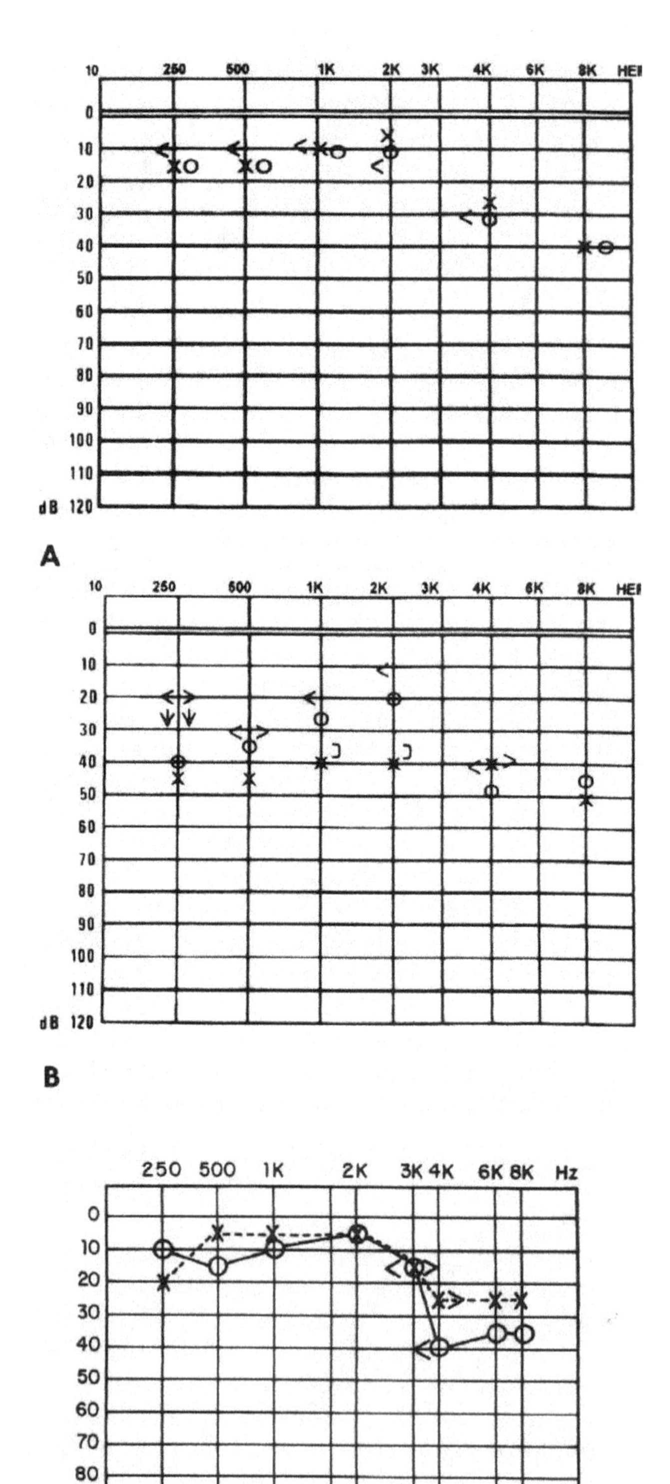

Figure 8. *Audiograms of the proband of the 1997 family. (A–C) Document fluctuating low tones sensorineural hearing loss. Reprinted with permission from Ref. [16].*

Proband	Age (y)	Sex	Audiometry
1	62	M	Bilateral moderate SNHL, downsloping on R, flat on L
2	43	F	Bilateral downsloping SNHL, moderate on R, severe on L
3	30	F	Normal
4	46	F	Normal
5	43	F	Flat moderate SNHL on R, normal on L
6	26	F	Normal
7	45	M	Bilateral moderate SNHL low and high tones, worse on L, middle tones normal
8	35	F	Moderate low-tone SNHL on L, normal on R

Speech discrimination score was compatible with pure tone loss in all patients.

SNHL — sensorineural hearing loss.

Reprinted with permission from Ref. [18].

Table 2. *Summary of audiometric findings in eight probands (2002 paper).*[*]

Probands	Affected Family Members	Age (y)	Sex	Tinnitus	Aural Fullness	Fluctuating Hearing Loss	Vertigo	Nausea	Vomiting	Audiometry	VENG	Scotoma	Photophobia	Atypical Headache	Hemicranial Headache	Pulsatile Headache
III-5		30	F	+	+	+	+	+	+	N	PIS R	+	+	–	+	+
(Family 3)	I-2	Deceased	F	+	+	+	+	+	–	ND	ND	+	+	–	+	+
	II-2	60	F	–	–	–	–	+	–	ND	ND	+	+	–	+	+
	III-6	16	F	+	–	+	+	–	–	SNHL bilat	PIS R	+	+	–	+	+
	III-8	37	F	–	–	–	–	+	–	ND	ND	–	+	–	+	+
	IV-1	10	M	+	+	+	+	–	–	N	N	–	–	+	–	–
III-2		46	F	+	+	+	+	+	+	N	PIS R	–	–	+	–	–
(Family 4)	II-2	60	F	+	–	–	+	–	–	N	N	–	+	–	+	+
	II-3	58	F	+	–	–	+	–	–	N	N	+	–	–	+	+
	II-4	65	F	+	+	–	+	+	+	N	PIS L	–	+	–	+	+
	III-3	43	F	–	–	–	+	–	–	N	PIS bilat	+	+	–	+	+
	III-7	33	F	–	–	–	–	–	–	ND	ND	–	+	–	+	+
	III-8	32	F	–	–	–	–	–	+	ND	ND	–	+	–	–	–
	IV-1	25	F	–	–	–	+	+	–	ND	ND	–	–	–	–	–
III-5		43	F	+	+	+	+	+	+	SNHL R	ND	+	+	–	+	+
(Family 5)	III-4	46	F	+	–	–	+	–	–	N	N	–	–	+	–	–
	IV-3	14	F	+	–	+	–	–	–	N	N	–	–	–	–	–
III-9		26	F	+	+	+	+	+	+	N	PIS bilat	+	+	–	+	+
(Family 6)	II-5	75	M	+	–	–	+	+	+	SNHL L	N	–	+	–	+	+
	III-8	32	F	+	–	–	+	–	–	ND	ND	–	+	–	+	+
	II-4	65	F	–	–	–	–	+	–	ND	ND	–	+	–	+	+
	III-2	46	M	–	–	–	–	–	–	ND	ND	–	+	–	–	–
	III-6	36	F	–	–	–	+	+	–	ND	ND	–	+	–	+	+
	II-1	40	F	–	–	–	–	+	–	ND	ND	+	+	–	+	–
	II-2	50	F	–	–	–	–	–	–	ND	ND	+	–	–	+	+
	II-4	52	F	–	–	–	–	+	+	ND	ND	–	+	–	+	+
II-22		45	M	+	+	+	+	+	+	SNHL L	N	–	–	–	–	–
(Family 7)	II-13	62	M	+	+	–	+	+	–	SNHL bilat	ND	+	–	+	+	+
	II-18	58	M	–	–	+	+	–	–	SNHL bilat	ND	–	–	–	–	–
	II-17	56	F	+	–	+	–	–	–	SNHL bilat	ND	+	–	+	+	+
	III-4	20	F	+	+	+	–	–	–	ND	ND	–	+	–	+	+
	III-5	12	F	–	–	–	–	–	–	N	N	–	+	–	+	+
III-5		35	F	+	+	+	+	+	+	N	PIS bilat	+	+	–	+	+
(Family 8)	II-5	54	F	+	–	+	–	+	–	ND	ND	+	+	–	+	+
	II-1	50	F	–	–	–	+	+	–	ND	ND	–	–	–	+	+

Tympanometric and stapedial reflex results were normal in all patients who had them done. Proband 1 had full-blown Meniere's syndrome and atypical headache. Proband 2 had both Meniere's and migraine symptoms.

VENG — vectoelectronystagmography, N — normal, PIS — peripheral irritative syndrome, ND — not done.

* *Reprinted with permission from Ref. [18].*

Table 3. *Summary of clinical, audiometric, and VENG findings in affected members of six families.*[*]

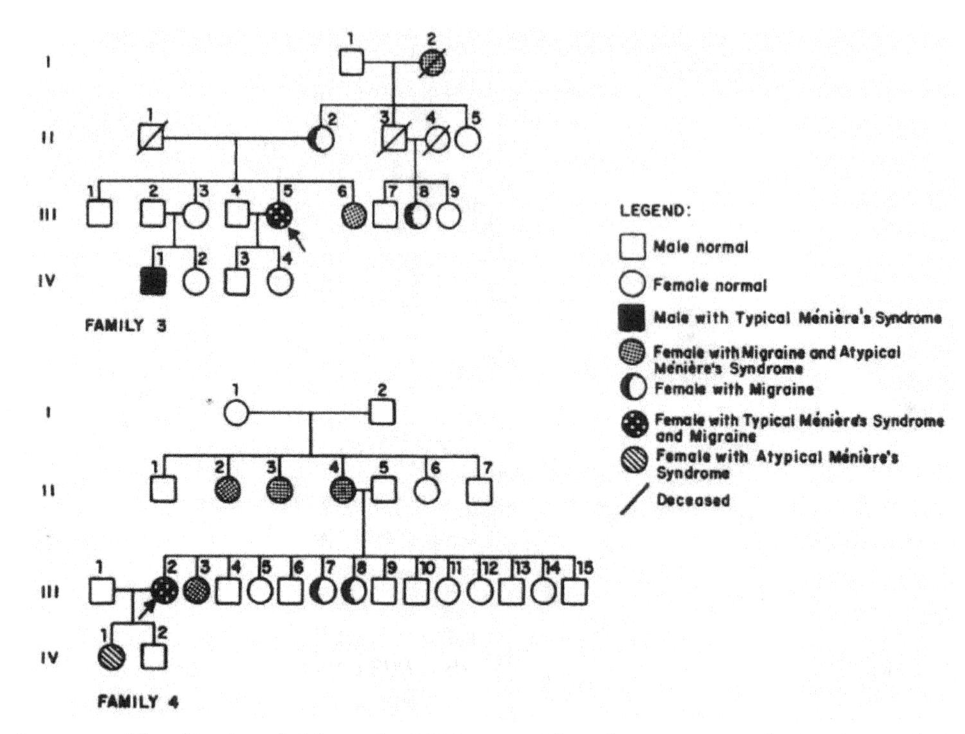

Figure 9. *Heredograms of families 3 and 4 from the 2002 paper. Note the spectrum of migraine and Menière's syndrome present in the affected siblings. Reprinted with permission from Ref. [18].*

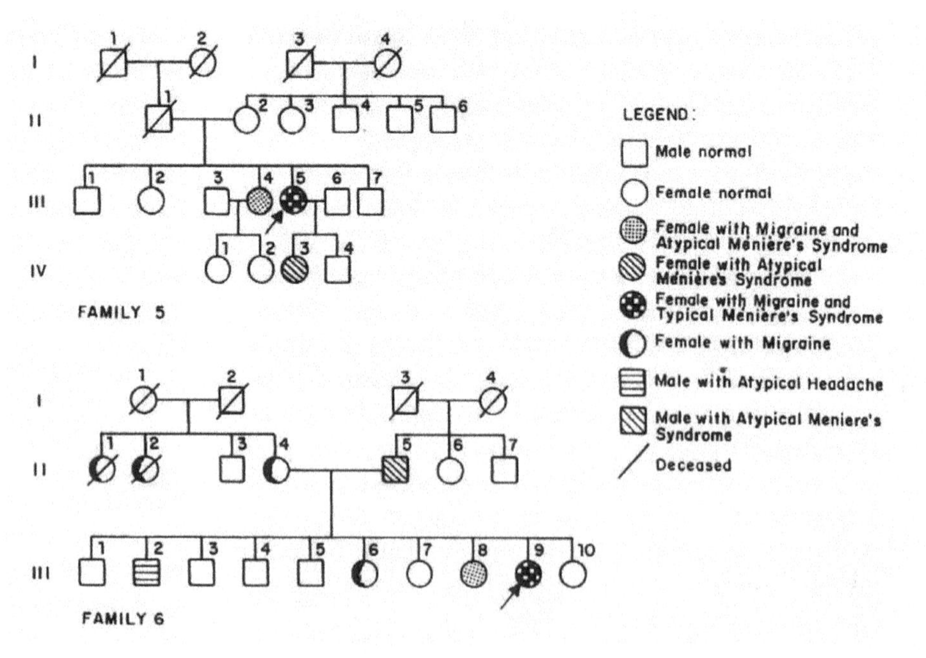

Figure 10. *Heredograms of families 5 and 6 of the 2002 paper. The pattern of symptoms distribution among the siblings are similar to the one present in families 3 and 4 above. Reprinted with permission from Ref. [18].*

From these data we reasoned that:

1. Typical Menière's syndrome is not very frequent in Brasília: during 2 years in a very buzzy Otology Clinic we collected only eight cases.

2. On the other hand, the occurrence of familial disease in patients with typi- cal Menière's syndrome

(Menière's disease) is quite high (six of eight index patients). If we consider Menière's syndrome all the spectrum of symptoms seen in these families then the disease is not so infrequent. In other words, we see incomplete Menière's syndrome much more often in our clinics than the typical syndrome. However, migraine can be associated with all the Menière`s spectrum of symptoms.

We wanted to ask: what happens to this spectrum of symptoms as time goes by?

The family we published in 1997 [17] lived in Brasília and we were able to follow them up from 1995 on for 10 years. The following paragraphs will refer to unpub- lished data from our group.

All affected and unaffected siblings in the heredogram in **Figure 7** were care- fully interviewed along the 10 years follow up. Twenty siblings had no qualitative changes in symptoms from 1995 to 2005. Four had changed from atypical headache in 1995 to typical migraine 10 years later. Two had migraine in 1995 and progressed to Menière's syndrome in 2005. Four siblings had vertigo and atypical headache in 1995 and progressed to vertigo and typical migraine in 2005.

Five unaffected siblings in 1995 had symptoms of the migraine—Menière's complex 10 years later: two with aural fullness, one with migraine, tinnitus, ver- tigo and hearing loss and two with migraine and vertigo. Three affected siblings had remarkable improvement in migraine and vertigo or complete remission of the symptoms.

Fifteen of the 38 affected siblings started out with migraine and the vestibular symptoms appeared in average 17.6 years later. Seven siblings continued with migraine only after 10 years follow up. Over time the intensity and periodicity of the migraine symptoms tended to diminish and the vestibular symptoms tended to become more frequent and intense (**Table 4** and **Figure 12**).

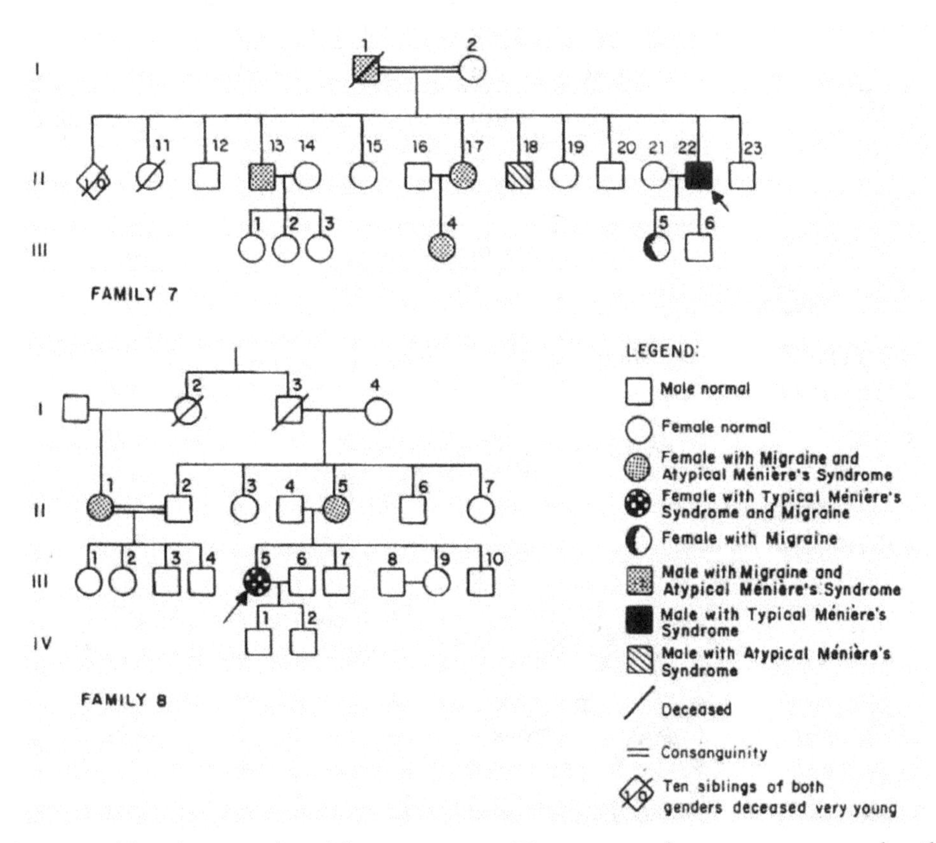

Figure 11. *Heredogram of families 7 and 8 of the 2002 paper. The pattern of symptoms among the siblings is similar to the families 3to 6. Reprinted with permission from Ref. [18].*

Patient	Age at the moment	Periodicity* (1995)		Periodicity* (2005)		Intensity (1995)		Intensity (2005)	
	(2005) (y)	**Migraine**	**Menière**	**Migraine**	**Menière**	**Migraine**	**Menière**	**Migraine**	**Menière**
1	81	2/w	1/w	1/w	1/w	9/10	Moderate	6/10	Severe
2	90	—	—	—	—	—	—	—	—
3	82	2/w	2/m	2/m	1/w	8/10	Moderate	6/10	Severe
4	87	1/w	1/m	1/m	1/w	6/10	Moderate	6/10	Severe
5	92	1/w	1/w	2/m	2/w	9/10	Severe	9/10	Severe
11	62	2/m	—	2/m	1/m	8/10	—	7/10	Severe
12	58	2/m	—	2/m	—	7/10	—	6/10	—
21	69	1/m	1/m	1/m	2/m	8/10	Moderate	5/10	Moderate
31	61	1/m	1/m	1/m	2/m	9/10	Moderate	6/10	Moderate
32	64	3–4/m	—	2/m	—	9/10	—	6/10	—
33	63	1/m	—	1/m	—	10/10	—	6/10	—
41	61	2/w	1/w	2/m	2/w	9/10	Moderate	7/10	Severe
51	68	1/m	1/m	1/m	2/m	9/10	Severe	8/10	Severe
52	66	1/m	—	1/m	—	8/10	—	8/10	—
53	54	1/m	2/y	1/m	4/y	7/10	Moderate	7/10	Severe
54	51	2/y	3/y	2/y	1/m	8/10	Moderate	8/10	Moderate
55	51	3/y	1/y	3/y	3/y	8/10	Moderate	6/10	Moderate
56	60	1/m	2/y	1/m	1/m	9/10	Moderate	8/10	Moderate
512	37	6/y	1/y	2/m	4/y	8/10	Moderate	8/10	Moderate
524	37	1/m	—	1/m	—	8/10	—	8/10	—
531	32	3/y	—	3/y	—	7/10	—	7/10	—
533	25	3/y	—	3/y	—	7/10	—	7/10	—
541	29	4/y	1/y	1/m	4/y	8/10	Moderate	8/10	Moderate

Unpublished observations.

Table 4. *Natural history of migraine and vestibular symptoms during 10 years follow-up (1997 family) (N = 23 affected siblings).**

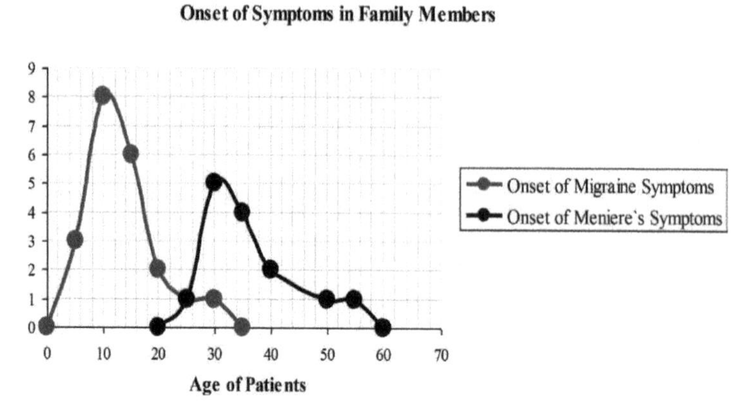

Figure 12. *Graphic representation of the natural history of this symptom complex during 10 years follow up of the 1997 family.*

Patient	Audiogram result (1995)	Audiogram result (2005)
1	Moderate to profound mixed hearing loss bilaterally	Profound mixed hearing loss bilaterally
2	Mild high frequency SNHL	Mild to moderate high frequency SNHL
3	Moderate high frequency SNHL	Moderate high frequency SNHL
4	Moderate mixed hearing loss bilaterally	Moderate mixed hearing loss bilaterally
5	Moderate high frequency SNHL bilaterally	Moderate to severe high frequency SNHL bilaterally
11	Normal	Normal
12	Normal	Normal
13	—	—
21	Normal	Normal
22	—	—
23	—	—
24	—	—
31	—	—
32	Normal	Mild high frequency SNHL bilaterally
33	—	—
41	Mild high frequency SNHL	Mild to moderate high frequency SNHL bilaterally
42	—	—
43	—	—
51	Moderate high frequency SNHL bilaterally	Profound high frequency SNHL bilaterally
52	Normal	Normal
53	Normal	Normal
54	Mild high frequency SNHL bilaterally	Mild to moderate high frequency SNHL bilaterally
55	Mild high frequency SNHL bilaterally	Mild to moderate high frequency SNHL bilaterally
56	Moderate high frequency SNHL	Profound high frequency SNHL bilaterally
511	—	—
512	Normal	Mild high frequency SNHL bilaterally
521	—	—
522	—	—
523	—	—
524	—	—
531	—	—
532	—	—
533	Normal	Normal
541	Normal	Normal
542	—	—
551	—	—
552	—	—
553	—	—

**Reprinted with permission from Ref. [19].*

Table 5. *Hearing loss during 10 years follow-up (N = 19).**

Hearing loss worsened in most patients. The loss was in high frequency tones and bilateral (**Table 5**). We were not able to document low tone fluctuating senso- rineural hearing loss during the crisis of vertigo/ migraine in all siblings but we did document this feature clearly only in the index patient (**Figure 8**).

Now we had the natural history of this complex of symptoms described. We were therefore able to organize the clinical data in order to define a phenotype of this syndrome in the large family from Brasília.

Our hypothesis was that this was a genetically determined symptom com- plex and the genetic transmission was monogenic with incomplete penetrance. Next step was to try to find the genetic locus for these symptoms. Because we were not able to document low tone sensorineural hearing loss in most of the siblings and the high frequency sensorineural hearing loss was bilateral in the majority of the siblings the clinical diagnosis of migrainous vertigo was adopted for these patients. The fact that some of them had typical Menière's syndrome including low tone sensorineural hearing loss was however pointed out in the final paper [18].

Twenty-three family members who were clinically and audiologically evaluated and had image studies also done had genome wide linkage analysis performed with Affymetrix GeneChip Human Mapping 10K microarrays. Genotyping of family members DNA with microsatellite markers was used to further assess candidate loci identified from the whole genome scan.

The results of vestibular testing and imaging studies were unremarkable. The genetic analysis defined a 12.0 MB interval on chromosome 5q35 between loci rs2448795 and D5S2073 that contained the disease gene (logarithm of odd score 4.21).

Molecular genetics studies were performed at the Molecular Genetics laboratory of Harvard Medical School headed by Professor Jonathan Seidman.

Discussion of above findings and correlation with current literature

Here we will blend our results with the current literature on the subject and formulate a new hypothesis.

It is important to acknowledge the recently described vertiginous migraine (VM) syndrome [19] which is now listed in the Barany Society and the International Headache Society classification of vestibular diseases [20]. This entity is very frequent, second only to benign paroxistic positional vertigo being probably present in 1% of the general population [8]. We are not going to describe in detail the VM symptoms but it is important to point out the differences between MD and VM.

One marked difference is the absence of hearing loss that fluctuates in the low frequencies in the beginning and that progresses to severe hearing loss along the life in Menière's disease but not in vertiginous migraine. Bilaterally of the symptoms seems to be more frequent in familial MD and VM than in sporadic MD but it is not different between these two syndromes.

There is a significant body of literature dealing with the interfaces of Menière's disease (DM) and VM. We will review briefly some papers on this subject.

Neuhauser et al. [21, 22] prospectively evaluated migraine in 200 patients from a dizziness clinic and 200 ones from a migraine clinic. Prevalence of migraine that satisfied the criteria of the International Headache Society (HIS) II was 38% in the dizziness clinic and 24% in sex and age matched controls ($p < 0.01$). Vertiginous migraine was present in 7% of patients in the dizziness clinic and 9% of the ones in the migraine clinic. In 15 of 32 patient's vertigo was always associated with migraine during the acute attacks. In 16 patients this association was sporadic and two patients never had both symptoms together.

Radke et al. [23] studied 78 patients (40 male and 38 female) aged 29–81 years all with idiopathic uni- or bilateral Menière's disease according to the AAO-HNS criteria. Lifetime prevalence of migraine with and without aura was 50% among these patients and 25% among normal control patients ($p < 0.001$). Furthermore 45% or the Menière's disease patients always experienced at least one migraine symptom (headache, photophobia, aura) during the acute attacks. They postulated a pathophysiologic link between migraine and MD.

Urkur et al. [24] studied VEMPs parameters in VM, MD and migraine patients and found very similar results for all these patients. Gazques et al. [13] published a paper on recent advances in the genetics of recurrent vertigo including familiar episodic ataxias and MD. They found that 20% of MD patients have positive family histories for this disease [25].

Cha et al. [27] described six families with index patients affected by MD and migraine. There were 56 affected siblings. Of these 26 (41%) met the HIS criteria for migraine. Fifty percent had migraine with aura. Three patients had typical aura without headache. Sixty-three family members had recurrent spells of spontane- ous vertigo. There were three twin pairs, two monos and one dizygotic. One of the homozygotic pair had migraine and MD while the other one had migraine and episodic vertigo without auditory involvement (VM).

Bertora and Bergman [38] using quantitative EEG (qEEG) studied 120 patients with MD and migraine and 85 patients with MD and no migraine. Eighty-five percent of MDs patients had hemodynamic brain variations like the ones found in migraine. Brain electric depolarizations and cortical irritative focuses are common to migraine and MD. However, MDs patients had important hyperactivity in the limbic lobe [28].

From this brief review of literature, we can say:

1. VM and MD are very often present in one single family and therefore have a common-genetic link.
2. Hearing involvement in MD and not in VM is the main clinical difference between these two syndromes.
3. Migraine is present in both syndromes.

Recently Welfang et al. [29] selected 30 classic MD patients and 30 patients with definite or probable VM matched by age and sex. Three-dimensional real inversion recovery magnetic resonance (3D real IR) was performed in these patients 24 hours after intratympanic gadolinium injection in order to assess endolymphatic hydrops (EH). Response rates, amplitudes, latency and response thresholds of cervical and ocular evoked myogenic potentials (c/o VEMP) were tested using air conducted sound. Pure tone audiometry was used to evaluate the level of hearing loss.

Different degrees of EH were observed in the cochlea and vestibule of MD patients. Some VM patients had 3D real—IR suspicious for cochlea EH and no EH was found in the vestibule of these patients. There was statistically significant cor- relation between EH and low tone sensorineural hearing loss. Response thresholds for c/o VEMP were no different in VM and MD patients.

Therefore, low frequencies sensorineural hearing loss correlate with EH on MD patients. 3R-real IR showed more severe degrees of EH in patients with MD but suggestion of EH in the cochlea of VM patients was showed. MD and VM patients behaved similarly in vestibular dysfunction and their transduction pathway (VEMP).

Ghawany et al. [30] treated 25 patients with typical MD following protocol to prophylactic migrainous treatment and showed marked improvement in quality of life in 92% of the patients. He states his results point to etiopathogenetic relation between MD and VM.

These results suggest a common etiopathogenesis for MD and VM and that VM may progress to MD as time goes by if EH develops in VM patients.

Conclusion

At this point we know that the spectrum of symptoms that goes from migraine alone to migraine with full blown MD including vertigo and migraine (VM), vertigo alone (atypical Menière's syndrome) has high familial incidence and is genetically transmitted in a monogenic autosomal dominant mode [16]. We have found that the locus for this spectrum of symptoms maps to chromosome 5q35 [18].

Studies using VEMP [26] and 3D real IR [27] have shown that EH is present in different degrees in both MD and VM. It may be that absence of low tone senso- rineural hearing loss in VM relates to the very small degree of EH present in this entity compared to MD.

Based on all this evidence we have up to now we believe that future efforts should be directed to isolate the gene in chromosome 5q35 and follow up longitudi- nally patients with VM with VEMP and 3D real IR MRI to test the hypothesis that VM and MD are different stages of the same process.

Sporadic MD and VM should be tested for the presence of the gene we are looking for after we have it isolated. Then we might also have a better idea about the etiology of MD and VM. Probably environmental factors [31] will be also important for the full development of the disease (multifactorial etiology).

We do believe that this research line should be taken to its future.

Etiopathogenesis of migraine—Menière's disease

Finally we must consider how migraine, a central syndrome relates to Meniere's disease a syndrome that originates in the periphery of the vestibular system.

Several authors [32–36] have shown that trigeminal vasomotor fibers innervate the inner ear (stria vascularis, cells of the ampullary crests) and through this pathway the vascular changes occurring in the central nervous system reach the peripheric vestibular system and bring about the symptoms of MD and EH. This certainly would occur in VM too.

Of course this theory needs experimental confirmation before it can be con- sidered proven. Nevertheless the anatomical pathways are in existence and this is factual evidence towards this theory. The natural history of the symptoms in our families supports it.

Dolowitz [37] has studied a big number of patients with MD and showed that headache is a nuclear symptom in sporadic MD but he did not characterize the headache as igraine so this must be done before we can say that migraine is a constant part of sporadic MD.

References

[1] Menière P. Memoires sur dês lesions de l`òreille interne donnant lieu a dês symptoms de congestion cerebrale apoplectiforme. GazMedicale de Paris. 1861;**15**:597-601

[2] Hallpike LS, Cairns H. Observations on the pathology of Meniere's syndrome. The Journal of Laryngology and Otology. 1938;**53**:625-655

[3] Yamakaua KJ. Pathologic changes in a Meniere's patient. Journal of Otolaryngology Society of Japan. 1938:2310-2312

[4] Hallpike LS, Wright HS. Histological findings in case of Menière's disease with remarks on pathologic anatomy and basis of this lesion. The Journal of Laryngology and Otology. 1940;**55**:59-66

[5] Lindsay JR. Histological studies of Menière's disease. Archives of Otolaryngology. 1994;**37**:853-867

[6] Altman F, Kornfeld M. LXXV histological studies of Meniere's disease. The Annals of Otology, Rhinology, & Laryngology. 1965;**74**:935-943

[7] Schuknecht HF. A critical evaluation of treatment for Meniere's disease. Journal of Contact Rd ORL Allergy. 1978;**40**:15-30

[8] Fraysse BG, Alonso A, House WF. Observations on the pathology of Meniere's syndrome. Annals of Otology, Rhinology and Laryngology. 1980;**89**(Suppl 6):2-22

[9] Rauch SD, Merchant SN, Thedinger BA. Menière's syndrome and endolymphatic hydrops. The Annals of Otology, Rhinology, and Laryngology. 1989;**98**:873-883

[10] HYS K. In: Nadol JB, editor. Second International Symposium on Meniere's Disease. Amsterdam: Kugler and Ghedini; 1989

[11] Merchant SN, Adams J, Nadol JB Jr. Pathophysiology of Menière's syndrome: Are symptoms caused by endolymphatic hydrops? Otology & Neurotology. 2005;**26**:74-81

[12] Oliveira CA. Thinking about tinnitus. The International Tinnitus Journal. 1995;**1**:1-4

[13] Oliveira CA, Braga AM. Meniere's syndrome inherited as an autosomal dominant trait. The Annals of Otology, Rhinology, and Laryngology. 1992;**101**:590-594

[14] Brown MR. Meniere's syndrome. Archives of Neurology and Psychiatry. 1941;**46**:561-565

[15] Brown MR. The factor of heredity in labyrinthine deafness and paroxysmal vertigo (Menière's syndrome). The Annals of Otology, Rhinology, and Laryngology. 1949;**58**:665-670

[16] Oliveira CA, Bezerra RL, Araujo MF, Almeida VF, Messias CI. Meniere's syndrome and migraine: Incidence in one family. The Annals of Otology, Rhinology, and Laryngology. 1997;**106**:823-829

[17] Bernstein JM. Occurrence of episodic vertigo and hearing loss in families. The Annals of Otology, Rhinology, and Laryngology. 1965;**74**:1011-1021

[18] Oliveira CA, Messias CI, Ferrari I. Occurrence of familial Meniere's syndrome and migraine in Brasília. 2002;**111**:229-236

[19] Bahmad F Jr, De Palma SR, Merchant SN, Bezerra RL, Oliveira CA, Seidman ES, et al. Locus for familial migrainous vertigo disease maps to chromosome 5q35. The Annals of Otology, Rhinology, and Laryngology. 2009;**118**:670-676

[20] Neuhauser H, Lempert T. Vestibular migraine. Neurologic Clinics. 2009;**27**(2):379-391

[21] Neuhauser H, Leopold M, von Brevern M, Arnold G, Lempert T. The interrelations of migraine, vertigo and migrainous vertigo. Neurology. 2001;**56**(4):436-441

[22] Lempert T, Olesen JF, Urlan J, Waterson J, Seemungal B, Carey J, et al. Vestibular migraine: Diagnostic criteria. Journal of Vestibular Research. 2012;**22**(4):167-172

[23] Radke A, Lempert T, Gresty MA, Brookes GB, Bronstein AM, Migraine NH. Meniére's disease: Is there a link? Neurology. 2002;**50**(11):1700-1704

[24] Urkur et al. Migrainous vertigo, Manière's disease and migraine. The Journal of International Advanced Otology. 2003;**9**(3):350-367

[25] Oliveira CA. Editorial. The International Tinnitus Journal. 2014;**19**:2-3

[26] Gazques I, Lopes Escames JA. Genetics of recurrent vertigo and vestibular disorders. Genomics. 2011;**12**(6):443-450

[27] Cha HI, Kane MJ, Baloh RHF. Familial clustering of migraine, episodic vertigo and Meniere's disease. Otology & Neurotology. 2008;**29**(1):93-96

[28] Oliveira CA. Letter to the editor. The International Tinnitus Journal. 2017;**21**(76)

[29] Welfang S, Guo P, Rent T, Wanda G. Magnetic resonance imaging of intratympanic gadolinium helps differentiate vestibular migraine from Meniere's disease. Laryngoscope. 2017;**127**:2382-2388

[30] Ghawani Y, Haiden YM, Moshtaghi O, Lin HW, Djalilian HD. Evaluating quality of life in patients with Meniere's disease treated as migraine. The Annals of Otology, Rhinology, and Laryngology. 2018;**125**:877-887

[31] Oniki J, Takahashi M, Wada R, Sato R. Comparative study of the daily lifestyle of patients with Meniere's disease and controls. The Annals of Otology, Rhinology, and Laryngology. 2005;**114**(12):927-933

[32] William HC. A review of the literature as to the physiologic dysfunction of Meniere's disease: A new hypothesis as to its fundamental cause. Laryngoscope. 1965;**75**:1661-1669

[33] Torok M. Etiology as a guide in the management of Menière's disease. Laryngoscope. 1982;**92**:237-238

[34] Vass Z, Steyger PI, Hordichok AJ, Taune DR, Jansen D, Nuttal AL. Capsaicin stimulation of the cochlea and electric stimulation of the trigeminal ganglion mediate vascular permeability in cochlear and vertebra-basilar arteries: A possible cause of inner ear dysfunction in headache. Neuroscience. 2001;**103**:189-201

[35] Vass Z, Shore SE, Nuttal AL, Miller JM. Endolymphatic hydrops reduces retrograde labeling of trigeminal innervations to the cochlea. Experimental Neurology. 1998;**151**:241-248

[36] Pondugula ST, Sanneman JD, Wangemann P, Milhaud Marcus DC. Glucocorticoids stimulates cation absorption by semicircular canal duct epithelium via epithelial sodium channel PG. American Journal of Physiology. Renal Physiology. 2004;**286**:1127-1135

[37] Dolowitz DA. Menière's—An inner ear seizure. Laryngoscope. 1979;**89**:67-77

[38] Bertora GO, Bergman JM. Menière's disease: Is it a special sort of migraine? Our experience. Archives of Sensology and Neurootology in Science and Practice. 2015. Available from: http:// www.neurootology.otg/ proceedings

16

Acupuncture Points Stimulation for Meniere's Disease/Syndrome: A Promising Therapeutic Approach

Jiaojun He, Liyuan Jiang, Tianqiang Peng, Meixia Xia, and Huade Chen

The Third Clinical Medical College of Zhejiang Chinese Medical University, Hangzhou, Zhejiang 310053, China

Correspondence should be addressed to Huade Chen; docchd@sina.com

Academic Editor: Paolo Roberti di Sarsina

ABSTRACT

Objective. This study aims to explore evidence for acupuncture points stimulation (APS) in treatment of Meniere's disease (MD). Method. A literature search was conducted in seven databases including EMBASE, Medline, Cochrane Library, Web of Science, CBM, CNKI, and WangFang database and the data analysis was performed by using the RevMan version 5.3. Results. 12 RCTs with 993 participants were acquired after the search. The quality of most eligible studies was very low which limited the value of the meta-analysis. Compared with western medicine comprehensive treatment (WMCT), the APS alone or in combination with WMCT had a significant positive effect in controlling vertigo; however, the result was negative in hearing improvement and DHI. No adverse events were reported in the studies. Conclusion. The APS might be a promising therapeutic approach for MD. However, the currently available evidence is insufficient to make a definitive conclusion for the poor quality of included studies. More highquality researches with larger sample size are urgently needed to assess the effectiveness and safety.

INTRODUCTION

Meniere's disease (MD), named after the French physician Prosper Meniere who firstly reported it in 1861 [1], is an idiopathic inner ear disorder characterized by episodic vertigo, fluctuating sensorineural hearing loss, tinnitus, and aural pressure. Some other complaints from patients including drop attack known as otolithic crisis of Tumarkin [2] and nausea [3, 4] always cooccur with the cardinal symptoms. The prevalence in reports ranged from 3.5 to 513 per 100,000 [5] with a slight female preponderance: about 1.89 : 1 in an American investigation [5, 6] and familial clustering, genetic heterogeneity [7, 8]. It is more common in people who are older and white [9] but rare in children [10].

Meniere's disease is a relentless illness [11], which means there would never be an ending through the whole life. The primary disability, vertigo, always accompanied by vomiting, makes the sufferers unable to keep normal posture [12]. Another predominant impact on the quality of life is impaired hearing. The hearing loss appeared in low-frequency at the earlier stage when it comes even without any prevision and goes and then gradually progressed to high-frequency until it developed to profound sensorineural hearing loss or singlesided deafness permanently [13, 14]. What the MD brings is not only physical dysfunction but also the mental problems consisting of anxiety and depression [15, 16]. It seems that there is a vicious cycle between them. The manifestations might be an origin of the unhealthy mental reaction and then the psychiatric comorbidity might well contribute to its pathology [17, 18].

Tons of endeavors have been devoted to the treatment ever since it was reported, but therapeutic progress was so frustratingly slow [19], which should be blamed on the complicated and exclusive mechanism. Until now, there has been no gold standard for treatment that can be adopted as the guideline and the strategies are needed to be individually tailored. The treatment, usually, starts with life-style change, and then there are the etiologic treatments including diuretics, betahistine, intratympanic gentamicin, intratympanic steroids, and surgery [20]. All available therapies, indeed, helped substantial patients. However, not all the sufferers were sensitive to the medications which might produce tolerance or side-effects after a long-term intake [21] or eligible to the surgery. Therefore, complementary and alternative therapy noticed by growing otolaryngology patients [22] might be a good choice for some people.

Acupuncture, a well-known complementary and alternative therapy, has been widely used in China. The symptoms of MD have been observed by Chinese antiquity and have been recorded in Huangdi Neijing [23]; however, the history that acupuncture, moxibustion, and massage were used in otorhinolaryngology could even date back to 5th century BC, much earlier than the time the masterpiece was written [24]. Nowadays, different acupuncture points stimulations (APS) are widely adopted in controlling the vertigo caused by various reasons including MD [25, 26] which made us wonder whether or not APS has some benefits to the sufferers. An analysis was carried out to explore evidence for the utilization of APS in MD.

Methods

Search Strategy. A strict research protocol was drafted before the work. According to the strategy, databases involving PubMed, EMBASE, Cochrane Library, Web of Science, Chinese BioMedical Literature Database (CBM), Chinese National Knowledge Infrastructure (CNKI), and WangFang data were searched. The studies were published before May 2015, regardless of the striation of language. The key words or free text words and the searching strategies were as follows: ("Meniere's disease" OR "Meniere's syndrome") AND ("acupuncture" OR "electroacupuncture" OR "acupoint" OR "meridian" OR "auricular therapy" OR "acupressure" OR "acupoint injection" OR "complementary medicine" OR "alternative medicine") AND ("clinical trial" OR "randomized controlled trial").

Criteria for Inclusion and Exclusion. Inclusion criteria were as follows: types of studies: randomized controlled trials; types of intervention and control: the main intervention for the experimental group is acupoints stimulations (including mammal acupuncture, scalp acupuncture, ear acupuncture, and auricular-plaster with vaccaria seed, moxibustion, acupoint injection, and acupressure which can be used alone or together) in combination with western medications comprehensive treatment (WMCT). The control group received western medications such as betahistine and other vasodilator, nutritional supports. Types of outcome assessments were the total effective rate assessed by the similar criteria and Dizziness Handicap Inventory (DHI).

Exclusion criteria included the following: (1) duplicated studies and animal experiments; (2) comparison between different acupuncture techniques or acupoints selection; (3) acupuncture in the junction with Chinese herbal medicine.

Data Extraction. According to the inclusion and exclusion criteria, two investigators (Jiaojun He and Liyuan

Jiang) independently screened the titles and abstracts and then downloaded the full text if they were potentially eligible for the analysis. The collection of information included the author(s), publish year, diagnostic criteria, sample size, disease course, the acupuncture intervention, control intervention, treatment course, main acupoints, effective criteria, and outcome measurement.

Quality of the Studies. The quality of the included trials was evaluated by two authors independently (Jiaojun He and Liyuan Jiang) in accordance with the risk of bias provided by Cochrane Handle Book 5 which consists of the following 7 items: random sequence generation, allocation concealment, blinding of participants and personnel, blinding of outcome assessment, incomplete outcome data, selective reporting, and other bias. All risks were evaluated as low, high, or unclear. Discrepancies reached an agreement after the discussion with the third reviewer (Huade Chen).

Data Synthesis and Analysis. Meta-analysis was performed by RevMan 5.3 of the Cochrane Collaboration. The outcome was presented as relative ratios (RRs) with 95% confidence intervals (CI) or mean difference with 95% CI. Before the data synthesis and analysis, heterogeneity test was done with the chi-squared test and the Higgins I^2 test [27]. Random effect models should be used if $I^2 > 50\%$; otherwise, a fixed effect model should be used. Begg's test and Egger's test were conducted to evaluate publication bias via a funnel-plot when the number of eligible studies was equal to or greater than 10.

Results

Literature Search. The detailed process of the search work was shown in the flowchart (Figure 1). A total of 473 articles we got form the initial search, and 323 of them were left after removing duplicates. And then 282 articles were excluded because they were nonrelevant ($n = 91$), case reports ($n = 167$), animals experiment ($n = 1$), and reviews ($n = 23$). 40 reports with control group remained. One of them was excluded because of lack of the diagnostic criteria, 9 of them were excluded because they were not RCT, 5 of them were excluded for the comparison between different acupuncture techniques, 10 of them were excluded for the junction with Chinese herbal medicine, and 3 of them were excluded for unavailable data and the small number of participants (less than 20). Finally, we included 12 studies for the meta-analysis.

The Basic Characteristics of Included Studies. The basic characteristics and main outcome of the 12 trials were summarized in Tables 1 and 2. All trials [28–40], in which the age range for participants was from 18 to 75 and the disease duration was several days to more than two decades, were conducted in China. The 12 RCTs with clear diagnostic criteria included 993 patients who had typical MD symptoms: 504 participants in the experimental group and 489 patients in the control group.

The interventions included traditional acupuncture, manual acupuncture (MA) in 3 studies [29, 33, 34, 36], MA coupled with moxibustion in two studies [28, 39], techniques in modern acupuncturology containing auricularstimulation in two reports [30, 37], scalp acupuncture in one study [32], acupoint injection in two trials [31, 38], acupressure in one report [40], or the combination between traditional and modern acupuncture in a study [35]. The main acupoints selected were Baihui (DU20), the top in the studies, Tinggong (SI19), and Fengchi (GB20). The mean treatment time was approximately 10 to 15 days once a day. Two studies [29, 36] mentioned Deqi, an indispensable element for MA, a sort of acid bilge feeling in patients and a sense in doctors which was vividly described as holding a float bobbing up and down when a fish was biting hook.

The follow-up time was 2 months in one report [29], 6 months in another two [28, 38], and 2 years in four articles [32–34, 36], and the rest even did not mention the follow-up. Clinical effective rates were the main outcome in 10 trials [28– 38] and the other two [39, 40] employed the DHI.

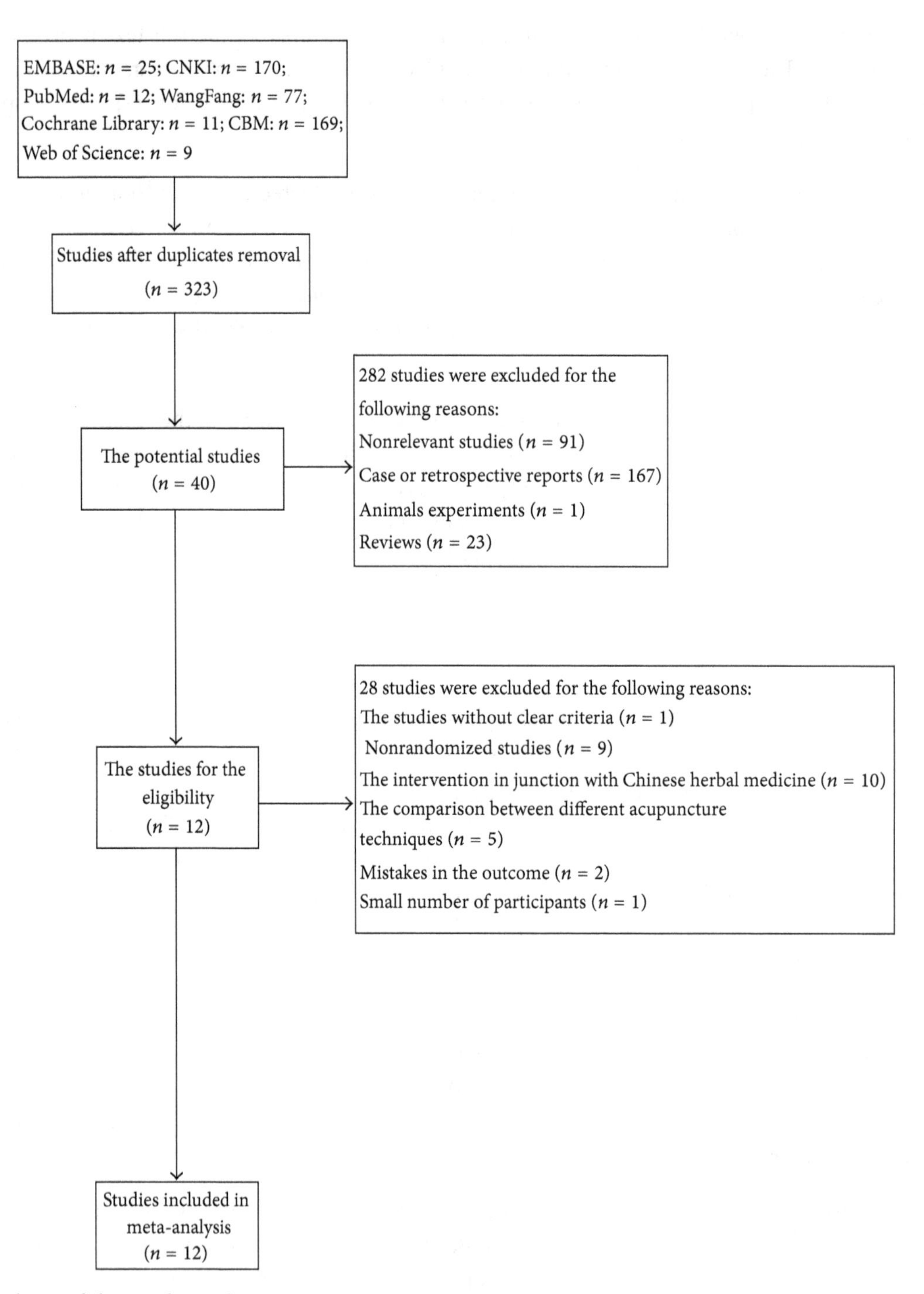

Figure 1: Flowchart of the studies selection process.

Risk of Bias Assessment. The risk of bias of the included RCTs was summarized in Figure 2.

All studies mentioned randomization; however, the bias, actually, in only 3 studies [32–34, 39] was considered low because of the right random sequence generation from random number table; two of them [28, 31, 38] were high for the visiting sequence, and the information in rest was not enough to make a judgement. One trial [39] used sealed envelope for allocation concealment and proper blinding to outcome, assessed by third party. There were some data missing in a trial [31], but the author did not give relevant reason; therefore the bias was considered high. No reports mentioned that the research was approved by ethics committee and was registered.

Table 1: The basic characteristics of included studies.

TABLE 1: The basic characteristics of included studies.

Study	Country	Study design	Sample size	Age	Disease duration	EC approval
Chen and Wu 2004 [28]	China	RCT	T: 34 C: 33	T: 28–65 C: 28–65	T: 5 days–10 years C: 5 days–10 years	Not reported
Mao et al. 2014 [29]	China	RCT	T: 30 C: 30	T: 25–49 C: 26–49	Not reported	Not reported
Zhang 2013 [30]	China	RCT	T: 50 C: 50	T: 25–63 C: 26–63	T: 3 days–2 years C: 3 days–2 years	Not reported
Xie and Wang 2014 [31]	China	RCT	T: 40 C: 40	T: 25–57 C: 26–63	T: 3 days–10 months C: 2 days–11 months	Not reported
Gao and Ni 2002 [32]	China	RCT	T: 58 C: 74	T: 16–76 C: 16–78	T: 3 days–7 years C: 2 days–7 years	Not reported
Zhu 2003 [33]	China	RCT	T: 40 C: 40	T: 18–76 C: 18–77	T: 2 days–9 years C: 3 days–9 years	Not reported
Huang et al. 2010 [35]	China	RCT	T: 30 C: 30	T: 20–63 C: 20–63	T: 3 months–3 years C: 3 months–3 years	Not reported
Wang et al. 2011 [36]	China	RCT	T: 40 C: 40	T: 20–60 C: 20–60	Not reported	Not reported
Zhang 2013 [37]	China	RCT	T: 100 C: 100	T: 45–76 C: 40–71	T: 3 days–11 years C: 3 days–11 years	Not reported
Mo 2010 [38]	China	RCT	T: 100 C: 100	T: 20–64 C: 20–64	Not reported	Not reported
Wu 2011 [39]	China	RCT	T: 30 C: 30	T: 28–65 C: 28–65	T: 2 years–20 years C: 2 days–20 years	Not reported
Sun et al. 2014 [40]	China	RCT	T: 16 C: 10	T: 20–70 C: 20–70	Not reported	Not reported

Note. RCT: randomized controlled trial; T: treatment group; C: control group; EC: ethical committee.

1.1. *Effect Estimates*

Total Effective Rate Assessed by TCM Effective Criteria 1994. Four trials adopted effective rate as the outcome by categorization of main symptoms improvement in four levels ((1) clinical cure, (2) markedly effective, (3) effective, and (4) inefficacious), a generally accepted rule in TCM which was performed in 1994. The total effective rate, the sum of the first three items, was the target of the analysis.

Four studies [28–31] compared APS alone with the western medicine comprehensive treatment (WMCT). With significant heterogeneity ($I^2 = 65\%$, $P = 0.04$), the result yields favours in the APS (RR = 0.21; 95% CI, 1.03–1.42; $Z = 2.27$; $P = 0.02$). Three trials [36–38] showed that APS plus WMCT was significantly better than WMCT ($I^2 = 47\%$, $P = 0.15$, RR= 1.26; 95% CI, 1.10–1.44; $Z = 3.34$; $P = 0.0008$) (see Figures 3 and 4).

Total Effective Rate Assessed by Chinese Medical Association of Otorhinolaryngology Criteria 1997. 3 RCTs [32–35] adopted efficacy standard made by Chinese Medical Association of Otorhinolaryngology, which contained the assessment of vertigo frequency and hearing. In a consequence, the metaanalysis was performed, respectively. As for the vertigo, the result of heterogeneity test showed that $I^2 = 0\%$ and $P = 0.45 > 0.05$, meaning that a fixed effects model should be used. The synthesis results indicated that the APS combined with WMCT had a better effect than WMCT alone (RR = 1.15; 95% CI, 1.06–1.24; $Z = 3.56$; $P = 0.0004$) (Figure 5). As for the hearing function, with significant heterogeneity ($I^2 = 79\%$; $P = 0.008$), meaning that a random model needed to be adopted, the data did not show significant difference between APS plus WMCT and WMCT alone in the improvement of hearing (RR = 1.07; 95% CI, 0.93, 1.24; $Z = 0.93$; $P = 0.35$) (Figure 6).

Table 2: Interventions and outcome assessment of included studies.

Study	Diagnostic criteria	T (main acupoints)	Control treatment	Treatment duration	Main outcome	Follow-up
Chen and Wu 2004 [28]	TCM effective criteria 1994	MA (DU20, GB8, SI19, GB2, SJ5, GB41, ST36) + moxibustion (DU20)	WMCT (niacin, VB6, ATP injection)	20 days Once a day 20 min	Effective rate	6 months
Mao et al. 2014 [29]	TCM effective criteria 1994	MA: sufficiency syndrome (DU20, GB20, LR3, PC6, SL19); deficiency syndrome (DU20, GB20, BL18, BL23); Deqi	WMCT (oral betahistine)	7 days Once a day 20 min	Effective rate	2 months
Zhang 2013 [30]	TCM effective criteria 1994	Ear acupuncture (kidney, spleen, ear shen men, internal ear)	WMCT (glucose, VB6 solution injection; chlorpromazine tablets, oral oryzanolum)	30 days Keeping for 7 days	Effective rate	Not reported
Xie and Wang 2014 [31]	TCM effective criteria 1994	Acupoint injection (PC6, LR3)	WMCT (niacin, oral VB6)	5 days Once a day	Effective rate	Not reported
Gao and Ni 2002 [32]	Criteria 1997	Scalp acupuncture (MS 6, MS 7) + WMCT	WMCT (buflomedil hydrochloride, hydrochloric acid, Danshen injection)	30 days Once a day Manual operation for 5 min and then a pause for 3 min, 3 times totally	Effective rate	2 years
Zhu 2003 [33]	Criteria 1997	MA (DU20, GB20, SI19) + WMCT	WMCT (glucose, ATP, Danshen injection)	30 days Once a day 30 min	Effective rate	2 years
Huang et al. 2010 [35]	Criteria 1997	MA (DU20, PC20, SI19, ST 36, SI19, SJ21) + moxibustion (DU20) + acupoint injection (GB34) + WMCT	WMCT (gastrodin injection, oral flunarizine)	10 days Once a day 20 min	Effective rate	2 years
Wang et al. 2011 [36]	TCM effective criteria 1994	MA (DU20, GB20, DU16, SJ17, SI19) + WMCT	WMCT (betahistine, Danshen injection), Deqi	30 days Once a day 30 min	Effective rate	2 years
Zhang 2013 [37]	TCM effective criteria 1994	Auricular-plaster (kidney, spleen, ear shen men, internal ear) + WMCT with vaccaria seed	WMCT (oral flunarizine)	12 days Once every two days	Effective rate	Not reported
Mo 2010 [38]	TCM effective criteria 1994	Acupoint injection (ST 40, ST36)	WMCT (anisodamine solution injection, chlorpromazine tablet, oral flunarizine)	Not reported Once a day	Effective rate	6 months
Wu 2011 [39]	DHI	MA (DU20, GB20, LR3, GB12, SJ4, GB2)	WMCT (oral sibelium)	6 days Once a day 30 min	DHI	Not reported
Sun et al. 2014 [40]	DHI	Acupressure (Diaoshi Jifa)	WMCT (Ginkgo injection)	1 day Once a day	DHI	No follow-up

Note. MA: manual acupuncture; T: treatment group; C: control group; WMCT: western medicine comprehensive treatment; Criteria 1997: Chinese Medical Association of Otorhinolaryngology criteria 1997.

DHI after the Interventions. The score from the questionnaire named DHI was the outcome in the remaining 2 trials [39, 40]. Compared with the WMCT group, the result failed to show a favour in APS group (MD = −21.26; 95% CI, −55.36, 12.84; $P = 0.22$) (Figure 7).

Publication Bias. The number of included studies in each part was less than 10, which was not enough to perform Begg's test, Egger's test, and funnel-plot.

Adverse Events. All the included studies did not describe adverse events during the progress of the treatment, a difficulty in evaluation of the safety of the APS.

	Random sequence generation (selection bias)	Allocation concealment (selection bias)	Blinding of participants and personnel (performance bias)	Blinding of outcome assessment (detection bias)	Incomplete outcome data (attrition bias)	Selective reporting (reporting bias)	Other bias
Chen and Wu 2004 [28]	−	?	?	?	?	?	?
Gao and Ni 2002 [32]	+	?	?	?	?	?	?
Huang et al. 2010 [35]	?	?	?	?	?	?	?
Mao et al. 2014 [29]	?	?	?	?	?	?	?
Mo 2010 [38]	−	?	?	?	?	?	?
Sun et al. 2014 [40]	?	?	?	?	?	?	?
Wang et al. 2011 [36]	?	?	?	?	?	?	?
Wu 2011 [39]	+	+	?	+	+	?	+
Xie and Wang 2014 [31]	−	?	?	?	−	?	?
Zhang 2013 [30]	?	?	?	?	?	?	?
Zhang 2013 [37]	?	?	?	?	?	?	?
Zhu 2003 [33]	+	?	?	?	?	?	?

Figure 2: The risk of bias assessment for each included study.

Discussion

To our knowledge, this is not the first time to find evidence for acupuncture used in the remedies of MD. The first one with the conclusion that acupuncture has potential benefits for the person with MD was published in 2011 [41]. Because of the language barrier, the authors just searched one Chinese database which was not very popular in China. After a more comprehensive search work, we made a meta-analysis, but we did not have much progress this time. In our analysis, the APS alone or plus WMCT displayed a positive effect in controlling vertigo but negative in hearing loss and DHI. However, the certain conclusion that APS is effective or is not effective for MD still cannot be settled down due to the poor quality of the included trials.

The quality of methodology in the included trials was very poor. Firstly, the vast majority of the studies failed to describe the details of the production of randomization and allocation concealment. Secondly, the lack of blinding among the patients and caregivers was a common problem in all the studies, which might lead to pronounced bias [42]. Finally, almost all the eligible studies were published in Chinese; if not, the experiment was also conducted in China. Moreover, the positive results highly exist in Chinese reports [43] which led to the publication bias. All the drawbacks might limit the value of the meta-analysis results.

Study or subgroup	Experimental Events	Experimental Total	Control Events	Control Total	Weight	Risk ratio M-H, random, 95% CI
Chen and Wu 2004 [28]	31	34	20	33	17.4%	1.50 [1.12, 2.02]
Mao et al. 2014 [29]	28	30	27	30	29.7%	1.04 [0.89, 1.21]
Xie and Wang 2014 [31]	39	40	34	40	31.1%	1.15 [1.00, 1.32]
Zhang 2013 [30]	43	50	32	50	21.8%	1.34 [1.06, 1.70]
Total (95% CI)		**154**		**153**	**100.0%**	**1.21 [1.03, 1.42]**
Total events	141		113			

Heterogeneity: $\tau^2 = 0.02$; $\chi^2 = 8.58$, df = 3 ($P = 0.04$); $I^2 = 65\%$
Test for overall effect: $Z = 2.27$ ($P = 0.02$)

Risk ratio M-H, random, 95% CI: 0.01 0.1 1 10 100; Favours [WMCT] Favours [APS alone]

Figure 3: The forest plot of APS alone on total effectiveness assessed by TCM effective criteria 1994.

Study or subgroup	Experimental Events	Experimental Total	Control Events	Control Total	Weight	Risk ratio M-H, fixed, 95% CI
Mo 2010 [38]	35	40	16	20	20.4%	1.09 [0.85, 1.40]
Wang et al. 2011 [36]	39	40	34	40	32.6%	1.15 [1.00, 1.32]
Zhang 2013 [37]	69	100	49	100	47.0%	1.41 [1.11, 1.79]
Total (95% CI)		**180**		**160**	**100.0%**	**1.26 [1.10, 1.44]**
Total events	143		99			

Heterogeneity: $\chi^2 = 3.78$, df = 2 ($P = 0.15$); $I^2 = 47\%$
Test for overall effect: $Z = 3.34$ ($P = 0.0008$)

Risk ratio M-H, fixed, 95% CI: 0.01 0.1 1 10 100; Favours [control] Favours [experimental]

Figure 4: The forest plot of APS plus WMCT on total effectiveness assessed by TCM effective criteria 1994.

Study or subgroup	Experimental Events	Experimental Total	Control Events	Control Total	Weight	Risk ratio M-H, fixed, 95% CI
Huang et al. 2010 [35]	29	30	25	30	22.8%	1.16 [0.98, 1.38]
Zhu 2003 [33]	35	36	25	32	24.2%	1.24 [1.03, 1.51]
Gao and Ni 2002 [32]	57	58	66	74	53.0%	1.10 [1.01, 1.20]
Total (95% CI)		**124**		**136**	**100.0%**	**1.15 [1.06, 1.24]**
Total events	121		116			

Heterogeneity: $\chi^2 = 1.60$, df = 2 ($P = 0.45$); $I^2 = 0\%$
Test for overall effect: $Z = 3.56$ ($P = 0.0004$)

Risk ratio M-H, fixed, 95% CI: 0.01 0.1 1 10 100; Favours [control] Favours [experimental]

Figure 5: The forest plot of APS plus WMCT on reducing vertigo frequency.

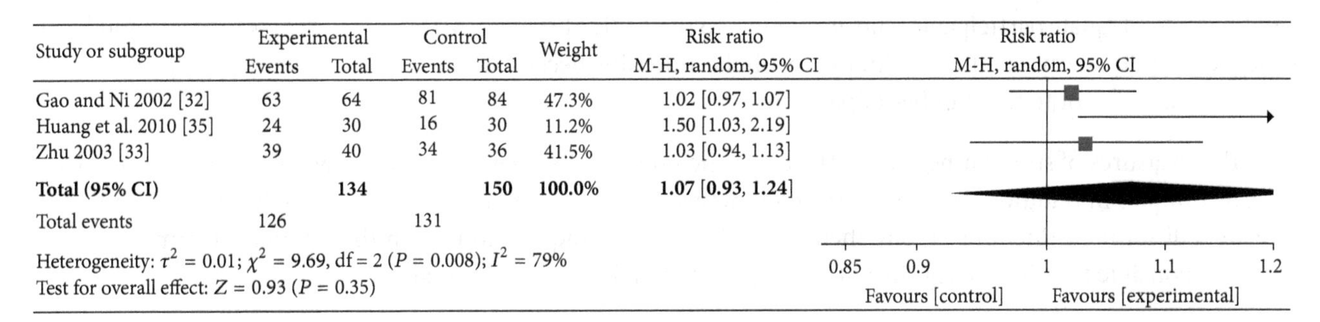

Figure 6: The forest plot of APS plus WMCT on hearing improvement.

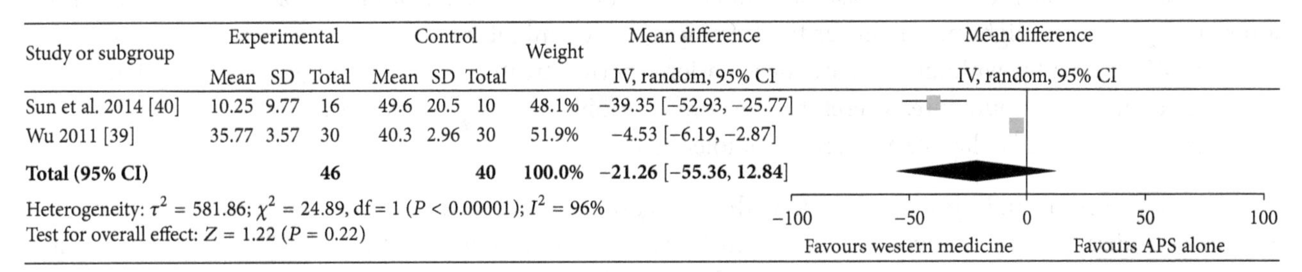

Figure 7: The forest plot of APS alone on DHI.

Currently, no special medical remedy can solve the problem of hearing loss very well. The APS was also ineffective in our result. According to our own observation and clinical experience, APS, indeed, had good effect in controlling the vertigo but it was not good in the hearing improvement. The negative result did not mean that APS was completely helpless in the treatment of MD. The negative result, meaning that APS was ineffective in hearing improvement, suggested that the hearing did not change much or even got worse. As long as it was not the worsening one, keeping the existing hearing or delaying the development of hearing loss was not a so bad result for patients.

Tinnitus, an easily negligible symptom, is also a terrible symptom which impacts the patients' quality of life [44]. It did not draw any attentions in our included studies. However, the application of acupuncture in the tinnitus has been in debate for over 40 years [45]. Several systematic reviews [46, 47] could not reach a definitive conclusion owing to the methodological flaws and risk bias. The similar phenomenon happened in our analysis again. Its major responsibility was the lack of proper blinding and sham acupuncture. What made the blinding and sham acupuncture hard to be put into practice was the acupuncture feature that was, naturally speaking, a sort of benign and minimally invasive therapy needed to be manipulated by a specialized doctor. In other words, blinding the performers to the intervention would be hardly possible in clinical trials. And then the blinding and sham acupuncture seemed to be not feasible to the patients who have already experienced acupuncture particularly in China where the population who did not know acupuncture is small. Supposing the blinding and sham acupuncture has been worked out, the assessment of APS for MD is still a hard nut to crack. Acupuncture as well as the other acupoints stimulation is a patient-centered therapy. The prescription is determined by the syndrome, the degree, and the physical conditions of patients. Consequently, the APS could not display the full capacity in the case of uniform treatment, a conflict with the strict methodology. The only solution to both is collecting the patients with the same disease and physical condition, but it sounds like a story in the Arabian nights.

The sample sizes in eligible trials were relatively small which is likely to overestimate the acupuncture efficacy. Moreover, the number of the included studies was limited and the results can be easily dominated by a single trial, which was a risk to the stability of our result. However, MD should be considered as a rare disease. Although the research focusing on the epidemiology was in blank in China, it was 50 per 100 000 in reports from Japan [48], an Asian nation too, which was much lower than cardiovascular disorders. As a consequence, it would be a very tough work to enroll adequate participants who are eligible to the RCT. Moreover, MD is a mysterious problem and hard to be diagnosed [49], always confused with the vestibular migraine because of the symptom overlap [50], which is also an unfavourable factor to the number of participants.

The measures of stimulating the points in our included studies were quite wide-range which involved near to all the techniques in traditional and modern acupuncture. Based on the same TCM theory, it has to be admitted that there are still some distinctions among them. The different techniques along with the different treatment duration may be responsible for slight or significant heterogeneity that existed in the analysis.

The interventions, combined with two or more techniques, were too complicated to analyze the exact effectiveness of each one. It was, obviously, an undeniable flaw in our meta-analysis. Looking at it, however, from another perspective, it might be a light for the treatment, which might be a daring idea from us or just might be nonsense. MD, currently, without any cure, needs a long-period treatment, which might produce tolerance even without exception to acupuncture. Therefore, the combinations, like the union medicine in hypertension, might strengthen the effects and delay the appearance of tolerance.

MD is a chronic and episodic disease with a remission between two attacks that means that the terrible symptoms can disappear themselves without any medical care. So the follow-up time plays a significant part in the effective assessment. However, the time in most included trials, less than 2 years, was too short to clarify where the effects came from, the effectiveness of APS or self-recovery. Moreover, most studies take the relief of self-reported symptoms as the effective standard rather than the AAO-HNS guidelines [51]. The results collected from self-reported symptoms can be easily affected by subjective emotion and judgement from both sides.

Considering the poor quality of present trials, more future rigorous randomized clinical trials are needed. Researchers should adopt right method of random sequence generation, allocation concealment, and blinding. The data statistics should be reasonable and the number of the dropouts, withdrawals, and the relevant explanations should be described clearly as well as the properly diagnostic and effective criteria and detail about the treatment progress.

Conclusions

In summary, the analysis results revealed a positive effect in controlling the vertigo but a negative effect in the hearing improvement and DHI. However, the currently available evidence is insufficient to make the conclusion that APS is effective or useless in the therapy of MD for the small scale of the included trials and for the poor quality. More rigorously designed trials are urgently needed to evaluate the validity of APS in the treatment of MD. This is not the first systematic review and also would never be the last one. What we desire is raising attentions to this nonpharmaceutical management, figuring out the shortcomings in present clinical trials, and providing some help to further trials.

Competing Interests

The authors declared no competing interests.

Authors' Contributions

Jiaojun He was responsible for conception and design, performed searches, appraised and selected trials, extracted data, performed analysis and interpretation of data, draft d the paper and revised it critically for important intellectual content, and was responsible for final approval of the version to be published. Liyuan Jiang performed searches, appraised and selected trials, extracted data, and performed analysis and interpretation of data. Tianqiang Peng and Meixia Xia performed searches, appraised and selected trials, and extracted data. Huade Chen was responsible for conception and design, appraised and selected trials, performed revision of the paper critically for important intellectual content, and was responsible for the final approval of the version to be published.

Acknowledgments

This research was supported by the National Natural Science Foundation of China (Grant no. 81373757, Beijing, China).

References

[1] P. Meniere, "Maladie de l'oreille interne offrant les sympto^ms de la congestion ce´re´brale apoplectiforme," *Gazette Me´dicale de Paris*, vol. 16, pp. 55–59, 1861.

[2] N. Perez-Fernandez, L. Montes-Jovellar, J. Cervera-Paz, and

E. Domenech-Vadillo, "Auditory and vestibular assessment of patients with Me´nie`re's disease who suffer Tumarkin attacks," *Audiology and Neurotology*, vol. 15, no. 6, pp. 399–406, 2010.

[3] C. Ha¨gnebo, G. Andersson, and L. Melin, "Correlates of vertigo attacks in Meniere's disease," *Psychotherapy and Psychosomatics*, vol. 67, no. 6, pp. 311–316, 1998.

[4] N. S. Longridge, "The value of nausea and vomiting due to Me´nie`re's disease—a theory," *Journal of Otolaryngology*, vol. 12, no. 6, pp. 403–404, 1983.

[5] T. H. Alexander and J. P. Harris, "Current epidemiology of Meniere's syndrome," *Otolaryngologic Clinics of North America*, vol. 43, no. 5, pp. 965–970, 2010.

[6] H. Shojaku, Y. Watanabe, M. Fujisaka et al., "Epidemiologic characteristics of definite Me´nie`re's disease in Japan. A longterm survey of Toyama and Niigata prefectures," *ORL: Journal for Oto-Rhino-Laryngology and Its Related Specialties*, vol. 67, no. 5, pp. 305–309, 2005.

[7] T. Requena, J. M. Espinosa-Sanchez, S. Cabrera et al., "Familial clustering and genetic heterogeneity in Meniere's disease," *Clinical Genetics*, vol. 85, no. 3, pp. 245–252, 2014.

[8] A. W. Morrison, M. E. S. Bailey, and G. A. J. Morrison, "Familial Me´nie`re's disease: clinical and genetic aspects," *The Journal of Laryngology & Otology*, vol. 123, no. 1, pp. 29–37, 2009.

[9] J. S. Tyrrell, D. J. D. Whinney, O. C. Ukoumunne, L. E. Fleming, and N. J. Osborne, "Prevalence, associated factors, and comorbid conditions for me´nie`re's disease," *Ear and Hearing*, vol. 35, no. 4, pp. e162–e169, 2014.

[10] Y. H. Choung, K. Park, C. H. Kim, H. J. Kim, and K. Kim, "Rare cases of Me´nie`re's disease in children," *Journal of Laryngology and Otology*, vol. 120, no. 4, pp. 343–352, 2006.

[11] M. T. Semaan and C. A. Megerian, "Me´nie`re's disease: a challenging and relentless disorder," *Otolaryngologic Clinics of North America*, vol. 44, no. 2, pp. 383–403, 2011.

[12] C. Fujimoto, N. Egami, M. Kinoshita, K. Sugasawa, T. Yamasoba, and S. Iwasaki, "Factors affecting postural instability in Meniere's disease," *Otolaryngology—Head and Neck Surgery*, vol. 149, no. 5, pp. 759–765, 2013.

[13] R. N. Samy, L. Houston, M. Scott et al., "Cochlear implantation in patients with Meniere's disease," *Cochlear Implants International*, vol. 16, no. 4, pp. 208–212, 2015.

[14] M. R. Hansen, B. J. Gantz, and C. Dunn, "Outcomes after cochlear implantation for patients with single-sided deafness, including those with recalcitrant me´nie´re's Disease," *Otology and Neurotology*, vol. 34, no. 9, pp. 1681–1687, 2013.

[15] J. Kanzaki and F. Goto, "Psychiatric disorders in patients with dizziness and Me´nie`re's disease," *Acta Oto-Laryngologica*, vol. 135, no. 5, pp. 447–450, 2015.

[16] M. Furukawa, T. Kitahara, A. Horii et al., "Psychological condition in patients with intractable Meniere's disease," *Acta Oto-Laryngologica*, vol. 133, no. 6, pp. 584–589, 2013.

[17] M. Sakagami, T. Kitahara, T. Okayasu et al., "Negative prognostic factors for psychological conditions in patients with audiovestibular diseases," *Auris Nasus Larynx*, 2016.

[18] K. C. Horner and Y. Cazals, "Stress hormones in Me´nie`re's disease and acoustic neuroma," *Brain Research Bulletin*, vol. 66, no. 1, pp. 1–8, 2005.

[19] C. A. Foster, "Optimal management of Me´nie`re's disease," *Journal of Therapeutics and Clinical Risk Management*, vol. 11, pp. 301–307, 2015.

[20] J. D. Sharon, C. Trevino, M. C. Schubert, and J. P. Carey, "Treatment of Menie`re's disease," *Current Treatment Options in Neurology*, vol. 17, article 14, 2015.

[21] O. Ba˘jenaru, A. M. Roceanu, S. Albu et al., "Effects and tolerability of betahistine in patients with vestibular vertigo: results from the romanian contingent of the OSVaLD study," *International Journal of General Medicine*, vol. 7, pp. 531–538, 2014.

[22] M. Shakeel, A. Trinidade, and K. W. Ah-See, "Complementary and alternative medicine use by otolaryngology patients: a paradigm for practitioners in all surgical specialties," *European Archives of Oto-Rhino-Laryngology*, vol. 267, no. 6, pp. 961–971, 2010.

[23] D. Huppert and T. Brandt, "Descriptions of vestibular migraine and Menie`re's disease in Greek and Chinese antiquity," *Cephalalgia*, 2016.

[24] L. Yap, V. B. Pothula, J. Warner, S. Akhtar, and E. Yates, "The root and development of otorhinolaryngology in traditional Chinese medicine," *European Archives of Oto-Rhino-Laryngology*, vol. 266, no. 9, pp. 1353–1359, 2009.

[25] N. Huang and C. Li, "Recurrent sudden sensorineural hearing loss in a 58-year-old woman with severe dizziness: a case report," *Acupuncture in Medicine*, vol. 30, no. 1, pp. 56–59, 2012.

[26] C. W. Chiu, T. C. Lee, P. C. Hsu et al., "Efficacy and safety of acupuncture for dizziness and vertigo in emergency department: a pilot cohort study," *BMC Complementary and Alternative Medicine*, vol. 15, article 173, 2015.

[27] J. P. T. Higgins and S. G. Thompson, "Quantifying heterogeneity in a meta-analysis," *Statistics in Medicine*, vol. 21, no. 11, pp. 1539– 1558, 2002.

[28] J. Y. Chen and H. Y. Wu, "34 Cases of Meniere's disease treated with acupuncture and moxibustion," *Modern Journal of Integrated Traditional Chinese and Western Medicine*, vol. 13, no. 10, p. 1315, 2004 (Chinese).

[29] L. Y. Mao, H. J. Lu, X. H. Shen et al., "Observation on therapeutic effect of acupuncture on Meniere's disease," *Shanghai Journal of Acupuncture and Moxibustion*, vol. 33, no. 6, p. 575, 2014 (Chinese).

[30] Y. H. Zhang, "50 Cases of Meniere's disease treated by auricular implantation," *Journal of Gansu College of Traditional Chinese Medicine*, vol. 30, no. 1, pp. 40–42, 2013 (Chinese).

[31] L. Xie and Y. Wang, "60 cases of Meniere's disease treatment by point injection with anisodamine," *Journal of Jiang Xi University of TCM*, vol. 26, no. 1, pp. 49–59, 2014 (Chinese).

[32] X. P. Gao and H. H. Ni, "Observation on therapeutic effect of scalp acupuncture on Meniere's disease," *Chinese Acupuncture & Moxibustion*, vol. 22, no. 9, pp. 583–584, 2002 (Chinese).

[33] H. X. Zhu, "36 cases of Meniere's disease patients treated with acupuncture," *Clinical Journal of An Hui Traditional Chinese Medicine*, vol. 12, no. 15, pp. 491–492, 2003.

[34] Q. Huang, "Fifty cases of vertebrobasilar ischemic vertigo treated by acupuncture," *Journal of Traditional Chinese Medicine*, vol. 29, no. 2, pp. 87–89, 2009 (Chinese).

[35] C. J. Huang, J. X. Zhou, and W. Y. Yin, "Observation on therapeutic effect of acupuncture combined with western medicine on Meniere's disease," *Chinese Journal of Modern Drug Application*, vol. 4, no. 8, pp. 146–147, 2010 (Chinese).

[36] X. Wang, D. K. Xia, Y. L. Cui et al., "The clinical observation about the Meniere's disease patients treated by acupuncture combined with western medicine," *Journal of Clinical Acupuncture and Moxibustion*, vol. 27, no. 5, pp. 32–33, 2011 (Chinese).

[37] W. Zhang, "Observation on effect of auricular points embedding in the combination with flunarizine on Meniere's disease," *Chinese Community Doctor*, vol. 13, no. 5, p. 63, 2013 (Chinese).

[38] L. B. Mo, "Observation on eff ct of acupoints injection with tian ma injection on Meniere's disease," *Journal of Chang Chun University of Traditional Chinese Medicine*, vol. 26, no. 8, p. 537, 2010 (Chinese).

[39] X. Wu, *Clinical research on traditional acupuncture manipulation combined with the moxibustion on BaiHui of Meniere's disease [M.S. thesis]*, Guangzhou University of Chinese Medicine, Guangzhou, China, 2011 (Chinese).

[40] Y.-X. Sun, Y. Wang, X. Ji et al., "A randomized trial of Chinese Diaoshi Jifa on treatment of dizziness in Meniere's disease," *Evidence-Based Complementary and Alternative Medicine*, vol. 2014, Article ID 521475, 7 pages, 2014.

[41] A. F. Long, M. Xing, K. Morgan, and A. Brettle, "Exploring the evidence base for acupuncture in the treatment of Me´nie`re's syndrome—a systematic review," *Evidence-Based Complementary and Alternative Medicine*, vol. 2011, Article ID 429102, 13 pages, 2011.

[42] A. Hro´bjartsson, F. Emanuelsson, A. S. S. Thomsen, J. Hilden, and S. Brorson, "Bias due to lack of patient blinding in clinical trials. A systematic review of trials randomizing patients to blind and nonblind sub-studies," *International Journal of Epidemiology*, vol. 43, no. 4, pp. 1272–1283, 2014.

[43] A. Vickers, N. Goyal, R. Harland, and R. Rees, "Do certain countries produce only positive results? A systematic review of controlled trials," *Controlled Clinical Trials*, vol. 19, no. 2, pp. 159–166, 1998.

[44] D. Stephens, I. Pyykko¨, T. Yoshida et al., "The consequences of tinnitus in long-standing Me´nie`re's disease," *Auris Nasus Larynx*, vol. 39, no. 5, pp. 469–474, 2012.

[45] M. Tassinari, D. Mandrioli, N. Gaggioli, and P. Roberti Di Sarsina, "Me´nie`re's disease treatment: a patient-centered systematic review," *Audiology and Neurotology*, vol. 20, no. 3, pp. 153–165, 2015.

[46] J. I. Kim, J. Y. Choi, D. H. Lee et al., "Acupuncture for the treatment of tinnitus: a systematic review of randomized clinical trials," *BMC Complementary and Alternative Medicine*, vol. 12, article 97, 2012.

[47] F. Liu, X. Han, Y. Li, and S. Yu, "Acupuncture in the treatment of tinnitus: a systematic review and meta-analysis," *European Archives of Oto-Rhino-Laryngology*, vol. 273, no. 2, pp. 285–294, 2016.

[48] H. Shojaku, Y. Watanabe, M. Fujisaka et al., "Epidemiologic characteristics of definite Me´nie`re's disease in Japan: a longterm survey of Toyama and Niigata prefectures," *ORL: Journal for Oto-Rhino-Laryngology and Its Related Specialties*, vol. 67, no. 5, pp. 305–309, 2005.

[49] A. Vassiliou, P. Vlastarakos, P. Maragoudakis, D. Candiloros, and T. Nikolopoulos, "Meniere's disease: still a mystery disease with difficult differential diagnosis," *Annals of Indian Academy of Neurology*, vol. 14, no. 1, pp. 12–18, 2011.

[50] J. A. Lopez-Escamez, J. Dlugaiczyk, J. Jacobs et al., "Accompanying symptoms overlap during attacks in Menie`re's disease and vestibular migraine," *Frontiers in Neurology*, vol. 5, article 265, 2014.

[51] American Academy of Otolaryngology—Head and Neck Foundation, "Committee on Hearing and Equilibrium guidelines for the diagnosis and evaluation of therapy in Meniere's disease," *Otolaryngology—Head and Neck Surgery*, vol. 113, no. 3, pp. 181– 185, 1995.

Permissions

All chapters in this book were first published by Hindawi & InTech Open Publishing Corporation; hereby published with permission under the Creative Commons Attribution License or equivalent. Every chapter published in this book has been scrutinized by our experts. Their significance has been extensively debated. The topics covered herein carry significant findings which will fuel the growth of the discipline. They may even be implemented as practical applications or may be referred to as a beginning point for another development.

The contributors of this book come from diverse backgrounds, making this book a truly international effort. This book will bring forth new frontiers with its revolutionizing research information and detailed analysis of the nascent developments around the world.

We would like to thank all the contributing authors for lending their expertise to make the book truly unique. They have played a crucial role in the development of this book. Without their invaluable contributions this book wouldn't have been possible. They have made vital efforts to compile up to date information on the varied aspects of this subject to make this book a valuable addition to the collection of many professionals and students.

This book was conceptualized with the vision of imparting up-to-date information and advanced data in this field. To ensure the same, a matchless editorial board was set up. Every individual on the board went through rigorous rounds of assessment to prove their worth. After which they invested a large part of their time researching and compiling the most relevant data for our readers.

The editorial board has been involved in producing this book since its inception. They have spent rigorous hours researching and exploring the diverse topics which have resulted in the successful publishing of this book. They have passed on their knowledge of decades through this book. To expedite this challenging task, the publisher supported the team at every step. A small team of assistant editors was also appointed to further simplify the editing procedure and attain best results for the readers.

Apart from the editorial board, the designing team has also invested a significant amount of their time in understanding the subject and creating the most relevant covers. They scrutinized every image to scout for the most suitable representation of the subject and create an appropriate cover for the book.

The publishing team has been an ardent support to the editorial, designing and production team. Their endless efforts to recruit the best for this project, has resulted in the accomplishment of this book. They are a veteran in the field of academics and their pool of knowledge is as vast as their experience in printing. Their expertise and guidance has proved useful at every step. Their uncompromising quality standards have made this book an exceptional effort. Their encouragement from time to time has been an inspiration for everyone.

The publisher and the editorial board hope that this book will prove to be a valuable piece of knowledge for researchers, students, practitioners and scholars across the globe.

List of Contributors

Jess Tyrrell and Sarah Bell
University of Exeter, Exeter, United Kingdom

Cassandra Phoenix
University of Bath, Bath, United Kingdom

Ting Liu, Ying Xu and Hongzhou Ge
Department of Otolaryngology, Qingdao Hospital of Traditional Chinese Medicine (Qingdao Hiser Hospital), Qingdao 266034, Shandong, China

Yujuan An
Department of Intravenous Infusion Center, Qingdao Hospital of Traditional Chinese Medicine (Qingdao Hiser Hospital), Qingdao 266034, Shandong, China

Mehmet Yilmaz
Yunus Emre Clinic, Turkey

Niraj Kumar Singh, Rahul Krishnamurthy and Priya Karimuddanahally Premkumar
All India Institute of Speech and Hearing, Mysore 570006, India

Maria Stella A. Amaral, Henrique F. Pauna and Miguel A. Hyppolito
Department of Ophthalmology, Otorhinolaryngology and Head and Neck Surgery, Ribeirão Preto Medical School—University of São Paulo, Ribeirão Preto, São Paulo, Brazil

Ana Claudia M.B. Reis
Department of Health Sciences, Ribeirão Preto Medical School—University of São Paulo, Riberão Preto, São Paulo, Brazil

Yuan F. Liu and Helen Xu
Department of Otolaryngology, Head and Neck Surgery, Loma Linda University Medical Center, Loma Linda, CA, USA

Barbara Colombo, Mimma Bianco and Angelo Corti
Division of Experimental Oncology, San Raffaele Scientific Institute, Milan, Italy

Marta Martinez-Lopez, Raquel Manrique-Huarte and Nicolas Perez-Fernandez
Department of Otorhinolaryngology, Clinica Universidad de Navarra, University of Navarra, Avenida P´ıo XII 36, 31008 Pamplona, Spain

Angelo Manfredi
Department of Internal Medicine and Division of Regenerative Medicine, Stem Cells & Gene Therapy, San Raffaele Scientific Institute, Universita` Vita-Salute San Raffaele, Milan, Italy

Ricardo Ferreira Bento and Paula Tardim Lopes
Department of Otorhinolaryngology and Neurotology, Hospital das Clínicas— University of São Paulo, São Paulo, Brazil

Norman A. Orabi, Brian M. Kellermeyer, Christopher A. Roberts and Stephen J. Wetmore
West Virginia University School of Medicine Department of Otolaryngology, Morgantown, WV 26506, USA

Adam M. Cassis
Arizona Hearing & Balance Center, 225 S Dobson Rd#1, Chandler, AZ 85224, USA

Esther Jiayi Lim
Novena Ent-Head & Neck Surgery Specialist Centre, 04-21/22/34, Mount Elizabeth Novena Medical Centre, 38 Irrawaddy Road, Singapore

Wong Kein Low
Novena Ent-Head & Neck Surgery Specialist Centre, 04-21/22/34, Mount Elizabeth Novena Medical Centre, 38 Irrawaddy Road, Singapore
Duke-NUS Graduate Medical School, 8 College Road, Singapore

Roberto Teggi, Matteo Trimarchi and Mario Bussi
ENT Division, San Raffaele Scientific Institute, Milan, Italy

Yongchuan Chai
Research Service, VA Loma Linda Healthcare System, Loma Linda, CA, United States
Loma Linda University School of Medicine, Loma Linda, CA, United States
Department of Otorhinolaryngology—Head and Neck Surgery, Shanghai Ninth People's Hospital, Shanghai Jiao Tong University School of Medicine, Shanghai, China
Ear Institute, Shanghai Jiao Tong University School of Medicine, Shanghai, China
Shanghai Key Laboratory of Translational Medicine on Ear and Nose Diseases, Shanghai, China

Hongzhe Li
Research Service, VA Loma Linda Healthcare System, Loma Linda, CA, United States
Loma Linda University School of Medicine, Loma Linda, CA, United States
Department of Otolaryngology—Head and Neck Surgery, Loma Linda University School of Medicine, Loma Linda, CA, United States

Yong-Xin Sun, Yuan Wang, Fei Yu, Wenbo Zhao and Jianping Jia
Department of Neurology, Xuan Wu Hospital of Capital Medical University, Beijing 100053, China

Xunming Ji
Department of Neurosurgery, Xuan Wu Hospital of Capital Medical University, Beijing 100053, China

Xiaoguang Wu
Evidence-Based Medicine Center, Xuan Wu Hospital of Capital Medical University, Beijing 100053, China

Yong Zhao
Department of Neurology, Wangjing Hospital, China Academy of Chinese Medical Sciences, Beijing 100102, China

Yuchuan Ding and Mohammed Hussain
Department of Neurological Surgery, Wayne State University School of Medicine, Detroit, MI 48201, USA

Yetkin Zeki Yilmaz, Begum Bahar Yilmaz and Aysegul Batioglu-Karaaltın
Istanbul University-Cerrahpasa Medical Faculty ENT, Istanbul, Turkey

Carlos A. Oliveira
Brasília University Medical School, Brasília, DF, Brazil

Jiaojun He, Liyuan Jiang, Tianqiang Peng, Meixia Xia and Huade Chen
The Third Clinical Medical College of Zhejiang Chinese Medical University, Hangzhou, Zhejiang 310053, China

Index

Printed in the USA
CPSIA information can be obtained
at www.ICGtesting.com
JSHW051356091023
49903JS00006B/162